MW01415637

Color Atlas of
ORAL PATHOLOGY

Color Atlas of
ORAL PATHOLOGY

Histology and Embryology • Developmental Disturbances
Diseases of the Teeth and Supporting Structures
Diseases of the Oral Mucosa and Jaws • Neoplasms

Robert A. Colby, D.D.S., M.S.
Consultant in Oral Pathology, U.S. Naval Dental School and Armed Forces Institute of Pathology; Formerly Chairman of the Department of Oral Pathology, U.S. Naval Dental School

Donald A. Kerr, D.D.S., M.S.
Professor of Oral Pathology, University of Michigan School of Dentistry; Professor of Pathology (for Dentistry), University of Michigan School of Medicine; Co-chairman, Department of Dentistry, University of Michigan Medical Center

Hamilton B. G. Robinson, D.D.S., M.S.
Dean and Professor of Dentistry (Oral Diagnosis and Pathology), University of Missouri-Kansas City School of Dentistry

THIRD EDITION

485 Figures in Color

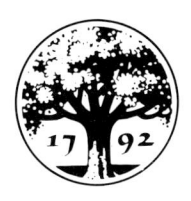

J. B. Lippincott Company
Philadelphia • Toronto

THIRD EDITION

COPYRIGHT © 1971, BY J. B. LIPPINCOTT COMPANY

COPYRIGHT © 1961, BY J. B. LIPPINCOTT COMPANY

This book is fully protected by copyright and, with the exception of brief excerpts for review, no part of it may be reproduced in any form by print, photoprint, microfilm or any other means without written permission from the publisher.

ISBN-0-397-50279-6

Library of Congress Catalog Card Number 73-147050

Printed in the United States of America

5 6

Preface to the Third Edition

In preparing this third edition the objectives of presenting a succinct but relatively comprehensive Atlas of Oral Pathology were continued. There is always a temptation to expand on one or another entity or area of oral pathology, but it was necessary to restrict discussions to the space available on each page containing the related illustrations or to change the entire format of the Atlas. Since the present format has been so well accepted, the authors decided to continue it.

For the third edition each section was carefully reviewed and the text revised wherever pertinent. Several new entities have been added with revision of the illustrations, and in other instances better examples have been substituted for those in previous editions. The International Classification of Disease was used wherever applicable (Application to Dentistry and Stomatology, ICD-DA, Dental Department, University Hospital, Copenhagen, 1969). Reference to the enlarged and updated bibliography affords a review of classical and current literature.

This Atlas does not attempt to illustrate all oral diseases and all oral manifestations of disease. For practical purposes concerned with the size and cost of production, this is not feasible.

This third edition, like previous editions, is essentially a collection of illustrations with terse descriptions. It is intended to serve as a quick, handy reference for students and practitioners of dentistry and medicine and not as an encyclopedic work. The reader should seek more detailed information in textbooks and in the current literature.

ROBERT A. COLBY
DONALD A. KERR
HAMILTON B. G. ROBINSON

Preface to the First Edition

The purpose of this book is to present in concise form the fundamental facts concerning oral disease. The volume is an atlas in the strictest sense—a book of pictures. The written material, which merely supplements the color plates, is confined to the page on which an entity is illustrated.

This Atlas is designed primarily for general practitioners, to help them achieve their main objective—arriving at a diagnosis so that treatment can be planned intelligently.

In general, diseases having similar causes have been grouped together, but when it appeared more logical they were arranged according to anatomic site. The amount of space allotted to an entity is not related to its frequency or importance, but rather reflects the number of pictures deemed necessary to depict salient points adequately. When appropriate, it has been the policy to illustrate the clinical, roentgenographic and microscopic appearance of lesions. Each disease has been designated by a preferred term, but commonly used synonyms are also given. The term "disease" has been used in its broadest sense, to denote any condition which is considered outside the zone of normality. Because a knowledge of histology and embryology is extremely important to the thorough understanding of pathology, a brief section on these two subjects has been included to provide a ready reference for the reader.

While the text is brief, as much pertinent information as possible has been condensed into the space available, including a precise definition of each entity and—where a systemic disease is under consideration—a discussion of the general as well as the oral aspects. No attempt has been made to cover oral pathology or oral diagnosis as academic subjects. Those readers desiring further information should refer to standard textbooks and to the periodical literature. To aid in locating such additional information, a brief list of articles relating to the various entities is included at the end of the book. Only papers which are written in English and appear in readily available publications have been selected. This suggested supplemental reading list in no way exhausts the available literature on any subject.

Pathology is not an exact science, and therefore it is to be expected that, through subsequent investigative procedures, some concepts presented in this Atlas may be proved incorrect. Care has been taken, however, not to perpetuate erroneous information. An effort has been made not to be dogmatic but to submit, when space permitted, various opinions regarding controversial subjects.

It is hoped that this book will be of value to those clinicians who seek further knowledge of oral disease as a background for formulating proper treatment.

Robert A. Colby
Captain (DC) USN
Head, Oral Pathology Division
U. S. Naval Dental School

Acknowledgments

Grateful acknowledgment is made to the United States Navy, under whose auspices the first edition of this Atlas was prepared, for relinquishing claims to the publication and releasing all Navy material to the three authors.

The color transparencies primarily are from the University of Michigan, the Ohio State University, the University of Missouri-Kansas City, the activities of the U. S. Navy and the personal collections of the authors. Twenty-eight of the illustrations came from other sources and the authors gratefully acknowledge the following contributions: Dr. R. L. Harding (21 *top*), Dr. H. L. Hubinger (24 *center*), Dr. W. M. Searcy, Jr. (38 *top*), Dr. A. E. Seyler (41 *center*), Dr. H. T. Hartsook (52 *top*), Drs. P. E. Boyle and N. Dinnerman (59 *top*), Dr. H. H. Scofield (59 *center*), Dr. H. A. Zander (68 *center and bottom*), Drs. H. Goldberg and P. Goldhaber (99 *bottom*), Drs. H. B. Marble and H. H. Scofield (154 *bottom*), Dr. P. J. Robinson (111 *top*), Drs. M. Moore and L. H. Jorsted (116 *top*), Dr. W. J. Carter (117 *bottom*), Memorial Hospital, New York City (24 *top*, 129 *top*, 134 *top and center*, 144 *top*, 146 *top and center*, 150 *top*, 155 *center*, 156 *top and bottom*, 160 *top*, 164 *top*) and Armed Forces Institute of Pathology (149 *center*, 161 *top*). These acknowledgments concern the pictures, and the contributors should not necessarily be considered responsible for the text. The sketches on pages 12 and 13 were prepared by Mrs. Warren Hedman and that on page 38 by Mrs. Helen F. Collison. Numerous other individuals contributed in many ways to the preparation of this Atlas. While they are not acknowledged individually, the authors hope they will realize that their assistance is deeply appreciated.

ROBERT A. COLBY
DONALD A. KERR
HAMILTON B. G. ROBINSON

Contents

1. **Histology and Embryology** 1
    Introduction 1
    Histology 2
        Skin 2
        Mucous Membrane 3
        Salivary Glands 4
        Tongue 5
        Enamel 6
        Dentin 6
        Periodontal Membrane and Cementum 6
        Pulp 7
        Cartilage and Bone 7
        Fibrous Connective Tissue 8
        Peripheral Nerve 8
        Inflammatory Cells 8
    Embryology 10
        Human Fetus 10
        Development of the Face 12
        Branchial Arches 12
        Development of the Tongue 12
        Thyroglossal Duct 13
        Tooth Development 14

2. **Developmental Disturbances** 17
    Introduction 17
    Clefts of the Lip and Palate 18
    Auricular Tags, Macrostomia and Lip Pits 18
    Brachygnathia (Micrognathia) and Pierre Robin Syndrome . . . 19
    Hemiatrophy 19
    Hygroma Colli Congenitum 19
    Branchial Cleft Cyst 20
    Preauricular Sinus 21
    Dermoid Cyst 21
    Epidermoid Cyst 21
    Thyroglossal Duct Cyst 22
    Lingual Thyroid 22
    Oral Tori 23
    Median Rhomboid Glossitis 24
    Bifid Tongue 24
    Ankyloglossia 24
    Macroglossia 25
    Hyperplastic Lingual Papillae 26
        Large Vallate Papillae 26
        Foliate Papillae 26
    Fissured Tongue 26

2. **Developmental Disturbances**—(*Continued*)

Fordyce Spots (Granules)	27
Median Palatine Cyst	28
Globulomaxillary Cyst	29
Nasoalveolar Cyst	29
Nasopalatine Duct Cyst	30
Dentigerous Cyst	31
Lateral Periodontal Cyst	32
Primordial Cyst	33
Periodontal Cyst	34
Calcifying Odontogenic Cyst	36
Gemination and Fusion	37
Dens Invaginatus (Dens in Dente)	38
Segmented Root	39
Dwarfed Roots	39
Microdontia and Macrodontia	40
Supernumerary Teeth	40
Ectodermal Dysplasia	41
Concrescence	42
Hypercementosis	42
Enamel Pearls	43
Dilaceration	43
Odontome (Odontoma)	44
Enamel Dysplasia	46
Defects of Dentin Formation	50
Dentinogenesis Imperfecta (Hereditary Opalescent Dentin)	50
Dentin Dysplasia	52
Odontodysplasia	53
Osteogenesis Imperfecta	53
Cleidocranial Dysostosis	54

3. **Diseases of the Teeth and Supporting Structures** 55

Introduction	55
Abrasion	56
Attrition	58
Erosion	58
Stains	59
Root Fractures	60
Internal Resorption	61
Apical Resorption	62
Cementoma (Cementosis)	62
Radiation Effect, Teeth	63
Dental Caries	64
Secondary Dentin Formation	68
Pulp Healing	68
Pulp Calcification	69
Pulpitis	70
Sequelae of Pulpitis	73
Normal Gingiva	76
Marginal (Simple) Gingivitis	76
Acute Herpetic Gingivostomatitis	77
Necrotizing Ulcerative Gingivitis (Vincent's Infection)	78

3. **Diseases of the Teeth and Supporting Structures**—(*Continued*)
   Gingival Enlargement 79
   Desquamative Gingivitis ("Gingivosis") 82
   Atrophic Senile Gingivitis 82
   Periodontitis 83
   Periodontal Pockets 84
   Periodontal Disease Involving Interradicular Areas 86
   Traumatism 87
   Fibrous (Fibroid) Epulis 89
   Giant Cell Epulis (Peripheral Giant Cell Reparative Granuloma) . . 90
   Granuloma Gravidarum (Pregnancy "Tumor") 90

4. **Diseases of the Oral Mucosa and Jaws** 91
   Introduction 91
   Cheek and Tongue Chewing 92
   Traumatic (Amputation) Neuroma 93
   Self-Inflicted Trauma During Anesthesia 94
   Hyperplasia from Denture Irritation 94
   Traumatic Bone Lesion 95
   Thermal Burns 96
   Chemical Burns 96
   Galvanism 97
   Nicotinic Stomatitis 97
   Pigmentation 98
   Radiation Effect, Soft Tissue and Bone 100
   Drug Idiosyncrasy 102
   Keratosis and Leukoplakia 104
   Solar Cheilosis 106
   White Sponge Nevus 107
   Mucous Retention Cyst (Mucocele) 108
   Sialolithiasis 109
   Sjögren's Syndrome 109
   Recurrent Herpetiform Lesions 110
   Exanthems 111
   Periadenitis Mucosa Necrotica Recurrens 111
   Tuberculosis 112
   Syphilis 114
   Histoplasmosis 116
   Actinomycosis 117
   Candidiasis 117
   Osteomyelitis 118
   Pyogenic Granuloma 119
   Lichen Planus 120
   Erythema Multiforme 122
   Pemphigus Vulgaris 123
   Lupus Erythematosus 123
   Geographic Tongue (Benign Migratory Glossitis) 124
   Black Hairy Tongue 124
   Varicose Veins, Tongue 125

4. **Diseases of the Oral Mucosa and Jaws—(*Continued*)**
    Hereditary Hemorrhagic Telangiectasia (Osler-Rendu-Weber Disease) . . . 125
    Vitamin B Complex Malnutrition 126
    Carotenemia 127
    Pernicious Anemia 128
    Mediterranean Anemia (Cooley's Anemia, Thalassemia) 128
    Agranulocytosis 128
    Primary Hyperparathyroidism 129
    The Histiocytoses 130
        Eosinophilic Granuloma of Bone 130
        Hand-Schüller-Christian Disease 130
    Scleroderma 131
    Fibrous Dysplasia 132
    Acromegaly 133
    Paget's Disease of Bone (Osteitis Deformans) 134

5. **Neoplasms** 135
    Introduction 135
    Benign Neoplasms 136
        Adenoma 136
        Papillary Cystadenoma Lymphomatosum (Warthin's Tumor) . . . 136
        Papilloma 137
        Fibroma 138
        Lipoma 139
        Myxoma 139
        Benign Tumors of Osseous Origin 140
        Neurilemoma 142
        Neurofibroma 142
        Myoblastoma 143
        Hemangioma 144
        Hemangioendothelioma 145
        Lymphangioma 145
        Neoplasms of Odontogenic Origin 146
        Benign Mixed Tumors of Salivary Gland Origin (Pleomorphic Adenoma) . . 150
    Malignant Neoplasms 152
        Malignant Salivary Gland Neoplasms 152
        Basal Cell Carcinoma 154
        Basal Cell Nevoid Syndrome 154
        Squamous Cell Carcinoma 155
        Carcinoma of the Nasopharynx 160
        Multiple Myeloma 161
        Malignant Lymphoma 162
        Leukemia 163
        Osteogenic Sarcoma 164
        Chondrosarcoma 164
        Fibrosarcoma 165
        Melanoma 166
        Metastasis to the Jaws 167

Bibliography 169

Index 201

Color Atlas of
ORAL PATHOLOGY

1
Histology and Embryology

INTRODUCTION

In order to recognize and understand the abnormal it is necessary to have an understanding of the normal. It is important to know the typical gross and microscopic appearance of various tissues and to be familiar with normal development. Many individuals have become frustrated in the study of pathology because they believe that their knowledge of histology and embryology is inadequate. While thorough knowledge in these two areas is of great advantage, one may begin to develop an understanding of disease adequate for the intelligent practice of dentistry on the basis of a reasonably limited background. The graduate of the modern dental school has been taught the basic information, and this section of the Atlas is designed to aid in reviewing that knowledge. It has not been planned as a replacement for standard textbooks in histology and embryology but only to present the essential information concerning the recognition of tissues and the development of the head and the neck that one should have in order to approach the study of pathology intelligently.

Before examining histopathologic material, it is necessary to be able to identify microscopically the following: skin and cutaneous appendages, oral and respiratory mucous membrane, salivary gland tissue, skeletal muscle, fibrous connective tissue, nerve tissue, cartilage, bone, enamel, dentin, cementum, pulp and the various inflammatory cells.

Rather than trying to memorize the appearance of a given cell, tissue or organ, one should learn the identifying characteristics of the various structures. Dependence on color to identify histologic entities is a bad practice. For example, if one attempts to find eosinophils by their red cytoplasm alone, they may be confused with Russell-Plimmer bodies. If, on the other hand, the characteristic reddish cytoplasm with coarse granules is used for identification, there should be no confusion. Similarly, under some circumstances mucous and serous acini may be confused if staining characteristics alone are considered.

In examining a tissue section, it is advisable to look at it first with the naked eye or a reversed eyepiece to learn the general characteristics of the section. When it is placed under the microscope, it should be studied first under low magnification (approximately $\times$ 30). At this magnification it is possible to determine the natural and artificial margins, the relation of one tissue to another, and any regions in which tissues vary from the normal. Areas that appear to be abnormal under low power should be examined further at a magnification of 100 or 200. Occasionally, it is necessary to investigate regional cellular detail with a magnification of 500. Oil immersion need be used only when searching for microorganisms. Some cells look nearly alike when viewed under very high power, and it is possible to identify them only by switching to a lower power and determining their arrangement and their relationship to other structures. Most histopathologic material may be evaluated without resorting to a magnification higher than 100, but it is a common error for those not familiar with tissue microscopy to make too great a use of the higher magnifications.

To learn the many details of the development of the head and neck requires concentrated and specialized study. For the practice of dentistry and the general understanding of oral pathology, it only is necessary to have a fairly detailed knowledge of tooth development and an understanding of the development of the tongue, palate, jaws and face.

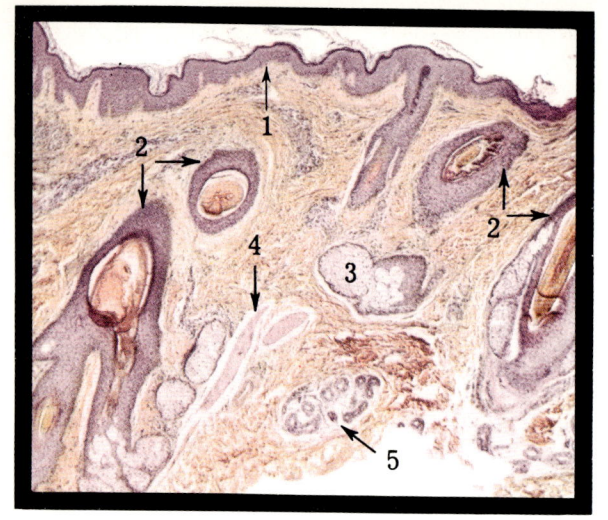

Skin   X 35

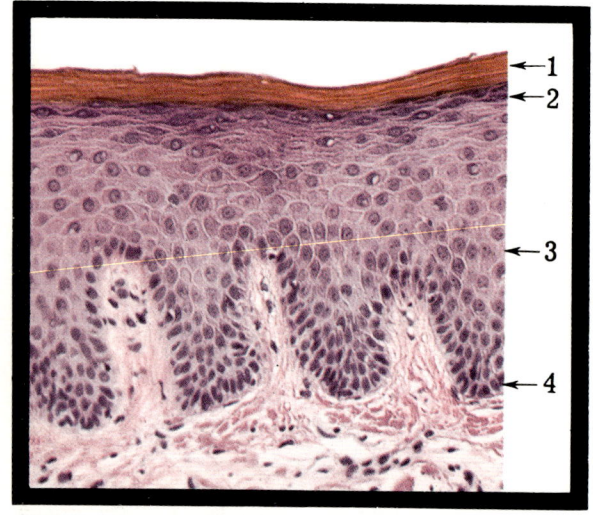

Stratified Squamous Epithelium   X 220

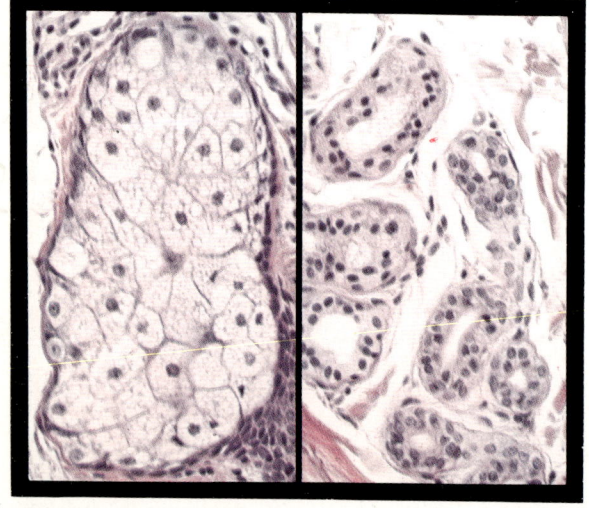

Sebaceous Gland   X 200   Sweat Gland   X 200

HISTOLOGY

Skin

(Top) The skin consists of epidermis (1), which is stratified squamous epithelium, and corium (dermis), which is mainly connective tissue. The corium supports the secondary skin structures, or cutaneous appendages: hair follicles (2), sebaceous glands (3), arrectores pilorum (4) and sweat glands (5).

(Center) Stratified squamous epithelium is composed of three main layers: stratum germinativum, stratum granulosum and stratum corneum. Stratum germinativum may be subdivided into the basal layer and the prickle cell layer. The basal cell layer (4) consists of a single row of dark-staining columnar cells which are perpendicular to the dermoepidermal junction. The prickle cell layer, or stratum spinosum (3), is composed of several rows of polyhedral cells which connect with each other by fine, spinous processes (intercellular bridges). Stratum granulosum (2) usually consists of two layers of flattened cells which contain dark-blue-staining keratohyalin granules. The stratum corneum, or horny layer (1), is made up of densely packed cells filled with keratin. The fingerlike processes of epithelium extending into the dermis are rete pegs. The connective tissue between two rete pegs is called a dermal papilla. The following terms refer to abnormalities of epithelium: acanthosis—hyperplasia of the prickle cell layer; pseudoepitheliomatous hyperplasia—benign overgrowth resembling carcinoma; hyperkeratosis—thickening of stratum corneum; parakeratosis—retention of nuclei in cells of the horny layer.

(Bottom) The sebaceous gland *(left)* is composed of large polyhedral cells having small, centrally placed nuclei and abundant, light-staining, vacuolated cytoplasm. The secretion, sebum, which usually is released into a hair follicle, becomes available when the individual cells rupture. The destroyed cells are replaced from the layer of squamous cells that surround the gland. Sweat glands *(right)* are coiled structures, but they appear in microscopic sections as nests of small cut tubules, each lined by a single row of cuboidal cells. At the periphery of the tubules a few spindle-shaped myo-epithelial cells may be seen.

Histology and Embryology

Mucous Membrane

Oral mucous membrane differs from skin mainly in lacking secondary skin structures in the subepithelial connective tissue (corium, lamina propria). Oral epithelium usually is thicker than epidermis with longer rete pegs. Most of the oral mucosa has a cornified surface layer, although in some individuals only parakeratosis is evident. Protected areas, such as the undersurface of the tongue and the floor of the mouth, are not cornified. A well-developed horny layer on the oral mucosa is demonstrated in the center picture on the opposite page. This photomicrograph, used to illustrate the layers of stratified squamous epithelium, is of a section from the palate.

(Top) This illustration demonstrates the transition zone between skin and mucous membrane on the lower lip. At the far left is an abrupt termination of the hair follicles and sebaceous glands. Above this point is the vermilion border of the lip, and below it is skin. The rete pegs extend progressively deeper into the corium as the oral cavity is approached.

(Center) Low- and high-power photomicrographs of the epithelial attachment on the lingual surface of a molar. Both the free and attached portions of the gingiva have long rete pegs which gradually diminish in size away from the free gingival margin. In higher magnification the epithelial attachment may be identified by the pale-staining cells. These, which have been separated from the cementum in preparation of the section, are derived from reduced enamel epithelium while the darker-staining cells are derived from the lining of the primitive mouth. The base of the gingival crevice is at the coronal end of the epithelial attachment. The sulcus epithelium is not hornified but the external gingiva may be fairly heavily hornified.

(Bottom) The nasal cavity proper and the paranasal sinuses are lined by pseudostratified ciliated columnar (respiratory) epithelium. This epithelium appears to be stratified because the nuclei are at different levels in the cells. The epithelium illustrated is from the maxillary sinus.

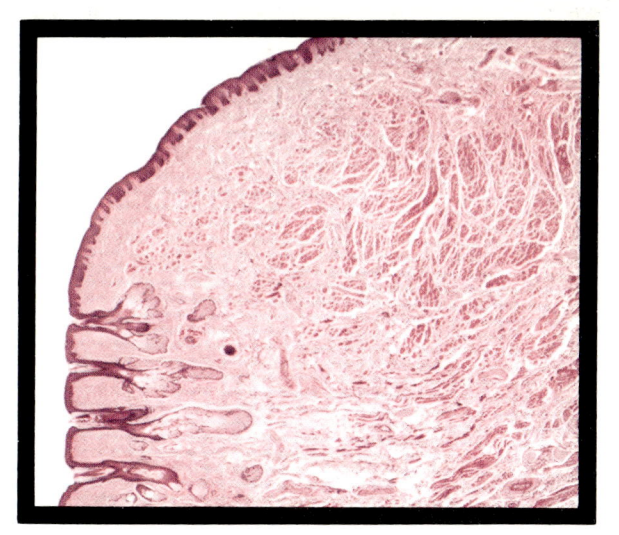

Mucocutaneous Junction, Lip   X 14

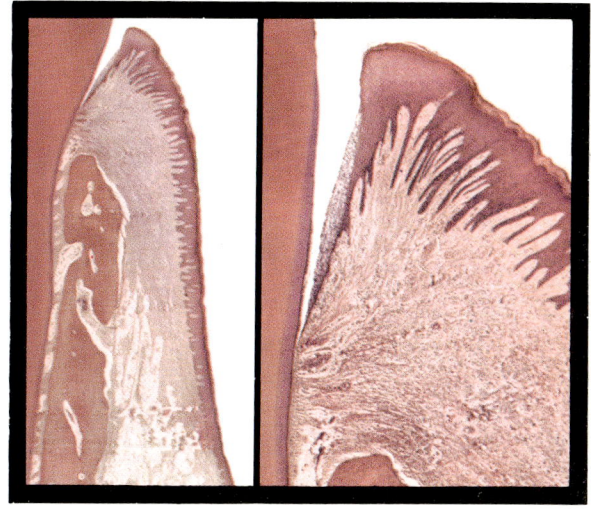

X 9   **Gingiva**   X 40

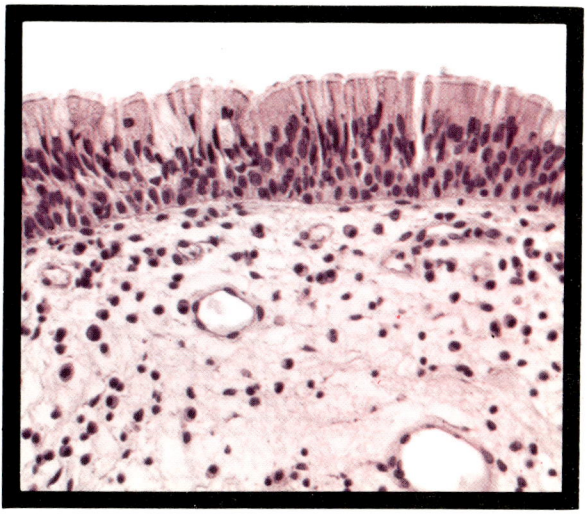

Pseudostratified Ciliated Columnar Epithelium   X 220

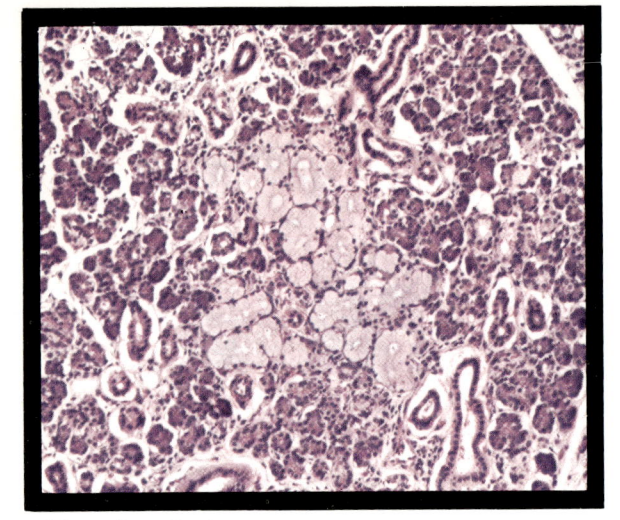

Submaxillary Gland   X 60

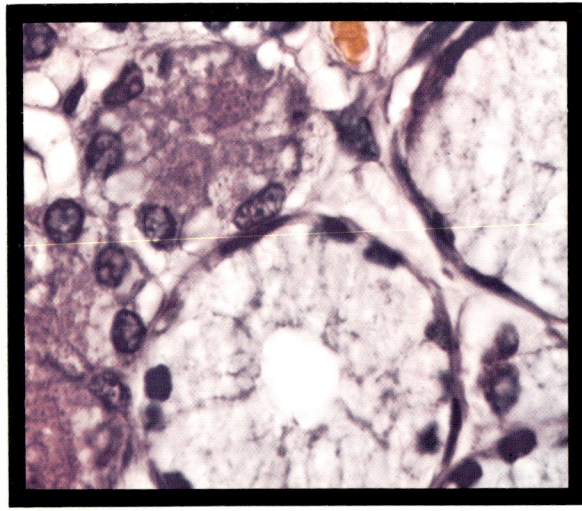

Serous and Mucous Acini   X 750

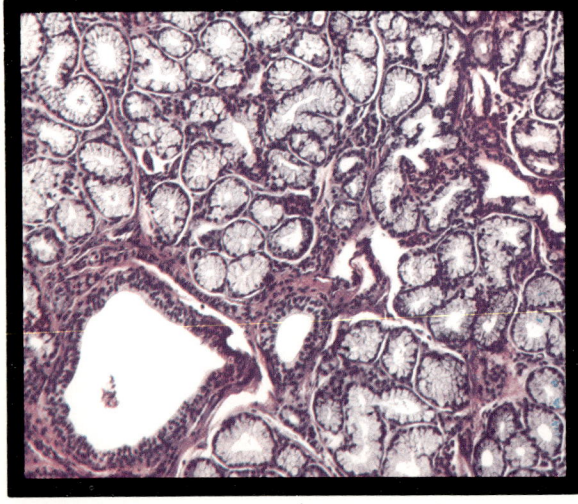

Accessory Salivary Gland   X 100

Salivary Glands

The major salivary glands are composed of serous and mucous cells in the following proportions: parotid—almost pure serous; submaxillary—almost 80 per cent serous; sublingual—usually more mucous than serous, but at least half mucous. Accessory salivary glands (located nearly everywhere in the oral mucosa but especially in the lips, palate, buccal mucosa and tongue) are predominately mucous except for the serous glands of von Ebner that open into the groove around each vallate papilla.

(Top) Salivary gland tissue composed mainly of serous acini, which at this magnification appear as groups of dark-staining cells. The light-staining units in the center of the field are mucous acini. The structures with the large lumina are ducts.

(Center) A mucous acinus (bottom of picture) is composed of triangular cells which are arranged in a circle, forming a distinct lumen. The nuclei of these cells are compressed against the basement membrane, and the cytoplasm is nearly colorless when stained with hematoxylin and eosin. A serous acinus (upper left) differs from the mucous type in that the nuclei of the individual cells are spherical, larger, and not compressed against the basement membrane, though they are situated near it. The cytoplasm of serous cells contains dark-blue-staining zymogen granules. Serous acini tend to be smaller than the mucous variety, and their lumina are rarely visible. A mixed acinus usually consists of a mucous unit partially surrounded by a cap of serous cells (serous demilune).

(Bottom) In this section of salivary gland tissue, which is from the lip, the acini are all of the mucous type. Ducts are evident near the lower border. The duct system varies in the different salivary glands, but in the main the peripheral ducts adjacent to the lobules of the gland are small and lined by a single row of short epithelial cells. Approaching the surface, the ducts become larger and are lined by taller cells. Close to the surface there is often a double row of cells. Finally, the last portion of the duct is lined by oral cavity epithelium.

Tongue

(Top) Histologic section through the tip of the tongue, demonstrating papillated dorsal surface and relatively smooth undersurface. The red-staining material that makes up the bulk of the tongue is voluntary muscle running in all directions. This complex musculature is peculiar to the tongue. The light-blue-staining areas (groups of mucous acini) constitute the anterior lingual gland.

(Center) Voluntary (skeletal) muscle fibers are extremely large, multinucleated cells composed of numerous myofibrils. The identifying features of skeletal muscle—cross striations and peripherally placed nuclei—are apparent in the photomicrograph of two longitudinally cut fibers. In cross section the fibers appear as eosinophilic islands, some of which have rounded nuclei situated just under the cell membrane.

(Bottom) There are three main types of lingual papillae—filiform, fungiform and vallate (circumvallate). The filiform papillae (upper left) are small, conical epithelial projections with rather thick cornified layers. The degree of tongue coating is reflected in the amount of cornification of these most numerous of papillae. The fungiform papillae (upper right) are scattered among the filiform papillae, being most numerous toward the sides and tip of the tongue. They are toadstool-like projections of connective tissue covered by relatively thin layers of epithelium. Clinically, these papillae appear as small red nodules because the thin epithelium does not mask the color of the underlying vascular connective tissue. The vallate papillae (lower), 8 to 12 in number, are arranged in an inverted V just anterior to the root of the tongue. The apex of the V is close to the foramen cecum. Each of these papillae (see p. 26, *top,* for the gross appearance) protrudes slightly and is surrounded by a deep groove. In some individuals rudimentary foliate papillae (see p. 26, *center*), which may be associated with lymphoid nodules, appear as parallel folds of mucosa on the lateral margins of the tongue posteriorly.

Taste buds (lower right) are seen as intraepithelial light-staining ovoid structures. While most common in the vallate papillae, they also are noted in the foliate and in some of the fungiform papillae.

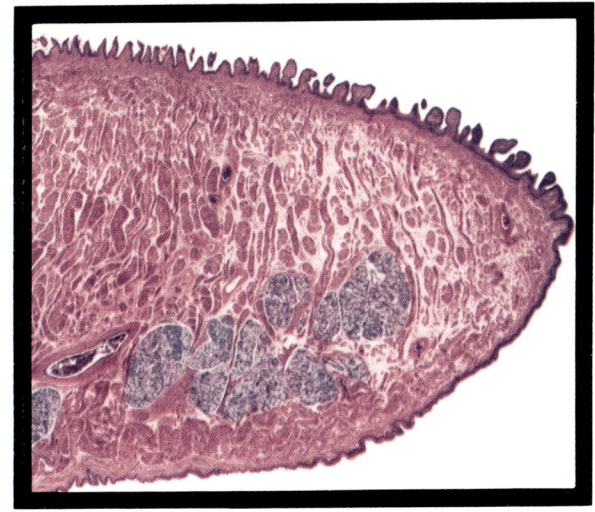

Tongue, Sagittal Section, Newborn Infant   X 11

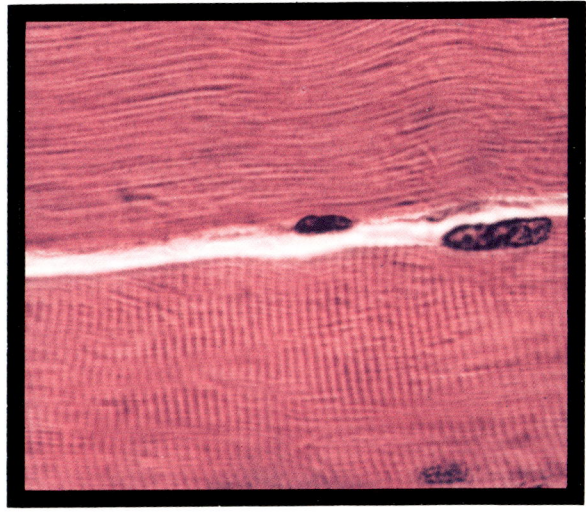

Voluntary Muscle   X 1080

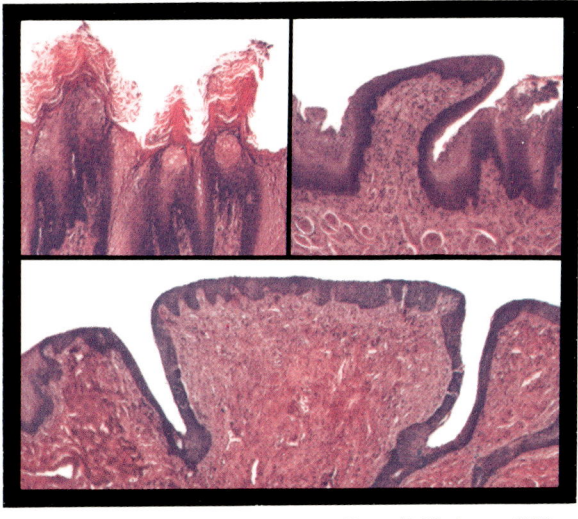

Lingual Papillae   Upper X 35, Lower X 28

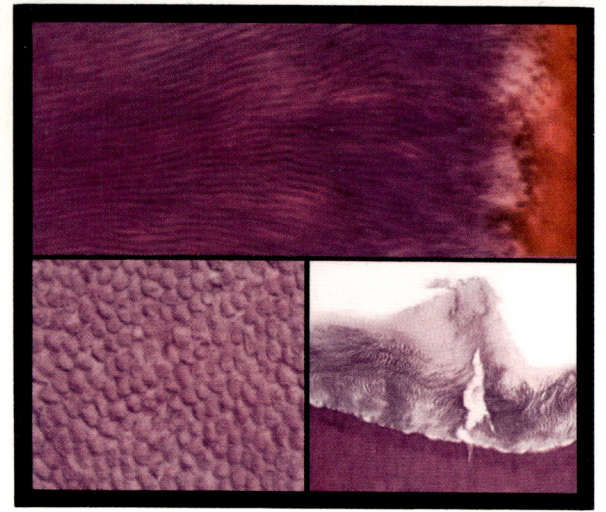

Enamel Upper X 427, Lower Left X 513, Lower Right X 100

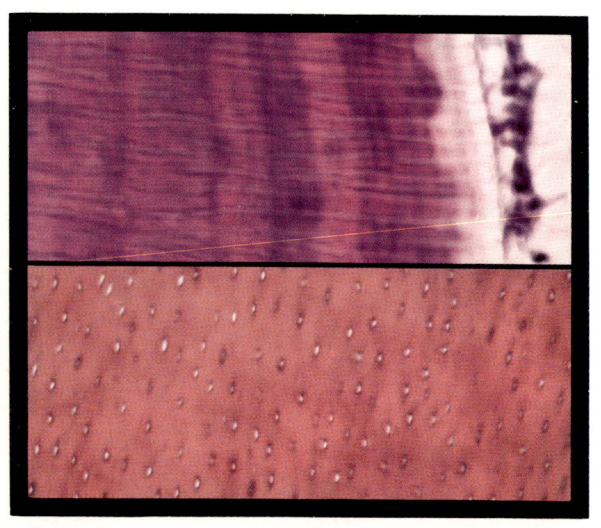

Dentin Upper X 550, Lower X 490

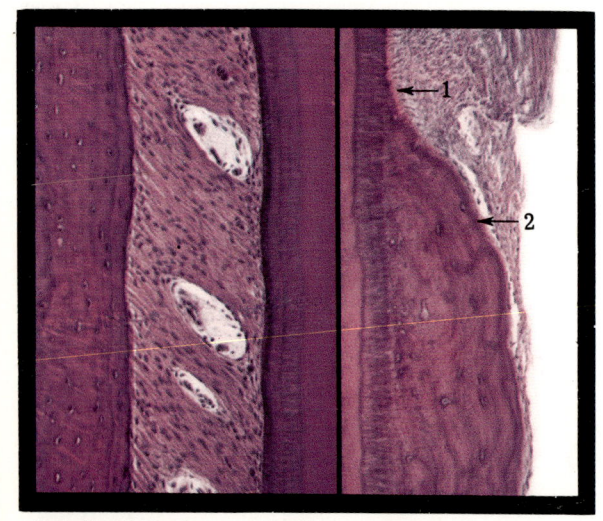

Periodontal Membrane X 100   **Cementum** X 100

Histology and Embryology

Enamel

(Top) Newly formed enamel matrix is demonstrated in the upper photomicrograph. A small area of dentin is seen at the right. Despite decalcification of this specimen, the enamel is well preserved because at this stage of development it has not undergone much mineralization. In the ground cross section of mature enamel (lower left) the ends of the enamel rods, as well as the interrod substance, may be seen. The appearance of rods cut in this plane has been likened to fish scales. In the lower right photomicrograph is a decalcified section of an erupted tooth. The dentin is at the lower border, and above this is a remnant of the acid-insoluble organic enamel matrix.

Dentin

(Center) In the upper half of the illustration, a row of odontoblasts is seen at the right. To the left of this region is a band of pale-staining predentin, and further to the left is calcified dentin. The light streaks that extend from the odontoblasts through the predentin and dentin are tubules which contain the dentinal (Tomes') fibers. The lower photomicrograph illustrates the dentinal tubules cut in cross section.

Periodontal Membrane and Cementum

(Bottom) In the center of the left photomicrograph are oblique fibers of the periodontal membrane which are attached to alveolar bone *(left)* and cementum *(right)*. The oval light-staining areas, between the bundles of principal fibers, are composed of very loose connective tissue in which are nerves, blood vessels and lymphatics. The right photomicrograph demonstrates acellular cementum (1) and cellular cementum (2). The first cementum deposited against the dentin is usually of the acellular variety. There is a slow but continuous formation of cementum throughout the life of the tooth which compensates for tooth movement and allows new fibers of the periodontal membrane to be embedded in the surface of the root.

Histology and Embryology

Pulp

(Top) Cross section of the coronal pulp of a third molar from a 21-year-old patient. The pulp consists of delicate, loose connective tissue in which there are numerous blood vessels, lymph vessels and nerves. Odontoblasts constitute the outermost portion of the pulp. In young pulp the fibroblasts, which are somewhat star-shaped, are quite numerous, but with age the pulp becomes less cellular and more fibrous.

Cartilage and Bone

(Center) Hyaline cartilage (left photomicrograph) is identified easily by its lavender-staining homogeneous matrix. In the matrix are spaces which contain 1 to 4 large cells with prominent centrally placed nuclei. In the upper portion of the illustration is a dense layer of fibrous connective tissue, the perichondrium, from which appositional growth takes place. The right photomicrograph is a low-power view to demonstrate compact bone (above) and trabecular bone (below). The relatively clear spaces enclosed by the trabecular bone are composed mainly of yellow or fatty marrow. Trabecular (spongy or cancellous) bone may be changed to the compact type by the deposition of layers of new bone on the sides of the trabeculae, so that finally the marrow spaces are reduced to small channels that contain only blood vessels. Bone is not a static substance, for its architecture is constantly changing (remodeling) in accordance with functional needs.

(Bottom) Osteoclasts are present at (1) and osteoblasts at (2) in the left photomicrograph. The osteoclasts (high power, upper right) are large multinucleated cells which are associated with bone resorption. Usually they are seen in small harborlike spaces (Howship's lacunae). Osteoblasts (high power, lower right) are spindle-shaped mesenchymal cells which secrete, or promote formation of, the organic intercellular substance of bone. Many of the osteoblasts become surrounded by this intercellular substance and remain in the bone as osteocytes. The vitality of bone is determined histologically by the presence of osteocytes.

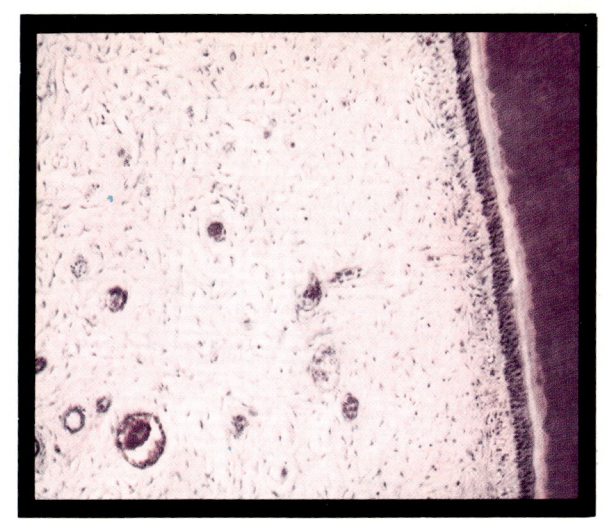

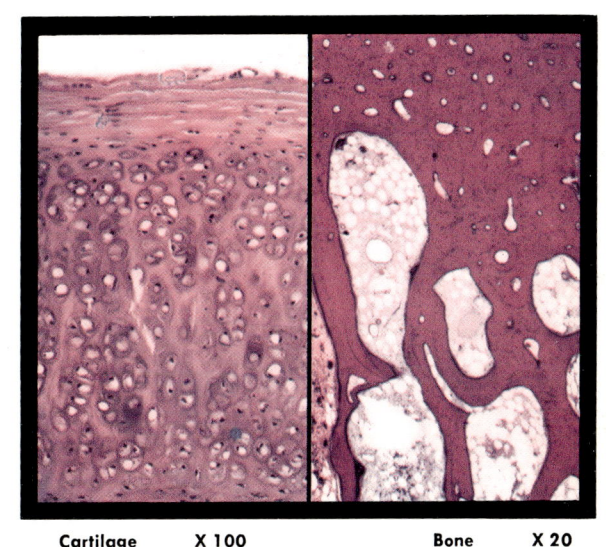

Pulp X 100

Cartilage X 100 Bone X 20

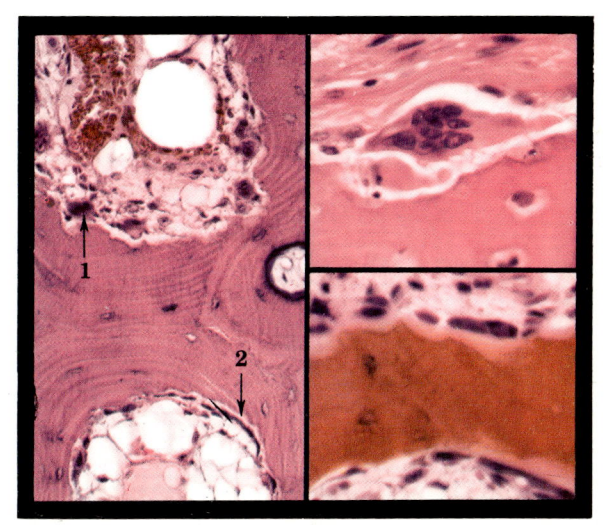

X 190 Osteoclasts and Osteoblasts
Upper X 456, Lower X 380

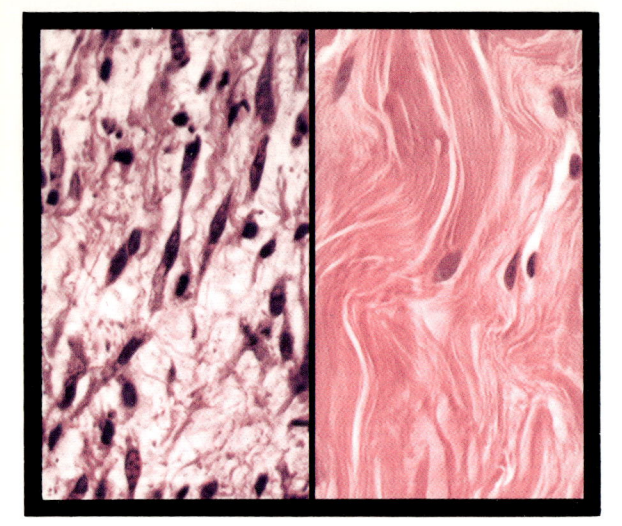

8 Histology and Embryology

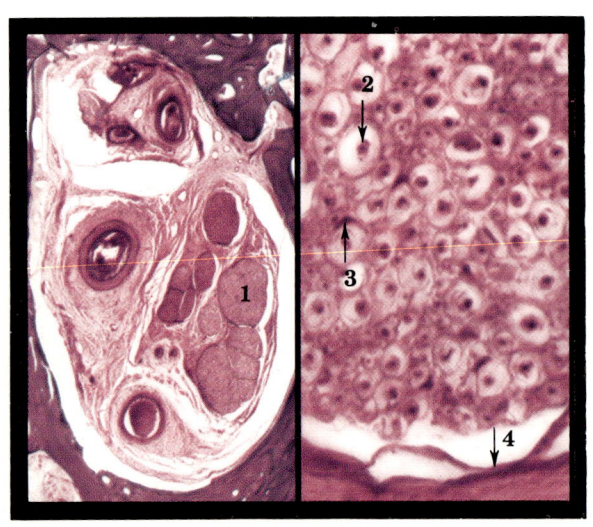

Fibrous Connective Tissue

(Top) Loose, immature connective tissue (left) has many young fibroblasts which have spindle-shaped nuclei and long cytoplasmic processes. Fibroblasts are associated with the production of the intercellular portion of connective tissue, but there is no general agreement as to the role they play. It seems certain, however, that the fibers are not extensions of these cells. Dense, mature fibrous connective tissue (right) has only a few fibrocytes, being composed mainly of eosinophilic collagenous fibers.

Peripheral Nerve

(Center) Cross section (left) through posterior portion of the mandibular nerve. One of the fasciculi of the nerve (1) is enlarged in the photomicrograph at right. An axis-cylinder is seen at (2), surrounded by a clear space which, before preparation of the specimen, was occupied by myelin. At the periphery of the myelin is the neurilemma (sheath of Schwann). A nucleus of a Schwann cell is apparent at (3). A connective tissue sheath, epineurium, surrounds the several fasciculi of a nerve. The perineurium (4) envelops each individual fasciculus. Connective tissue extending into fasciculi is termed endoneurium.

Inflammatory Cells

(Bottom) The following types of inflammatory cells, with their distinguishing characteristics, are shown: Polymorphonuclear neutrophils (upper left)—finely granular cytoplasm staining light bluish pink; nuclei with 3 to 5 lobes. Lymphocytes (upper right)—varying in size; very thin rim of cytoplasm around circular deep-purple-staining nucleus. Eosinophils (lower left)—coarsely granular reddish cytoplasm; 1- or 2-lobed nuclei. Plasma cells (lower right)—eccentrically placed nuclei, having appearance of cartwheel or clock face because of clumped arrangement of chromatin; lavender cytoplasm, often pale near nucleus, producing halo-like effect. The size of these various cells may be judged by comparison with erythrocyte (7.6 microns) in lower right picture.

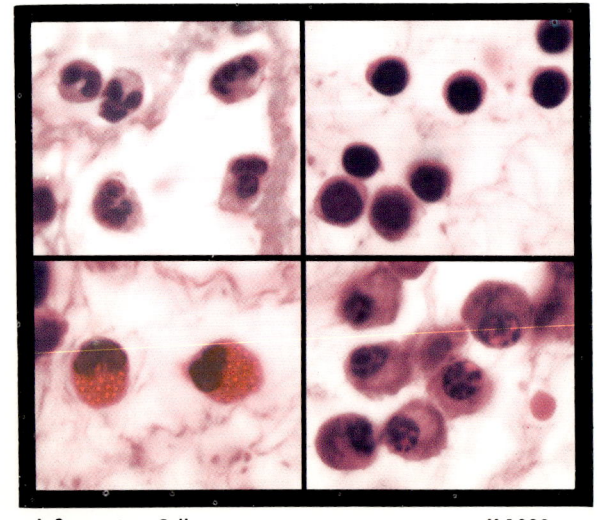

Histology and Embryology

Inflammatory Cells (Cont.)

Inflammation is the body's response to any irritant which kills or injures cells. The neutrophils, which come from the blood, are the first cells to arrive in an injured area. They ingest bacteria and provide proteolytic enzymes, which liquefy injured cells. Macrophages, which are the second line of defense, assist the neutrophils in the ingestion and the digestion of bacteria. They phagocytize tissue debris, thus preparing the area for repair. These scavenger-type cells may be from the blood (large mononuclears) or from the tissues. Those of histogenous origin are known by various names, such as histocytes, endothelial leukocytes, resting-wandering cells, clasmatocytes, polyblasts, and cells of the reticuloendothelial system. Some lymphocytes are from the blood, while others migrate from lymphoid tissue in the area. They are present in all stages of inflammation but are most numerous in chronic types; their functions in the process are not positively known. Plasma cells are usually prominent in chronic oral lesions; both their function and their origin are controversial, but they may be related to antibody formation. The eosinophils are probably all from the blood. They are slightly phagocytic and are numerous in inflammations of an allergic nature, in parasitism and in certain long-standing chronic processes.

(Top) Large lipid-containing macrophages (upper section). The nuclei have been pushed to one side, and the cytoplasm consists of vacuoles, the fat having been lost during processing of the specimen. Neutrophils have been engulfed by the macrophage in the lower left picture. A hemosiderin-containing macrophage is seen in lower right section.

(Center) A foreign body giant cell *(left)* with numerous haphazardly situated nuclei. At right is a similar cell surrounding suture material.

(Bottom) Numerous lens-shaped slits *(left)* formerly occupied by cholesterol crystals. Enlargement *(right)* shows foreign body giant cells in close apposition to a crystal. Cholesterol crystals may be found wherever there has been tissue disintegration; they are common in walls of periodontal cysts.

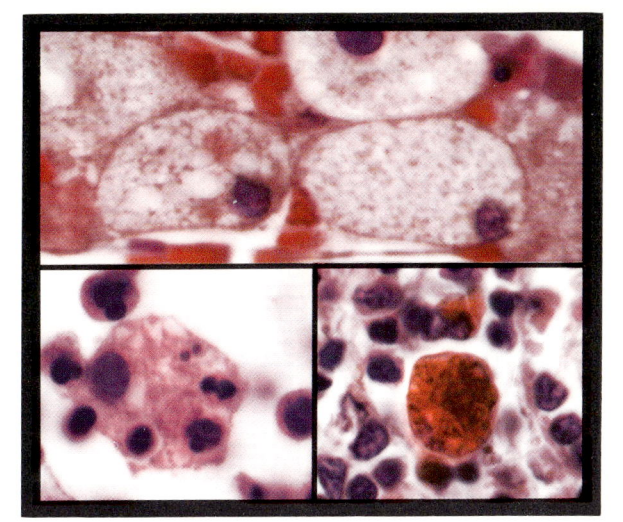

Macrophages   X 1080

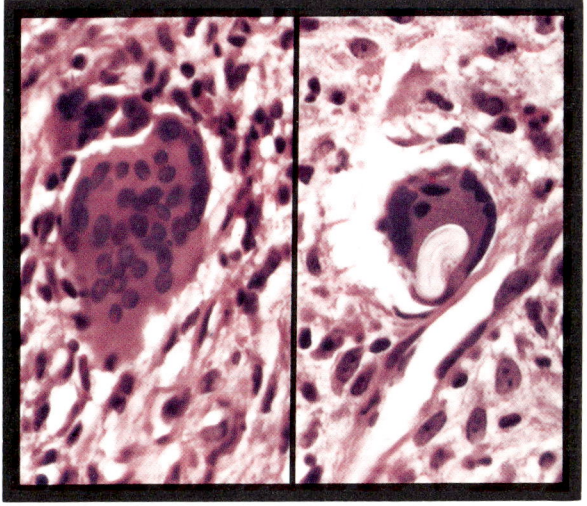

Foreign Body Giant Cells   X 490

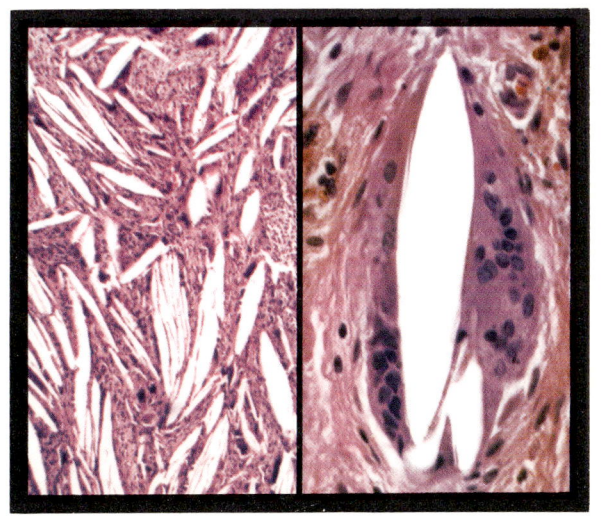

X 62   Cholesterol Slits and Foreign Body Giant Cells   X 387

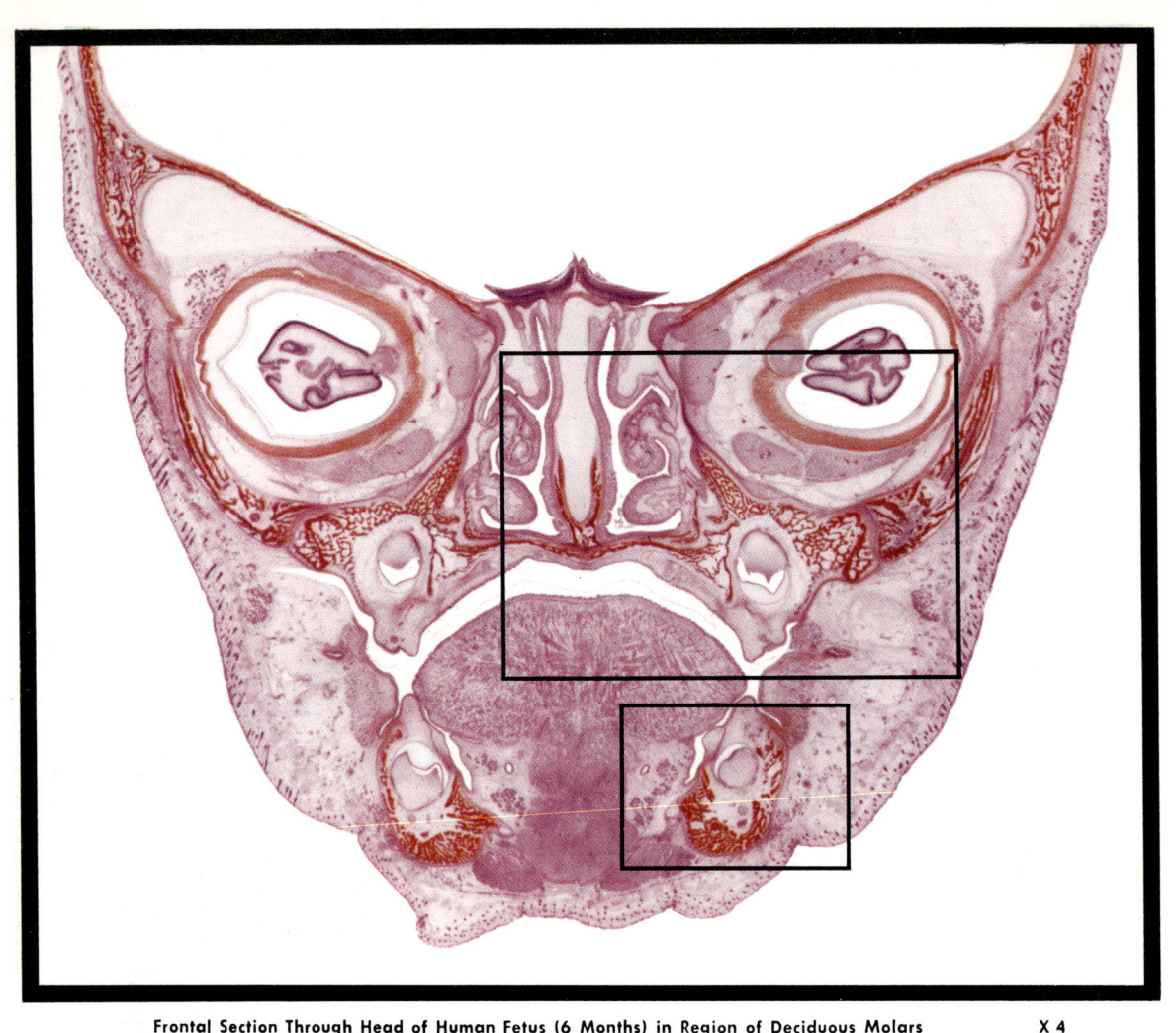

Frontal Section Through Head of Human Fetus (6 Months) in Region of Deciduous Molars   X 4

EMBRYOLOGY

Human Fetus

In the enlargements (opposite page) of the blocked areas shown above, the following structures are demonstrated:

1. Developing eye
2. Optic nerve
3. Extrinsic eye muscles
4. Infra-orbital nerve
5. Inferior, middle and superior conchae
6. Respiratory epithelium
7. Nasal cavity
8. Nasal septum
9. Maxillary bone
10. Dorsal surface of tongue
11. Palatal glands
12. Developing teeth
13. Zygomatic bone (malar)
14. Parotid duct
15. Buccinator muscle
16. Tongue muscle
17. Dental lamina
18. Oral epithelium
19. Submaxillary gland duct (Wharton's)
20. Sublingual gland
21. Meckel's cartilage
22. Mylohyoid muscle
23. Anterior belly of the digastric muscle
24. Bone of mandible
25. Mandibular nerve
26. Mandibular vessels
27. Platysma muscle
28. Epidermis of the face
29. Lanugo hair follicle

Frontal Section Through Head of Human Fetus

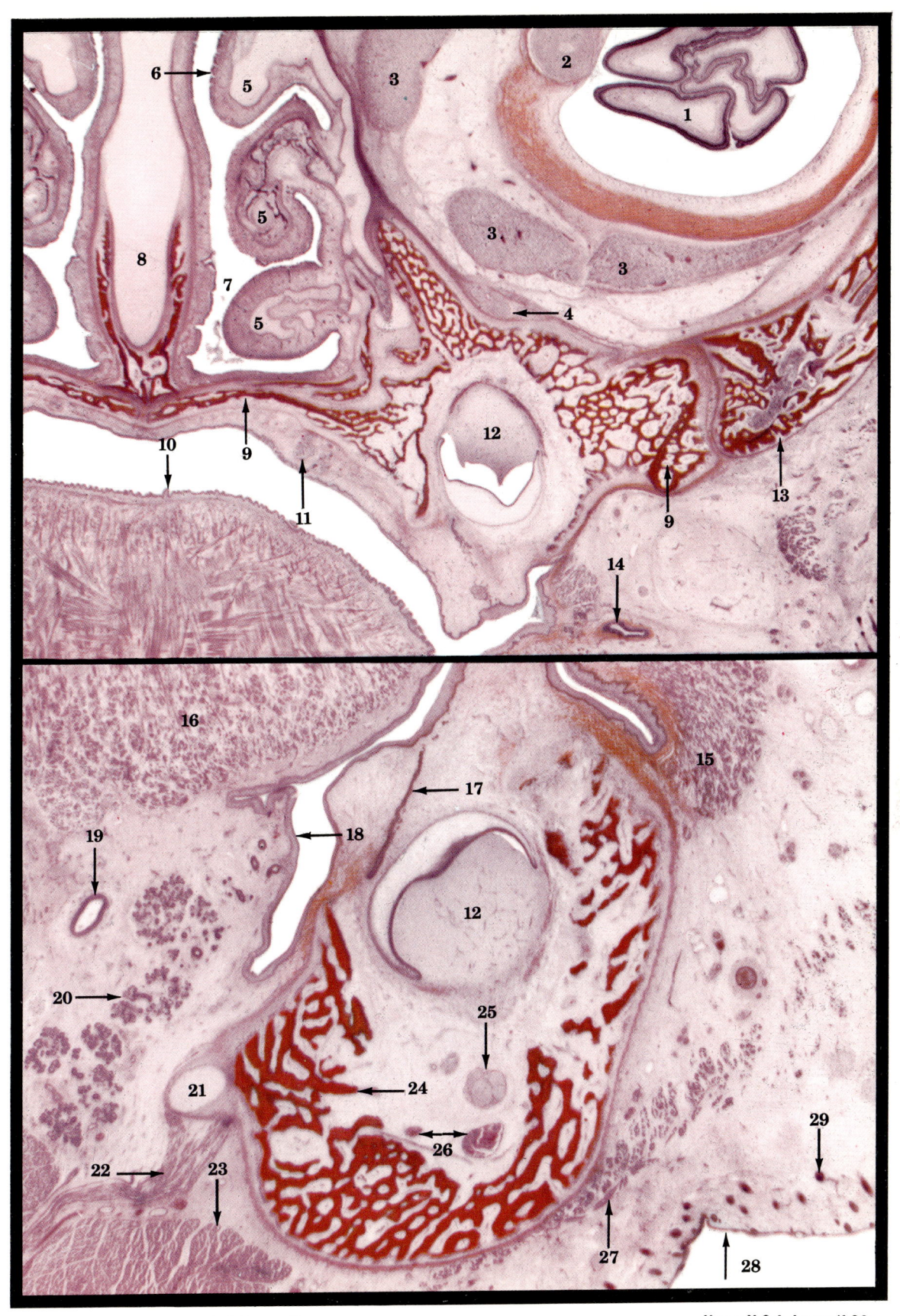

11

Upper X 9.6, Lower X 20

Histology and Embryology

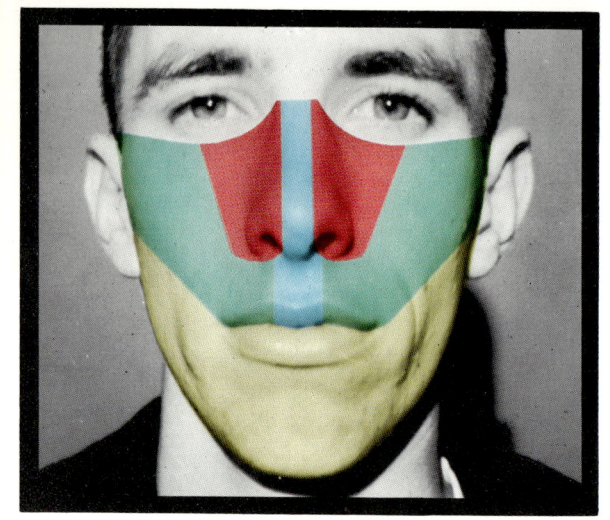

Embryonic Derivations of Various Parts of the Face

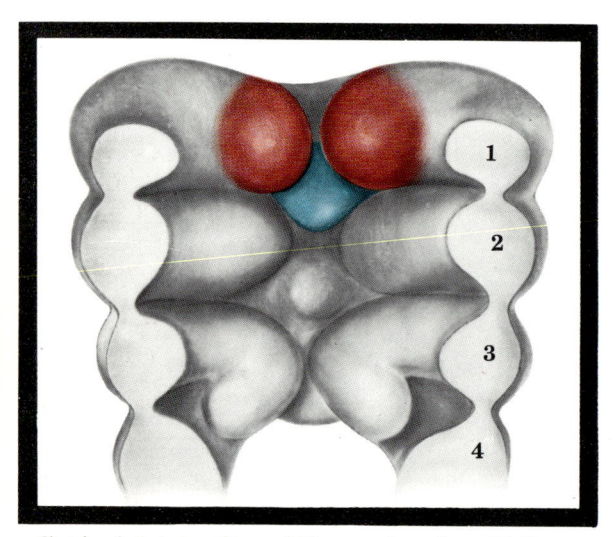

Sketch of Anterior View of Pharynx, Seen from Within, Human Embryo (3 Weeks)

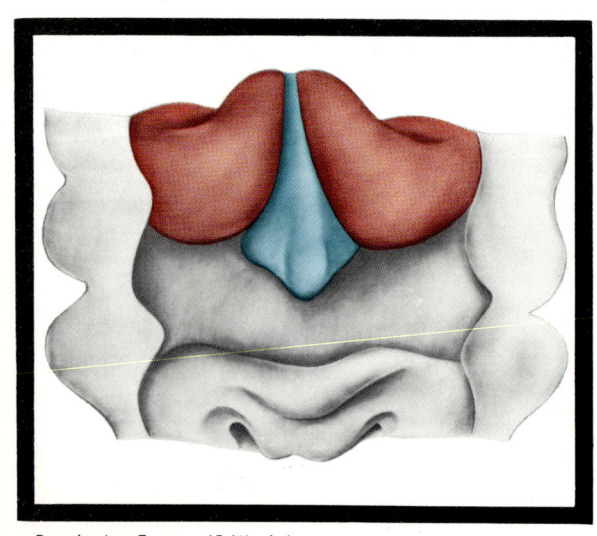

Developing Tongue (5 Weeks)

Development of the Face

(Top) The colors superimposed on the adult face designate areas derived from the following embryonic structures: mandibular arch (yellow), maxillary processes (blue green), medial nasal process (blue), lateral nasal processes (red).

Branchial Arches

(Center) The external depressions between the branchial bars or arches (1 through 4) are branchial clefts, while the furrows on the inside are termed pharyngeal pouches. The clefts and the external surfaces of the arches are bordered by ectodermal epithelium, while the pouches and internal surfaces of the arches (except the 1st) are bordered by entodermal epithelium. At a certain stage the epithelium of the pouches on the inside meets the epithelium of the external clefts, with no mesoderm between them. In lower animals, like the fish, this double epithelial membrane ruptures, and gill slits result, but in man the arches merge by the process of mesenchymal tissue proliferation, which pushes the epithelia of the pouches and clefts inward and outward, finally presenting smooth inner and outer surfaces. The pouches are the origin of numerous structures, among which are the middle ear (1st pouch), palatine tonsil (2nd pouch) and parathyroid glands (3rd and 4th pouches).

Development of the Tongue

(Center) The tongue develops from the internal surfaces of the 1st, 2nd and 3rd branchial arches by 4 nodular swellings. The anterior portion, or body, is formed from the 1st arch by 2 lateral prominences (red) and 1 medial prominence, the tuberculum impar (blue). The posterior portion, or root, is formed from the copula, which is the nodule seen just below the blue-colored tuberculum impar.

(Bottom) The 3 prominences forming the anterior part of the tongue (same colors as in the center picture) are about equal in size at this stage. As development progresses, the tuberculum impar (blue) stops growing and partially degenerates, allowing the 2 lateral prominences to grow over it and meet in the midline.

Histology and Embryology 13

Development of the Tongue (Cont.)

(Top) The two lateral halves of the tongue have now united (line of fusion shown in black). The diamond-shaped area (broken blue line) represents the final position of tuberculum impar beneath the surface of the tongue. Small circle indicates foramen cecum. (This picture and the three on p. 12 modified after Sicher and Tandler.)

Thyroglossal Duct

The thyroid gland develops from an epithelial-lined tube (thyroglossal duct) which arises from an area between the copula and the tuberculum impar. (See center picture, opposite page.) This tube grows downward through the tongue and through a region that later will become hyoid bone to a point in the midline of the neck, where the thyroid gland is formed from it. After forming the thyroid gland the duct should involute. Its point of origin on the tongue is indicated permanently by an enlarged pit, the foramen cecum. (See top picture.)

(Center) Low-power photomicrograph *(left)* illustrates that at this stage of development the embryo still has a marked dorsal convexity, with the large head curved forward and the short mandible lying tight against the chest. A small channel may be seen extending into the primitive oral cavity, which at this stage is occupied mostly by the tongue. Just below the oral opening is the heart. The large organ near the bottom of the picture is the liver. Enlargement *(right)* of blocked area *(left)* shows base of tongue, oral cavity, pharynx, esophagus and trachea. The thyroglossal duct can be seen extending from the foramen cecum (arrow) through the tongue to a region just in front of developing hyoid bone. At this age the duct should begin to involute.

(Bottom) Frontal section through tongue in region of the foramen cecum. The persistent thyroglossal duct, lined by stratified squamous epithelium, extends almost to the hyoid bone. Nonlingual remnants of the duct usually consist of pseudostratified columnar epithelium.

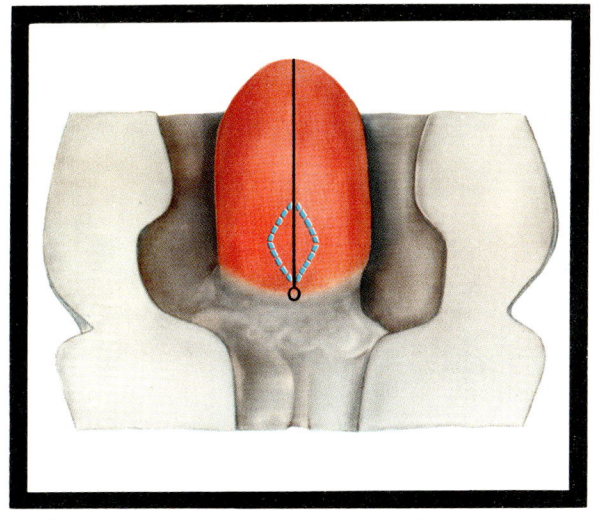

Sketch of Anterior Part of Tongue, Human Embryo (6 Weeks)

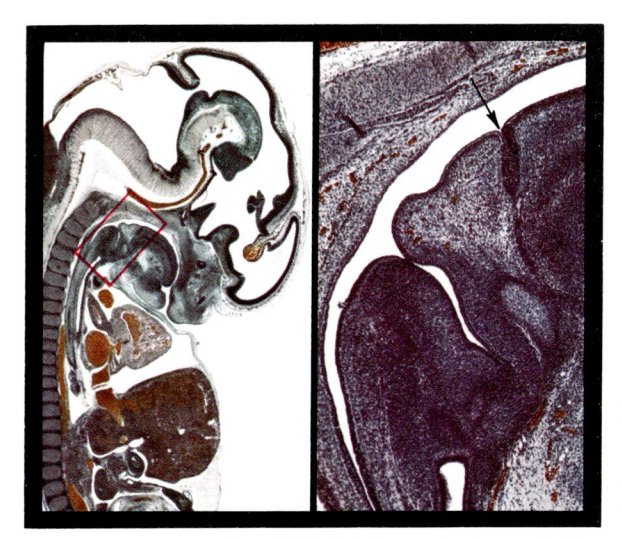

X 7   **Human Embryo (7 Weeks), Sagittal Section**   X 40

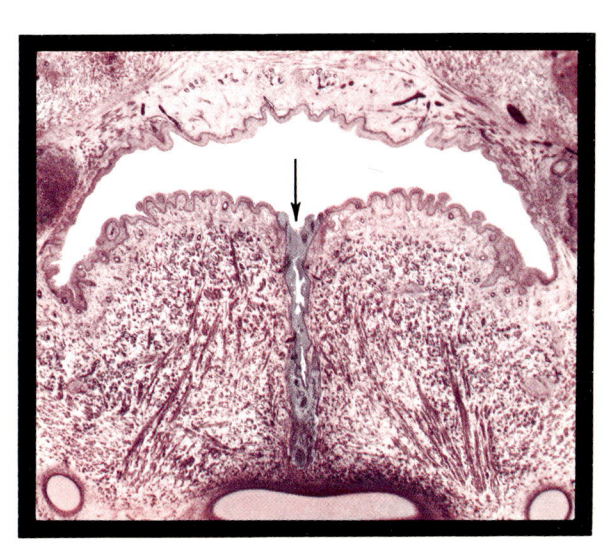

Persistent Thyroglossal Duct, Human Fetus (5 Months)   X 14

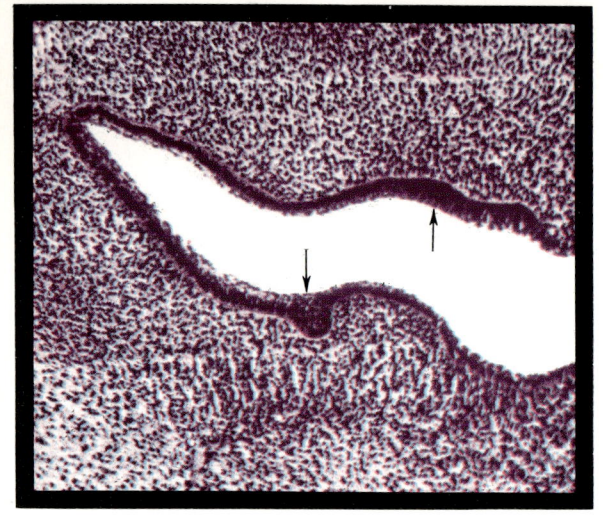

Initiation of Tooth Development, Frontal Section, Human Embryo (6 Weeks)

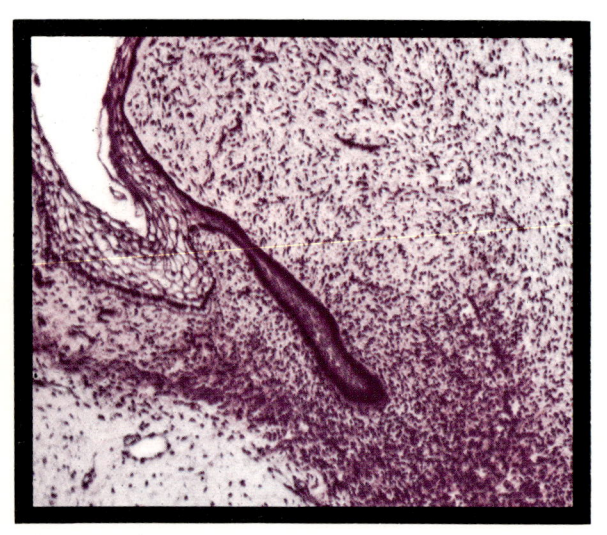

Dental Lamina

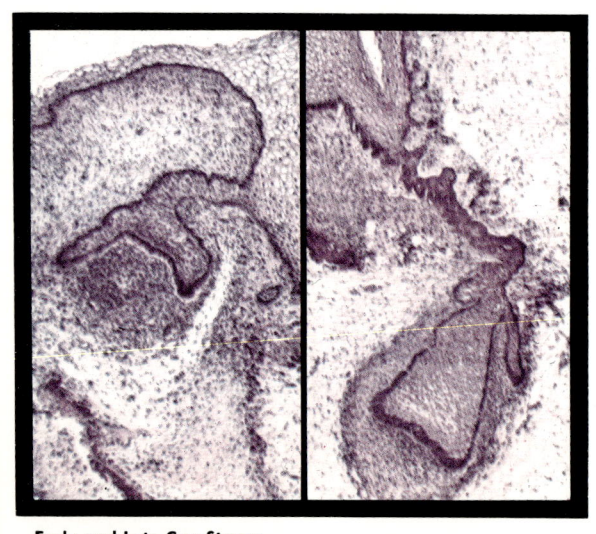

Early and Late Cap Stages

Tooth Development

Tooth development comprises the following physiologic processes: stimulation of certain cells to multiply (initiation and proliferation); establishment of tooth pattern (morphodifferentiation); differentiation of cells to perform special functions (histodifferentiation); formation of dentin and enamel matrix (apposition); influx of mineral salts and their subsequent crystallization (calcification and maturation); emergence of the crown into the oral cavity (eruption).

(Top) Human tooth development begins, usually between the 35th and 42nd days in utero, by a thickening of the primitive oral epithelium (arrows) in areas that are destined to become the maxillary and mandibular ridges. This epithelial thickening, which extends along the length of both jaws, is termed the dental lamina.

(Center) In 10 locations along each jaw the dental lamina proliferates into the primitive connective tissue. One of these extensions is shown. Eventually, cells of this epithelial structure will form the enamel portion of the tooth, while cells derived from the surrounding mesenchymal tissue will form dentin, pulp, cementum, periodontal membrane and alveolar bone.

(Bottom) Each proliferating epithelial extension becomes large at the end, developing a concave lower surface which somewhat resembles a cap (left picture). The mesenchymal tissue within the confines of the cap changes its character by becoming quite cellular. Eventually, this portion of connective tissue will be the dental pulp. As development progresses *(right),* the epithelial cells at the lower portion of the enamel organ become columnar (inner enamel epithelium), while the remaining peripheral cells are cuboidal (outer enamel epithelium). The epithelial cells in the central portion of the enamel organ begin to separate, initiating the formation of the stellate reticulum. The mesodermal tissue surrounding the whole structure becomes condensed, forming the connective tissue follicle, or dental sac. The epithelial extension seen near the right border of the picture is the primordium of a succedaneous tooth.

Tooth Development (Cont.)

(Top) At this stage of development the dental lamina is just beginning to disintegrate. The inner enamel epithelium (ameloblastic layer) has become stabilized, thus establishing the future dentino-enamel junction, which reflects the ultimate shape of the tooth (morphodifferentiation).

(Center) In an enlargement of the blocked area from above, the outer enamel epithelium (1) meets the inner enamel epithelium (4) to form the cervical loop, the tip of which proliferates apically to become Hertwig's sheath after the enamel is fully apposed. The stellate reticulum (2) resembles young, loose connective tissue but actually is composed of star-shaped epithelial cells which, except for fine, threadlike connections, are widely separated from each other by a mucoid substance. The stratum intermedium (3) consists of a few rows of cells which are believed to be important in enamel maturation. The dental papilla is identified at (5).

(Bottom) High-power view *(right)*, from side of enamel organ, identifies the stellate reticulum (1), stratum intermedium (2), ameloblasts (3), odontoblasts (4) and dental papilla (5). The ameloblasts at the bottom of the low-power photomicrograph *(left)* have large, centrally placed nuclei, and adjacent to them is a clear, cell-free area in the dental papilla. The ameloblasts near the middle of the picture have elongated at the expense of the clear area, and their nuclei are situated at the stratum intermedium end. These tall ameloblasts have influenced cells of the dental papilla to become odontoblasts, some of which have already participated in the formation of dentin (orange). After dentin is formed, the ameloblasts again become short. Now they must receive their nutrient supply from the dental sac, for their former source (the dental papilla) is blocked by dentin. At the upper border *(left)* the enamel matrix appears as a thin black line between the ameloblasts and the dentin. Connective tissue cells do not differentiate into odontoblasts without the organizing influence of the ameloblasts, and the ameloblasts do not commence amelogenesis until laying down of dentin has begun.

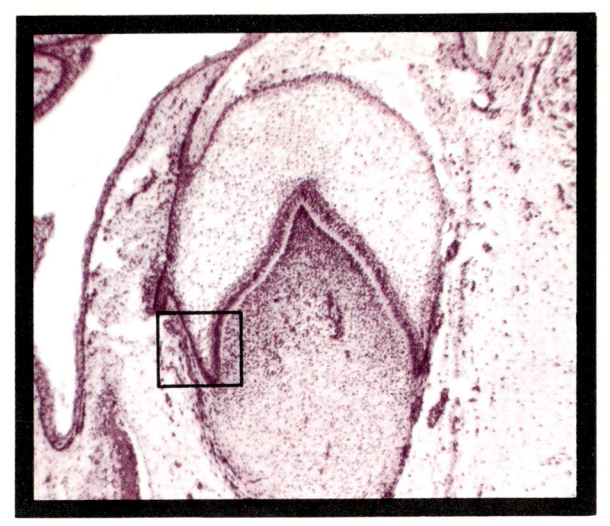

Advanced Bell Stage

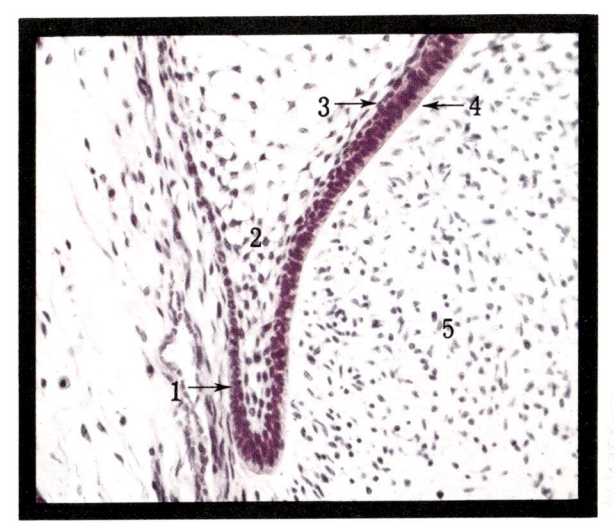

Cervical Loop

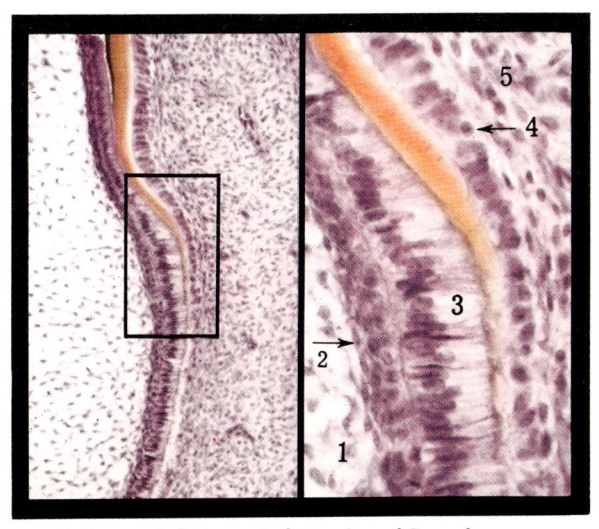

Cell Changes Relative to Early Dentin and Enamel Formation

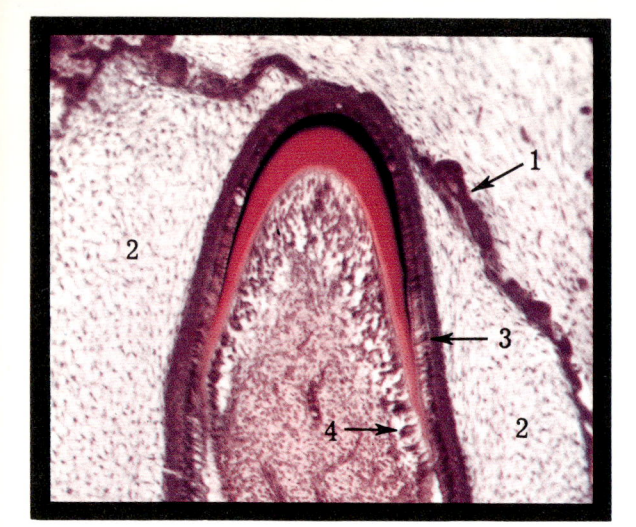

Histology and Embryology

Dentin and Enamel Formation

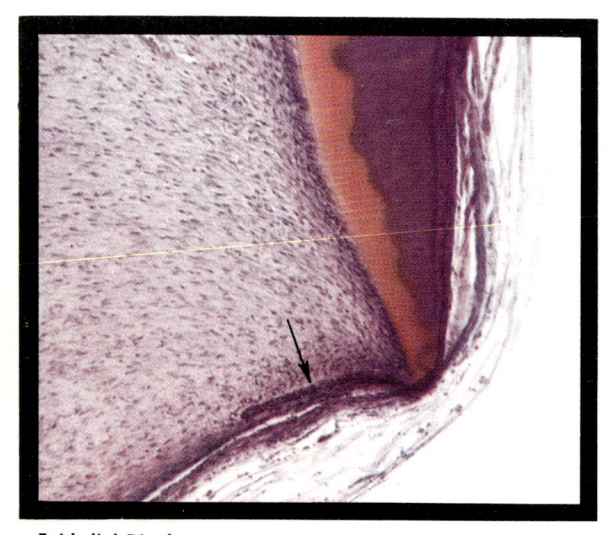

Epithelial Diaphragm

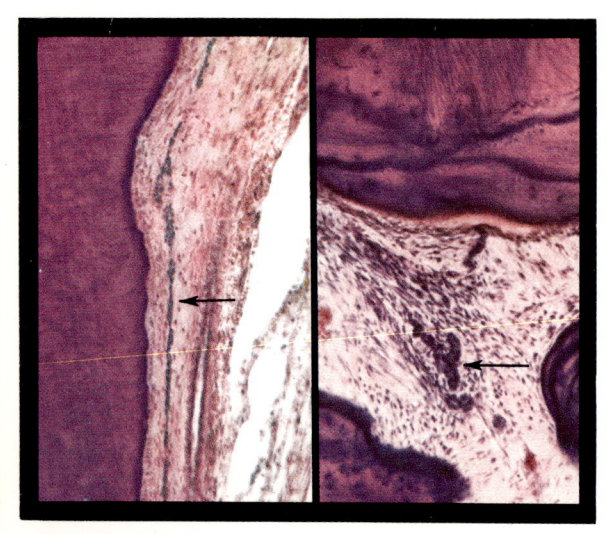

Remnants of Hertwig's Sheath

Tooth Development (Cont.)

(Top) The incisal tip is capped by enamel matrix (black) and dentin matrix (red). The outer enamel epithelium is at (1), the stellate reticulum at (2), the ameloblastic layer at (3) and the odontoblasts at (4). Near the top of the picture the stellate reticulum has disappeared, and the cells of the outer enamel epithelium are in contact with the stratum intermedium. After enamel formation is completed the stratum intermedium, outer enamel epithelium, and the ameloblastic cells, now reduced in height, fuse and persist until the tooth emerges into the oral cavity. As the tooth approaches the surface, the reduced enamel epithelium and the oral epithelium fuse. After eruption the epithelium attached to the tooth surface forms the epithelial attachment. The transformation of enamel matrix into hard enamel begins with the influx of minerals in an organic state. The process whereby the proper crystalline structure of the enamel is gradually developed by the conversion of these minerals to an inorganic form is termed maturation.

(Center) Hertwig's sheath, which consists of inner and outer enamel epithelium, is responsible for root shape and for initiating the formation of root dentin. This double row of epithelial cells proliferates apically from the future cemento-enamel junction and abruptly turns inward to form the epithelial diaphragm (arrow). The inner enamel epithelium induces adjacent pulpal cells to become odontoblasts, and dentinogenesis begins. As root dentin is formed, the tooth migrates coronally, allowing the continuously proliferating epithelial diaphragm to remain in its original relationship.

(Bottom) Immediately after root dentin begins to form in any given area, connective tissue of the dental sac grows inward and perforates Hertwig's sheath, obliterating much of it. The dental sac becomes the periodontal membrane, and its innermost cells form cementum while its outermost cells form the alveolar bone. Remnants of Hertwig's sheath (debris of Malassez) are seen near the lateral surface of a root (arrow, left picture) and in periapical tissue (arrow, *right*). Varying amounts of epithelial debris are probably present in all periodontal membranes.

2
Developmental Disturbances

INTRODUCTION

Developmental disturbances may be classified as variations, anomalies, malformations and monstrosities, each being of increasing severity. Variations are quite minor deviations from normal (e.g., large oral orifice); anomalies are more severe but do not interfere with function (e.g., enamel hypoplasia, peg laterals); malformations are even more severe and interfere with function (e.g., cleft lip); and monstrosities are extreme deviations which severely interfere with function (e.g., agnathia, dicephalus).

Some abnormalities result largely from intrinsic factors (heredity, metabolic dysfunction, mutations); others largely from extrinsic factors (physical or chemical agents, living agents, nutritional deficiency, stress). In some instances both intrinsic and extrinsic factors play a part.

Certain developmental disturbances are apparent at birth (congenital); others, though determined before birth, may not be evident until later. Some noncongenital developmental defects result entirely from postnatal environmental influences on structures still developing.

Many developmental defects of the head-and-neck region result from failure of embryonic processes to unite properly. These failures may cause clefts of the face, the lips, the alveolus, or the hard or soft palate. Incomplete union of the maxillary and mandibular processes produces a very large oral orifice (macrostomia), while union extending too far anteriorly causes a small oral opening (microstomia). If the two lateral halves of the tongue fail to unite anteriorly, a bifid tongue results.

Because much of the intricate development of the head-and-neck region involves epithelium, many opportunities are afforded for the enclavement of epithelial cells. These residual epithelial cells then become potential sources of cysts (closed epithelial-lined spaces), sinuses (epithelial-lined spaces opening onto a body surface or into a natural cavity) and fistulae (epithelial-lined tracts opening upon 2 surfaces). Epithelium trapped during the uniting of embryonic processes either by faulty merging or faulty fusion may form branchial cleft, epidermoid, dermoid, globulomaxillary or median palatine cysts. Incomplete involution of Hertwig's sheath, the dental lamina, the nasopalatine ducts or the thyroglossal duct may leave epithelium to form cysts in the respective regions. Every individual has some residual epithelium in the head-and-neck region, but only a small percentage develop cysts from it, for cyst formation is dependent upon proliferation of the residual epithelium. Inflammation is definitely known to cause periodontal cysts, but for most of the other cysts the exciting cause seldom is apparent.

Auricular tags, Fordyce spots, lingual thyroid and enamel pearls are examples of normal tissues developing in abnormal sites.

Primordial cysts form because of regressive changes in tooth buds, and a similar process is responsible for the formation of dentigerous cysts at a later stage of odontogenesis. Failure of the tuberculum impar to involute is, in part, the cause of median rhomboid glossitis.

Hygroma, tori, macroglossia, hypercementosis, supernumerary teeth and some of the odontomas are examples of excessive growth.

Among the disturbances resulting from underdevelopment are micrognathia, dwarfed roots, microdontia, anodontia, enamel hypoplasia and enamel hypocalcification.

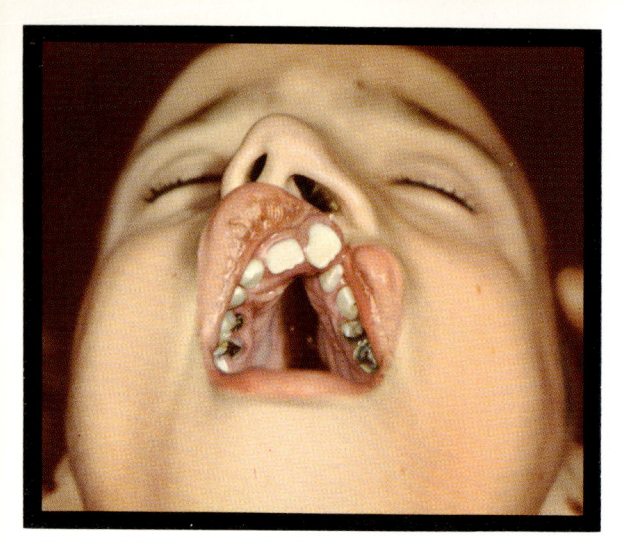

Unilateral Cleft Lip and Cleft Palate

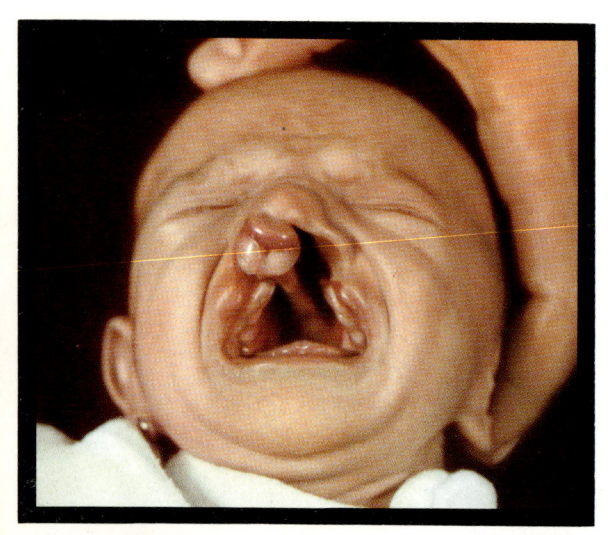

Bilateral Cleft Lip and Cleft Palate

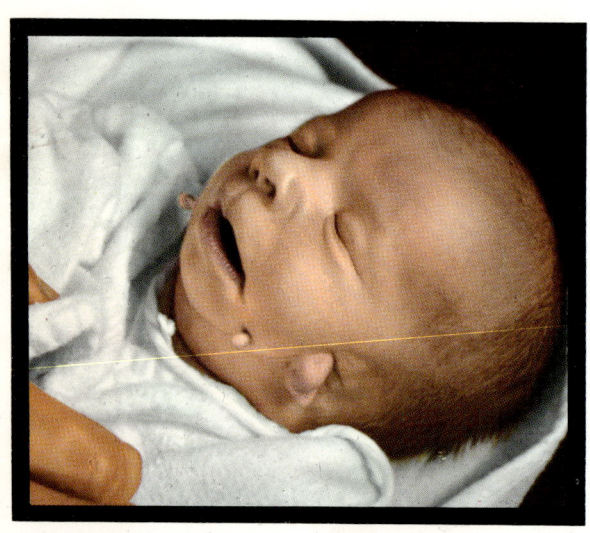

Auricular Tags and Macrostomia

18   *Developmental Disturbances*

CLEFTS OF THE LIP AND THE PALATE

Clefts of the lip and palate are often genetic in origin. Some degree of these disturbances has been reported as occurring once in every 800 births. Clefts of the upper lip are either unilateral or bilateral, midline clefts appearing rarely in the lower lip. These malformations may not be due to failure of fusion of epithelium primarily, but rather to failure of mesenchymal tissue on either side to unite. Clefts may be limited to the lips (cheiloschisis), the alveolus (gnathoschisis), the soft palate (staphyloschisis) or the hard and soft palate (staphylo-uranoschisis), or may present various combinations involving these structures.

(Top) The unilateral cleft of the lip and the alveolar process is due to failure of the median nasal and the maxillary processes to unite. The left and right palatine processes have not met or united in the midline, resulting in cleft palate (staphylo-uronoschisis).

(Center) An extensive bilateral cleft of lip and jaw combined with a midpalatine cleft caused by failure of development of palatine processes. The globular mass is the premaxilla which developed from the median nasal process but did not fuse with the maxillary processes.

AURICULAR TAGS, MACROSTOMIA AND LIP PITS

(Bottom) The external auditory canal develops from the 1st branchial cleft and the auricle from a group of nodules on the external surfaces of the 1st and 2nd branchial arches. The malformed external ear illustrated has no meatus, and accessory rudimentary appendages (auricular tags) containing cartilage are present anteriorly on each cheek quite remote from the normal position of the ear. The maxillary and mandibular processes have not fused completely, and there is some degree of macrostomia. Faulty union of these processes also may result in blind epithelial-lined tubes at the corners of the mouth (commissural lip pits—incidence 12-21%). Other congenital pits may be found as paired, paramedian collapsed structures, often exuding mucin, on the vermilion of the lower lip. The origin of these paramedian clefts is under discussion with varying viewpoints, but their formation may be related to failure of the bilateral grooves on the mandibular arch to fuse during early developmental life.

Developmental Disturbances

BRACHYGNATHIA (MICROGNATHIA) AND PIERRE ROBIN SYNDROME

(Top) An example of acquired brachygnathia in which the heads of the condyles were damaged during forceps delivery. The growth centers for the mandible are the hyaline cartilages in the condylar heads, and injury to these areas with or without ankylosis results in cessation of development. In severe congenital micrognathia the infant may experience respiratory distress from glossoptosis and from having the tongue caught in a cleft uvula (Robin, Pierre Robin syndrome). Inability to masticate, extensive speech defects, periodontal disease and psychological maladjustment are complications of acquired as well as congenital micrognathia.

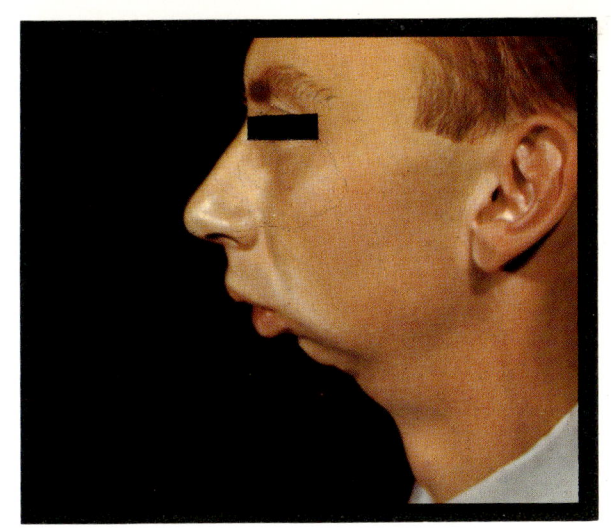

Brachygnathia

HEMIATROPHY

In hemiatrophy one half of the face or the head or an entire side of the body may diminish in size. The atrophy, usually of neurogenic origin, is progressive, and the region previously of normal size becomes smaller. It should not be confused with other facial asymmetries due to unilateral underdevelopment (hypoplasia) or unilateral overdevelopment (hyperplasia).

(Center) A few years previously this individual's face was of normal contour. Now the entire right side is flattened, and the eye is deeply set. Maxillary, mandibular and malar bones as well as the facial and masticatory muscles show evidence of atrophy unilaterally.

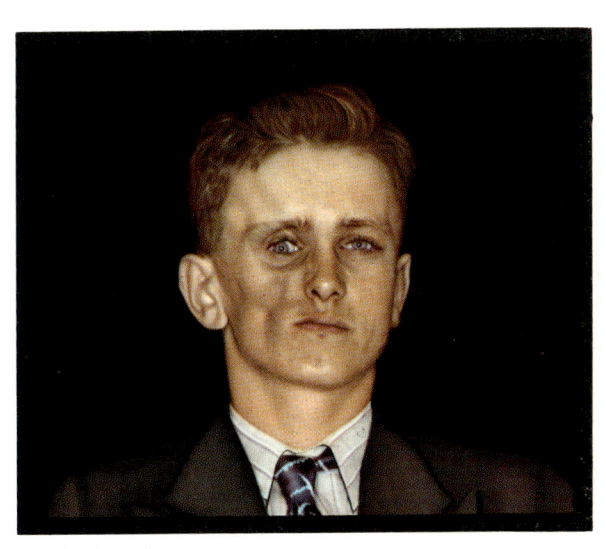

Hemiatrophy

HYGROMA COLLI CONGENITUM

(Bottom) An example of a so-called watery tumor of the neck that extends bilaterally. This anomaly may be present at birth but may not develop to a noticeable degree until several months thereafter. Occasionally it may be of such size that swallowing and breathing are impaired. This lesion, which is a cystic type of lymphangioma, consists of numerous large lymph-filled, noncommunicating spaces lined by endothelium. The tumor is produced by growth, dilatation and coalescence of embryonic lymph sacs in the neck, in some instances it extends into the mediastinum. A similar type of lesion may occur in the axillary and the inguinal regions.

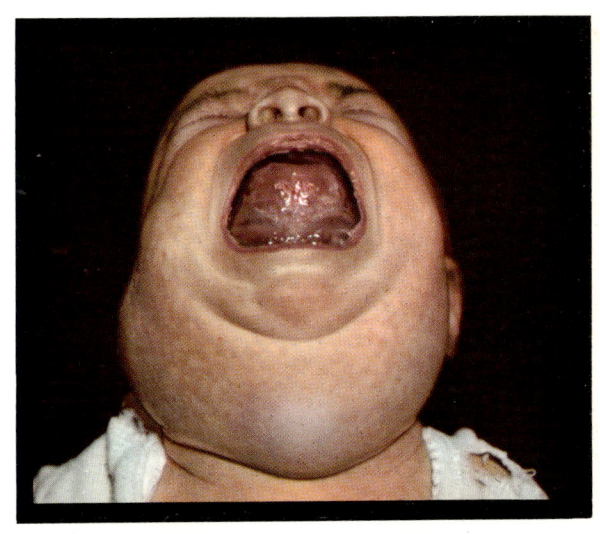

Hygroma Colli Congenitum

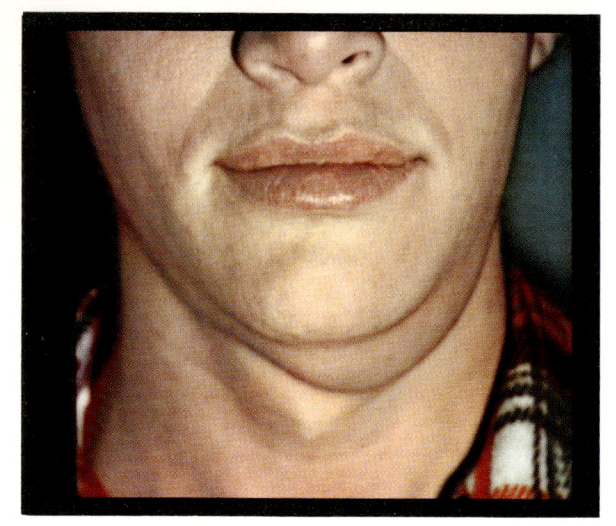

Branchial Cleft Cyst, Neck

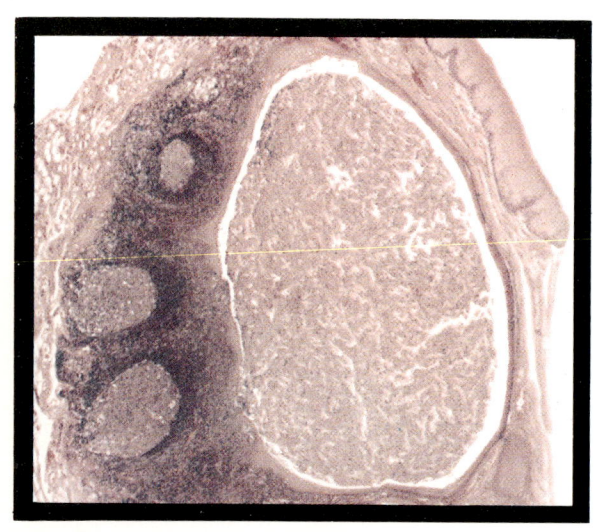

Branchial Cleft Cyst, Floor of Mouth   X 35

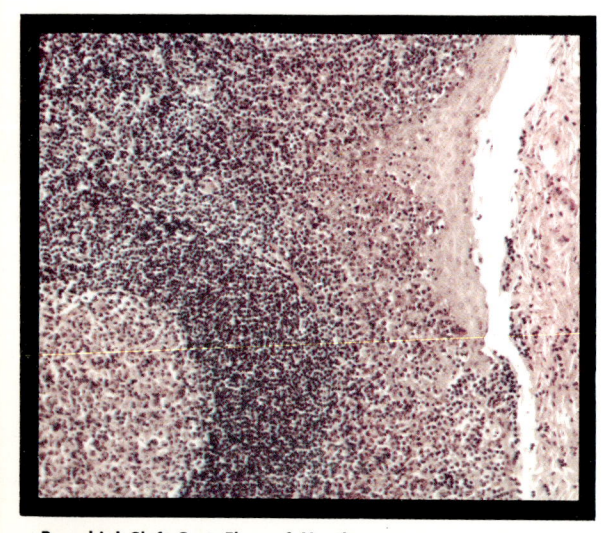

Branchial Cleft Cyst, Floor of Mouth   X 100

BRANCHIAL CLEFT CYST

(Top) A branchial cleft cyst is manifest clinically as a painless, fluctuant swelling, either on the lateral aspect of the neck, as illustrated, or in the floor of the mouth. It is never in the midline. This developmental anomaly originates from epithelium that is entrapped between branchial arches. As shown on page 12, the branchial clefts are lined by ectodermal epithelium, and the pharyngeal pouches by entodermal epithelium. Therefore, it is possible, depending on which cells are entrapped, that these cysts may be lined by stratified squamous epithelium which originally was destined to become skin, by stratified squamous epithelium which would have become mucous membrane, or by pseudostratified ciliated columnar epithelium. In the course of development of the neck, the 2nd branchial arch or bar outgrows the rest of the arches in a caudal direction and overlaps them. This makes a recess on the side of the embryonic neck that is lined by epithelium and is called the lateral cervical sinus. Because of this formation, the epithelium from the 2nd branchial cleft is entrapped more often than the epithelium from the other clefts. Branchial cleft cysts derived from the region in which faucial tonsils are developed often have lymphoid tissue in their walls. Sometimes these are designated as tonsillocysts because of their resemblance to dilated tonsillar crypts.

(Center) A branchial cleft cyst from the floor of the mouth. Beneath the mucosa shown at the upper right there is a flattened stratified epithelium lining a large oval cystic area containing desquamated keratinized cell remnants. At the far left there is lymphoid tissue with three germinal centers.

(Bottom) Higher magnification of above cyst wall, lining and contents. It has been suggested that cysts with lymphoid tissue in their walls may develop from epithelial inclusions in lymph nodes, and that some cysts of this type within the mouth may result from plugging of the crypts of small accessory oral tonsils.

Developmental Disturbances

PREAURICULAR SINUS

(Top) A sinus just anterior to the external ear is identified by a probe. The scar tissue resulted from a previous infection of the tract. Cysts and sinuses in this area are due to defective closure of the 1st branchial cleft. Pits found in the pinna of the ear probably are the result of faulty coalescence of the 6 nodules from which the auricle originates.

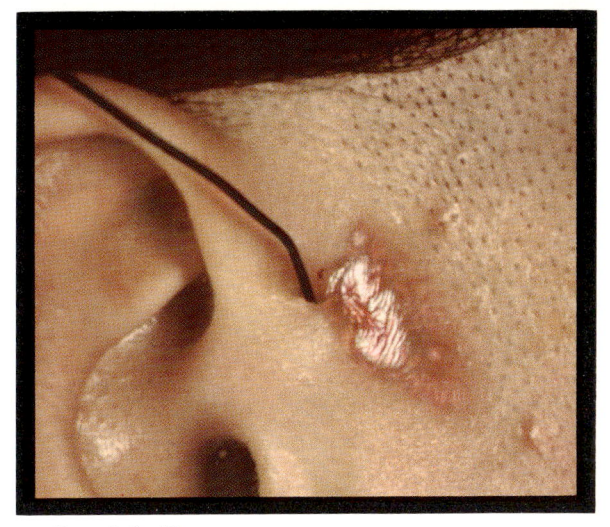

DERMOID CYST

A dermoid cyst is lined by stratified squamous epithelium and has in its wall one or more secondary skin structures. It arises from epithelium left in the tissue upon closure of embryonic processes or from traumatic implantations. When this type of cyst occurs in the oral cavity, it is usually found in the anterior portion of the floor of the mouth. Because of its location and clinical appearance it may be mistaken for a ranula, but a dermoid cyst usually has a thicker wall and is less distended. The lesion discussed here is not to be confused with a teratomatous dermoid cyst.

(Center) At the extreme left is a clear space which is the cystic cavity. Next is the stratified squamous epithelial lining with keratin exfoliating from its outer surface. The rest of the photomicrograph shows the cyst wall, in which there are 4 sebaceous glands.

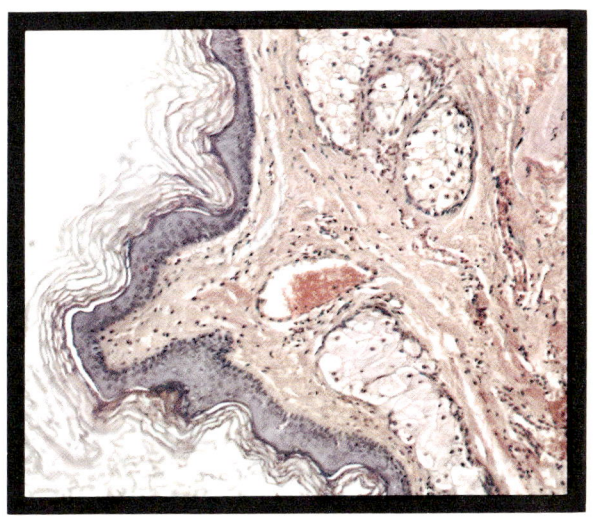

EPIDERMOID CYST

(Bottom) The lower half of the photomicrograph shows a portion of a cyst filled with keratin and lined by flattened stratified squamous epithelium. This is an epidermoid cyst because no cutaneous appendages are present in the cyst wall. Like the dermoid cyst, this type may originate from epithelial remnants or from implanted epithelium. The cyst illustrated was removed from the vermilion portion of the lower lip, just lateral to the midline. In one stage of the development of the lower lip there are 3 furrows, one in the midline and one on each side of it. This cyst probably developed from misplaced islands of epithelium when one of these lateral furrows was obliterated. Paramedian lip pits may have the same origin.

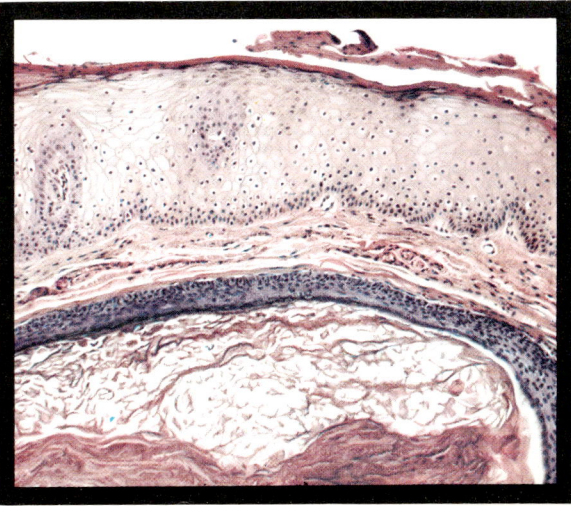

Preauricular Sinus

Dermoid Cyst   X 100

Epidermoid Cyst   X 100

Developmental Disturbances

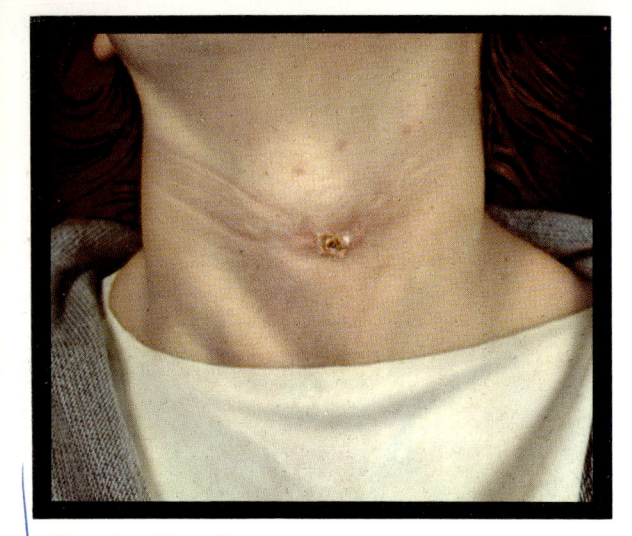

Thyroglossal Duct Sinus

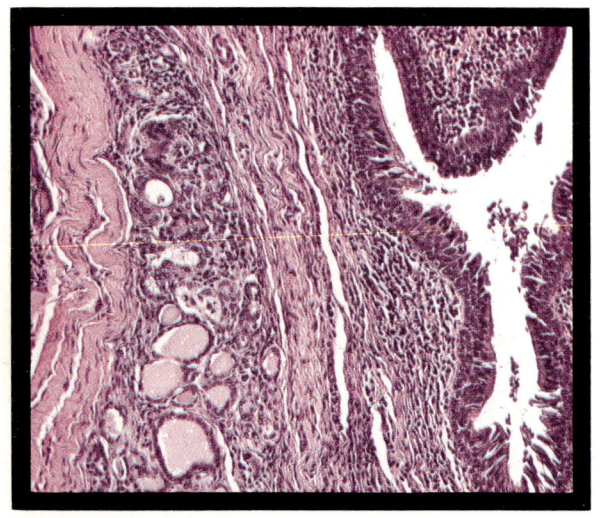

Thyroglossal Duct Cyst   X 100

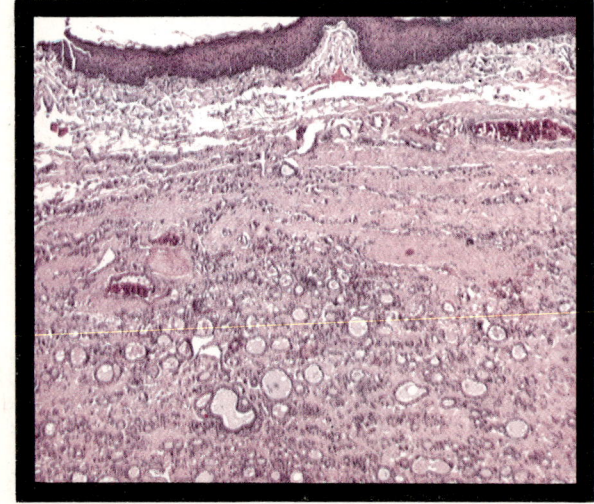

Lingual Thyroid (Lingual Goiter)   X 30

THYROGLOSSAL DUCT CYST

The thyroglossal duct (see p. 13) is an epithelial-lined tube that originates on the anterior surface of the primitive pharynx at a point between sites of origin of the anterior and the posterior parts of the tongue. This duct during its transitory existence grows downward through the tongue and the hyoid bone area to a predetermined point in the anterior aspect of the neck, where it bifurcates to form the thyroid gland. After its function is performed, it should involute, but portions of it may persist and give rise to cysts or sinuses. As residual cells from the upper third of the duct tend to develop into stratified squamous epithelium and those from the remainder into pseudostratified columnar epithelium, the resultant cysts may be lined by either or both types.

(Top) The defect illustrated was preceded by a thyroglossal duct cyst that appeared as a large, fluctuant midline swelling. Spontaneous rupture of the cyst resulted in this thyroglossal duct sinus. Thyroglossal duct defects may develop anywhere along the course of the duct. They are always close to the midline and usually become apparent in early adult life.

(Center) The clear area at the right is a portion of the cyst cavity, which is lined by pseudostratified ciliated columnar epithelium. The circular areas in the connective tissue wall that are bordered by cuboidal cells and filled with a pink-staining, homogeneous, amorphous material are thyroid acini. Aberrant thyroid tissue, as seen here, is found frequently in the wall of thyroglossal duct cysts, sinuses and fistulae.

LINGUAL THYROID

(Bottom) This is a section of a mass which was removed from the undersurface of the tongue because it interfered with deglutition. In the lower portion of the photomicrograph are numerous thyroid acini of an embryonic type. This anomaly is possible because the thyroglossal duct passes through the posterior part of the tongue, and its lining cells have the potentiality for forming thyroid tissue at any point.

ORAL TORI

A hyperostosis occurring in the midline of the hard palate is termed torus palatinus, while one located on the lingual aspect of the mandible in the canine-premolar region is designated torus mandibularis. Other localized, nonneoplastic, external bony overgrowths are frequently associated with the maxillary buccal plate, but these hyperostoses usually are not classified as tori.

(Top) Torus palatinus of the lobular type with a well-defined midline groove. Palatal exostoses may be of various sizes and patterns. They consist of excess bone which bulges into the oral cavity from the slow, continued overgrowth of the medial margins of both palatine processes. The cause of this growth stimulus is not known. There is no need for removal of these bony protuberances unless they interfere with speech or the fitting of dentures. The mucosa overlying tori is usually very thin, blanched and easily traumatized. This condition occurs in about 20 per cent of the total population, being more frequent in adults than in children. It appears to be more common in Mongoloid peoples than in members of either the Caucasian or Negroid groups. This bony overgrowth should not be confused with a mixed tumor. Such tumors are extremely firm, yet lack a characteristic bony hardness; they are rarely found directly in the midline. The torus palatinus is very hard and appears as a radiopacity in an occlusal radiograph.

(Center) Bilateral lingual tori in the cuspid and first bicuspid regions. The thinness of the overlying mucosa is well demonstrated. Mandibular tori may be a source of annoyance if they are of such a configuration as to allow food debris to collect beneath them. It is usually necessary to remove them before constructing a denture. They occur less frequently than palatal tori, being found in 7 per cent of the general population except for some Eskimo tribes. They usually are bilateral but may be unilateral.

(Bottom) A histologic section from a mandibular torus that is composed entirely of laminated cortical bone. The deeper portions of larger tori may contain spongy bone.

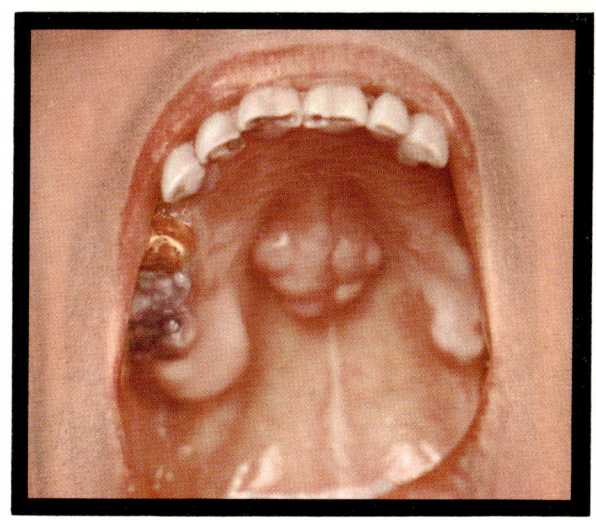

Torus Palatinus

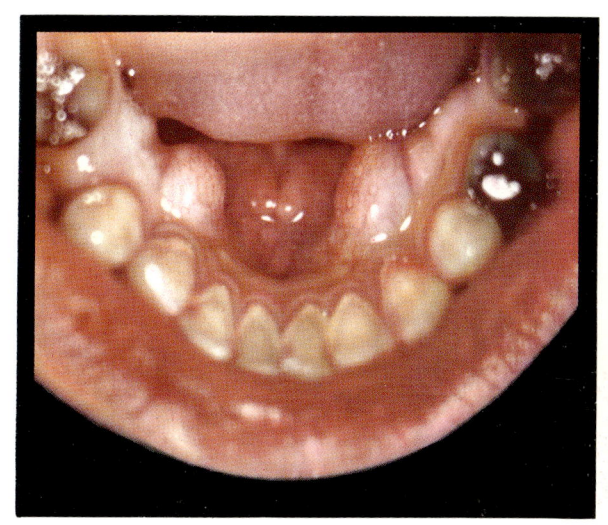

Mandibular Tori

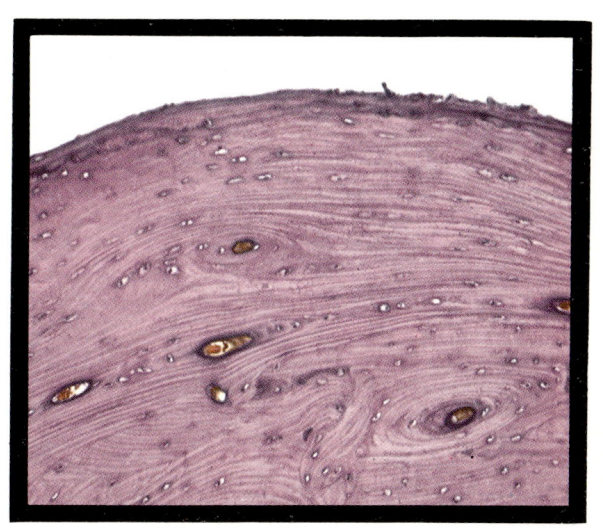

Torus   X 100

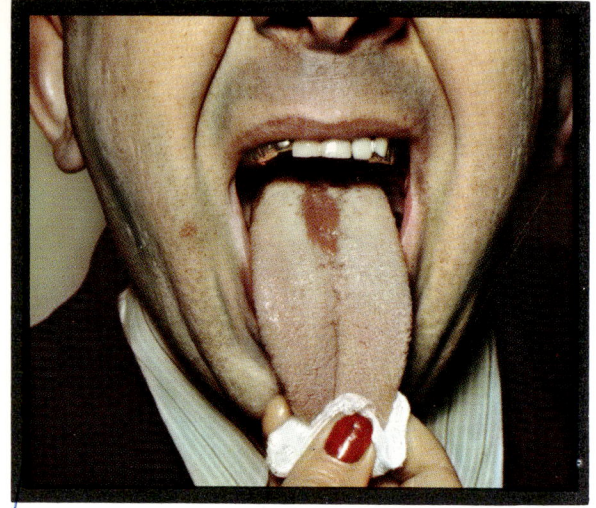

Median Rhomboid Glossitis

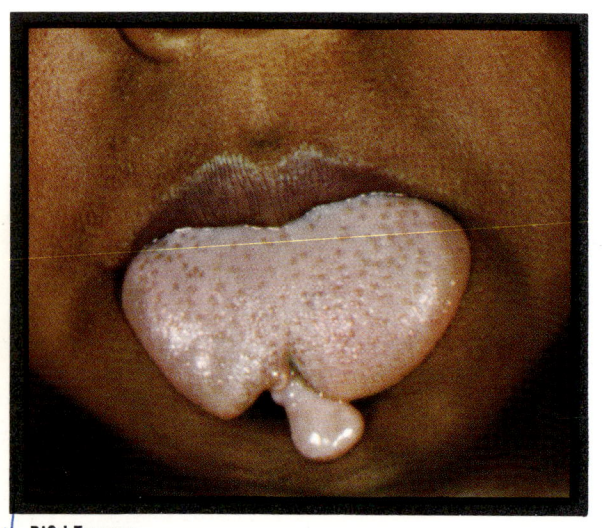

Bifid Tongue

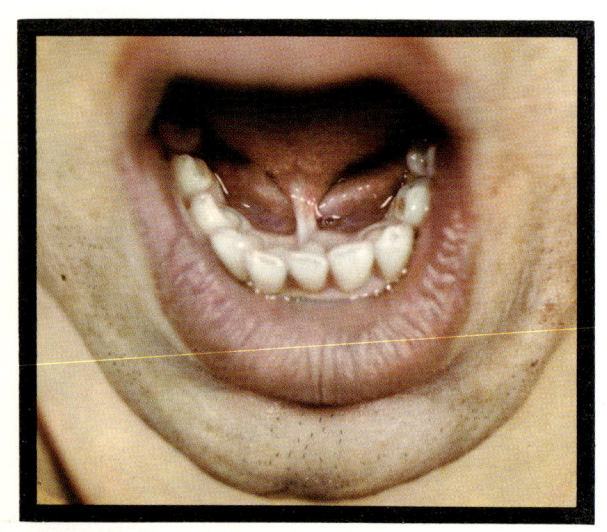

Ankyloglossia

MEDIAN RHOMBOID GLOSSITIS

Median rhomboid glossitis is a minor developmental disturbance of the tongue and not an inflammation, as the suffix "itis" would imply. As shown on pages 12 and 13, the anterior part of the tongue develops from the 1st branchial arch by 2 lateral prominences and a medial one. Early in development the 3 prominences are about equal in size, but later the medial one, tuberculum impar, ceases to enlarge and finally is depressed into the body of the tongue and overgrown by the 2 lateral prominences, which unite in the midline. When glossogenesis is faulty, the tuberculum impar may appear on the surface just anterior to the foramen cecum as a diamond-shaped wedge between the 2 lateral halves of the tongue. The persistence of the tuberculum impar, which does not develop papillae, results in the anomaly median rhomboid glossitis.

(Top) In this example there is a smooth, slightly raised rhomboid area just anterior to the foramen cecum. The redness is due not to inflammation but to lack of papillae. Sometimes the anomaly is polypoid in character and is located further anteriorly. This congenital defect, often undiscovered until adult life, has no clinical significance and should not be confused with carcinoma, which is extremely rare in this location.

BIFID TONGUE

(Center) A midline cleft that divides the tip of the tongue into 2 parts. The tag of tissue seen in the bifurcation consists of muscle, apparently formed in an effort to obliterate the defect. This fairly rare anomaly is the result of the failure of the 2 lateral halves of the tongue to fuse completely in the midline.

ANKYLOGLOSSIA

(Bottom) An abnormally broad, short lingual frenum which is attached near the tip of the tongue. Tongue-tie of this degree markedly limits the movement of the tongue and may interfere greatly with proper enunciation. This anomaly can be corrected by surgery.

MACROGLOSSIA

Macroglossia (large tongue) may be congenital or acquired. Congenital macroglossia may be idiopathic or the result of developmental disturbances such as angiomas and neurofibromas. Acquired macroglossia may be due to cretinism, myxedema, mongolism, acromegaly, amyloidosis, true muscular hypertrophy or edema from cortisone therapy. Individuals who have been edentulous for many years may develop large tongues because of muscular hypertrophy due to the marked use of their tongues to aid in mastication of food. If the patient is able to wear dentures, the tongue muscle may regress with reduction in the size of the tongue.

(Top) At birth the tongue was enlarged without apparent cause and increased in size with growth. It more than fills the interarch space, and the resulting pressure produced decubital ulcers on the tongue, expansion of the arch with spacing of the teeth and facial deformity.

(Center) Congenital macroglossia due to hemangioma. A 20-month-old girl is unable to retract her tongue into her mouth. The dark crusted tip is continuously exposed. A large tongue was noted at a few days of age, gradually increasing in size with continuously greater exposure. Less frequently similar changes are produced by lymphangioma. Congenital neurofibroma also produces macroglossia, but the tongue is usually more firm than when enlargement is on a vascular basis and there is no alteration in color. When hemangioma is the cause, the tongue is bluish in color; with lymphangioma it is pink or brownish.

(Bottom) This tongue with the serrated border due to pressure from contacting the teeth is a typical form of enlargement. It may be the result of fluid retention in association with generalized disease or may be due to muscular hypertrophy in patients who have the habit of pressing the tongue against the teeth. Recognition of tongue habits denied by the patient may be achieved by observing these changes in the tongue. Recognition of such tongue habits is important in patients with periodontal disease and in patients who are candidates for dentures.

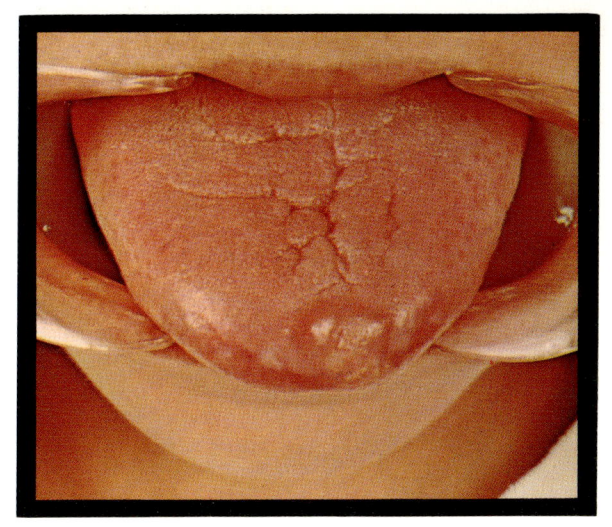

Congenital Idiopathic Macroglossia

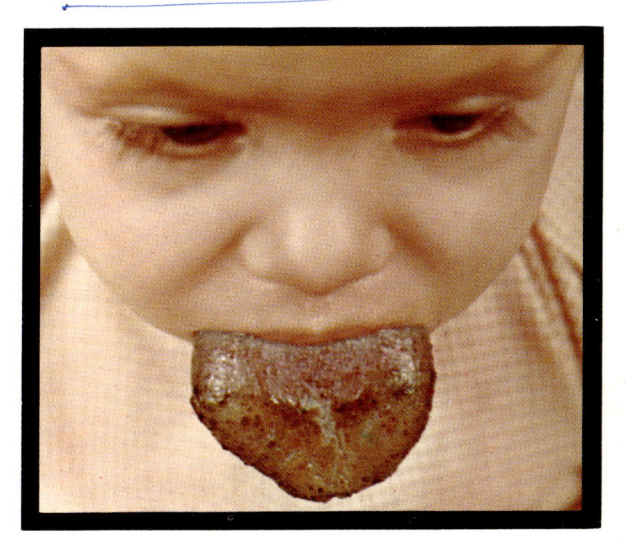

Congenital Macroglossia (Hemangioma)

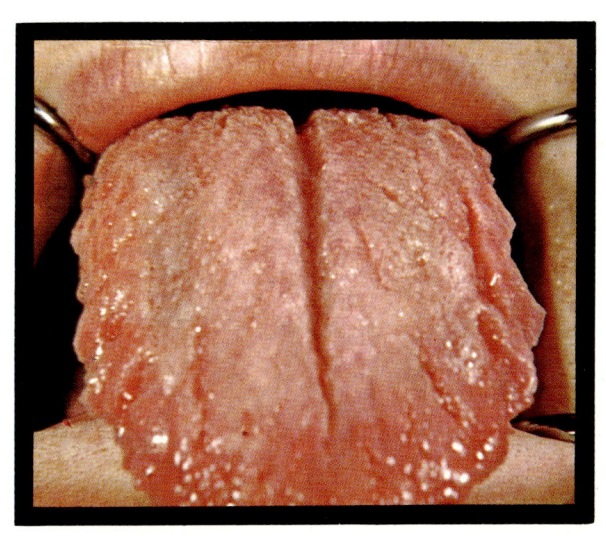

Acquired Macroglossia

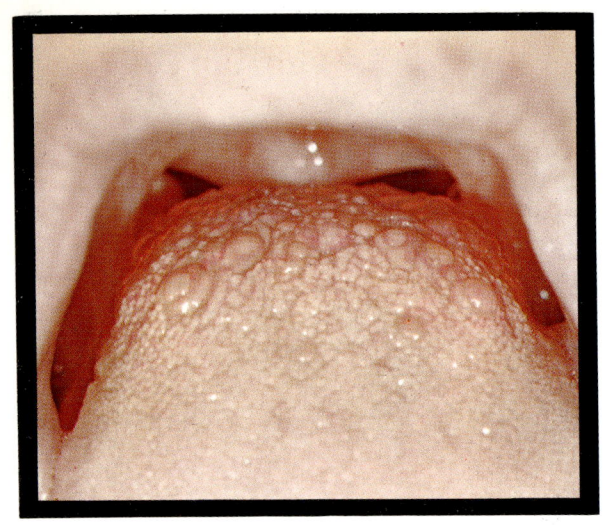

Large Circumvallate Papillae

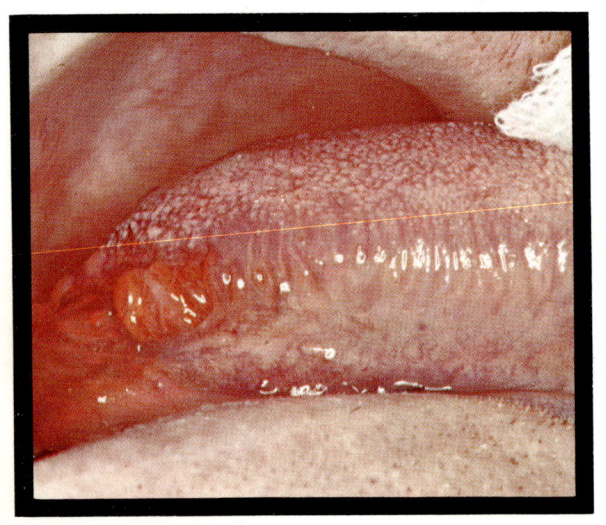

Inflamed Foliate Papillae

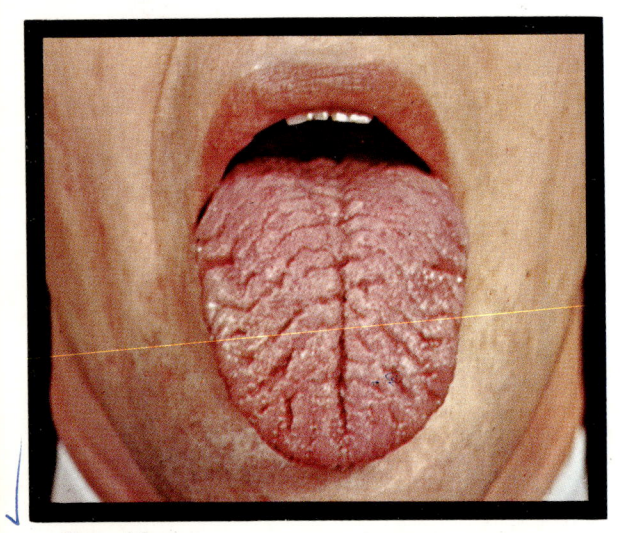

Fissured Tongue

26 Developmental Disturbances

HYPERPLASTIC LINGUAL PAPILLAE

Large Vallate Papillae

(Top) Overdeveloped circumvallate papillae (compare normal, p. 5) are plainly visible as large nodules on the dorsum of the tongue. Circumvallate papillae vary greatly in size, but because they are so far to the posterior, they are not readily visualized unless the tongue is pulled forward.

Foliate Papillae

(Center) The foliate papillae (p. 5), generally vestigial in man, may sometimes be seen as vertical folds of mucosa posteriorly on the lateral borders of the tongue. They contain varying amounts of lymphoid tissue. The most posterior ones, which generally are the largest, are believed by some to be ectopic lingual tonsils. Due to lymphoid hyperplasia associated with upper respiratory infection, these papillae may become enlarged, red and tender, as shown here. The lingual changes, which may create a burning sensation, frequently remain after pharyngeal symptoms subside. Any persistent unilateral lesion should be excised to confirm or dispute the clinical impression (see p. 156). Following repeated attacks it may be advisable to destroy the entire foliate papilla by cautery or excision.

FISSURED TONGUE

(Bottom) This abnormality is found in varying degrees in approximately 5 per cent of the population and is designated as folded, grooved or scrotal tongue. It is rarely congenital but may appear in childhood or early adult life. Prevalence progressively increases in each decade of adult life. This change is of little significance except when the fissures become irritated due to retention of debris. The pattern of the fissuring varies from symmetrical configurations to irregular haphazard distribution. This illustration demonstrates a tongue with closely adapted deep folds of symmetrical pattern. Visualization is accomplished by having the tongue fully extended and stretched.

Developmental Disturbances

Fissured Tongue (Cont.)

(Top) This picture illustrates an irregular fissured pattern with deep branching grooves. The fungiform papillae are prominent at the borders of the fissures where filiform papillae are absent. The enlarged fungiform papillae are subject to irritation and may become tender. The smooth lighter area on the right lingual margin posteriorly is known to be a healing lesion of benign migratory glossitis (see p. 124). Fissuring of the tongue sometimes is associated with vitamin B complex deficiency.

FORDYCE SPOTS (GRANULES)

(Center) The numerous small, light-yellow macular areas in the right buccal mucosa and the upper lip are Fordyce spots. They are ectopic sebaceous glands that are in close relation to the covering epithelium. These spots, which are without clinical significance, are found in 82 per cent of the general population. They are seen less frequently in children because, although the sebaceous glands may be present in this abnormal position, they are small and undeveloped; at the age of puberty they become activated and are more prominent and easily observed. Fordyce spots (granules) are usually few in number and discrete, but when they are confluent and involve the whole buccal mucosa, they give it the appearance of chamois skin with a nodular surface. They are found most commonly in the buccal mucosa, the retromolar region and the lip, but they sometimes occur in the gingiva and the palate. Close inspection of the involved areas will occasionally reveal duct openings from which a greasy substance, sebum, may exude.

(Bottom) Section from the buccal mucosa of an individual having clinical evidence of Fordyce spots. At the top of the section is stratified squamous epithelium. Below it in the lamina propria and submucosa are 4 sebaceous gland lobules. Sebaceous glands are normally located in the dermis of skin. (See p. 2.)

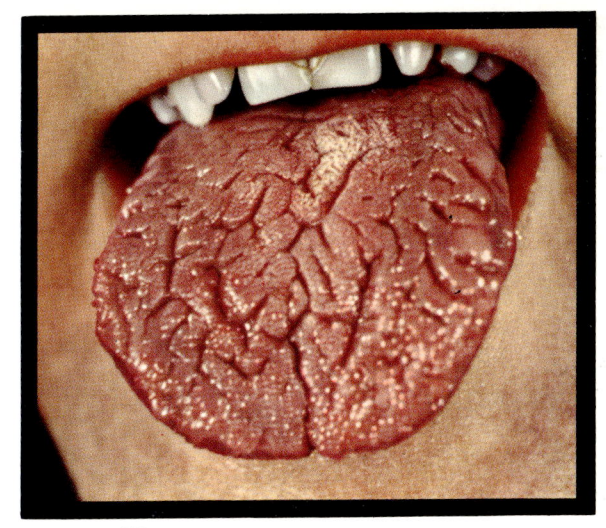

Fissured Tongue

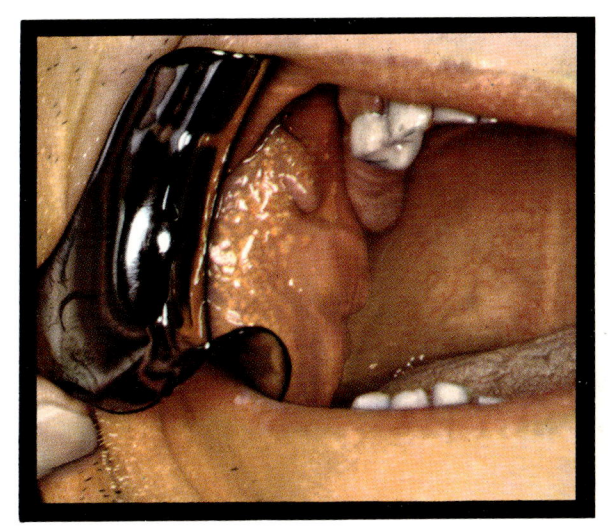

Fordyce Spots

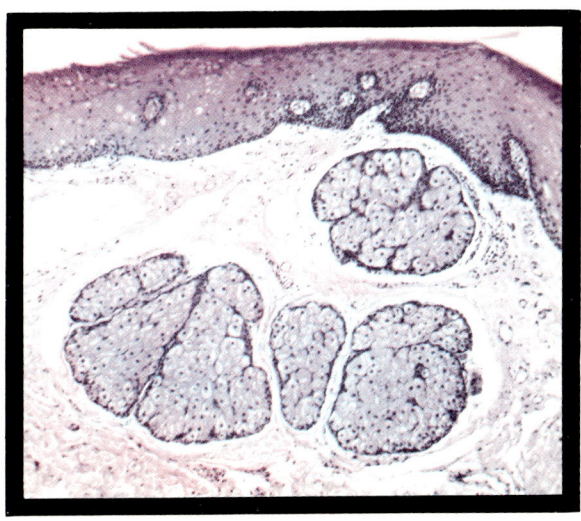

Ectopic Sebaceous Glands   X 80

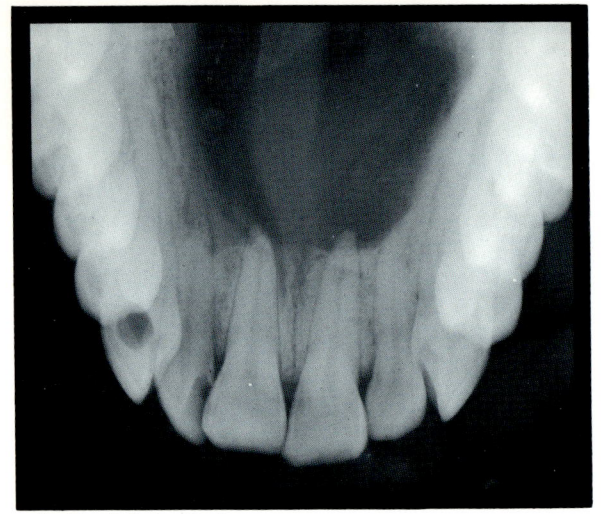

Median Palatine Cyst

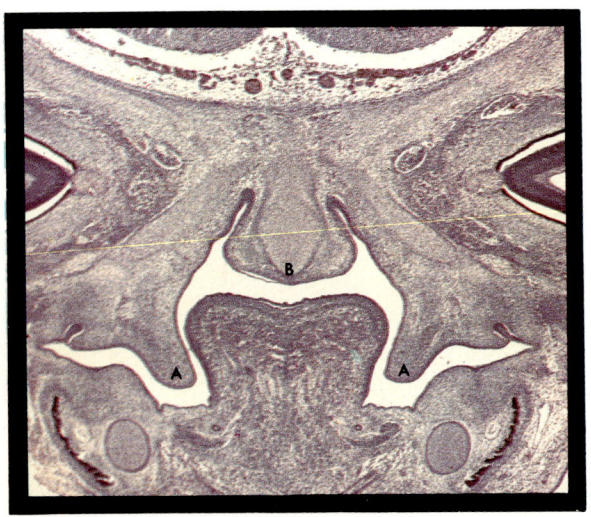

Developing Palate, Human Embryo (8 Weeks)   X 30

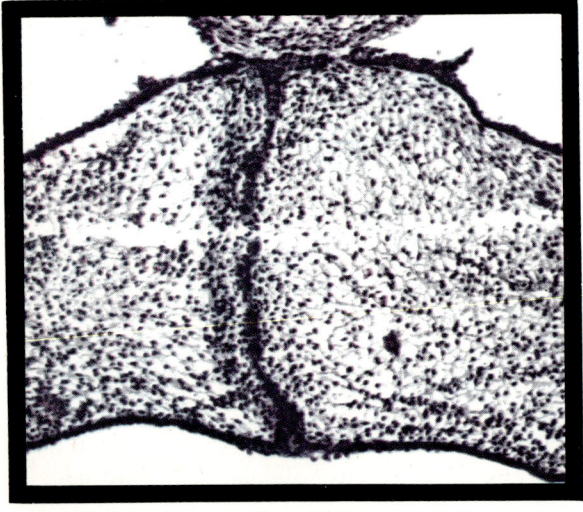

Fused Palatine Processes, Human Embryo (10 Weeks)   X 100

MEDIAN PALATINE CYST

A median palatine cyst is a fissural cyst originating from epithelium persistent in the embryologic fusion line of the 2 palatine processes. Its location is in the midline of the palate posterior to the premaxilla.

(Top) Median palatine cyst revealed in the radiograph as a large, circular radiolucent area in the center of the hard palate. All maxillary teeth in this case tested vital. This cyst bulged into the oral cavity, but many examples of the entity are not evident clinically and are not discovered until routine radiographs are taken. A median palatine, globulomaxillary or nasopalatine duct cyst, evidenced by radiolucency in a periapical film, may be misdiagnosed as a periodontal lesion unless further diagnostic procedures are conducted.

(Center) A frontal section through the head of an 8-week-old human embryo showing that the oral and nasal cavities communicate. The tongue is seen at the bottom of the picture. The palatine processes (A) have not as yet united with each other or with the nasal septum (B).

(Bottom) Section from a 10-week-old embryo cut in the same plane as the one in the center picture, showing a later stage of development. The palatine processes have now joined with each other and with the nasal septum above. The vertical line of union in the center of the photomicrograph consists of a double row of dark-staining embryonic epithelial cells. On each side of this line is lacelike primitive mesenchymal tissue which should perforate and obliterate the epithelium, making the union complete. If any of the epithelial cells remain in the midline, they may give rise to a median palatine cyst. The upper portion of this epithelium has the potentiality of differentiating into pseudostratified ciliated columnar epithelium, the lower portion into the stratified squamous variety. Therefore a cyst developing in this region may be lined by either or both types, depending on which epithelial cells are entrapped.

GLOBULOMAXILLARY CYST

A globulomaxillary cyst is a fissural type of cyst that may occur on either side of the upper jaw between the roots of the lateral incisor and cuspid teeth. Its lining is derived from epithelium that is enclaved in the fusion of the globular portion of the medial nasal process with the maxillary process. It may be lined by either respiratory epithelium or the oral type (stratified squamous), depending on the potentiality of the residual cells.

(Top) Globulomaxillary cyst represented in an occlusal radiograph as a radiolucent area between the roots of the lateral incisor and cuspid teeth. Normal vitality of the lateral and cuspid and divergence of their roots are diagnostic points in differentiating this type of cyst from the periodontal (radicular) type. When a globulomaxillary cyst is removed, it may not be necessary to sacrifice the adjacent teeth.

(Center) Photomicrograph of a portion of a globulomaxillary cyst. The cyst cavity, upper left, is lined by stratified squamous epithelium. In some areas, however, the epithelium has certain characteristics of the respiratory type in that a few light-blue-staining mucous cells are evident. Diagnosis of a globulomaxillary cyst cannot be made from histologic evidence alone.

NASOALVEOLAR CYST

(Bottom) A nasoalveolar cyst is a fissural cyst formed from epithelium entrapped at the junction of the medial nasal, the lateral nasal and the maxillary processes. It is found above the cuspid-lateral region, usually on the surface of the maxilla. This cyst may cause a bulge in the floor of the nose or on the face. It may be misdiagnosed as an extension of a dentoalveolar abscess from a lateral incisor or cuspid tooth or as an abscess formed from an infected hair follicle within the naris. The diagnosis of nasoalveolar cyst can be confirmed by aspirating the fluid, replacing it with radiopaque media and radiographing.

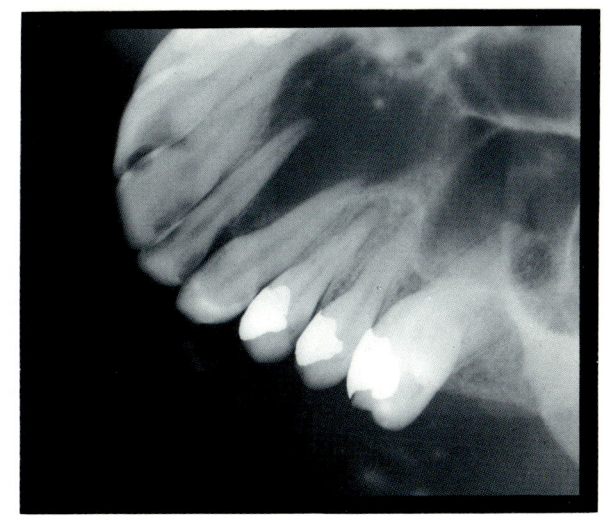

Globulomaxillary Cyst

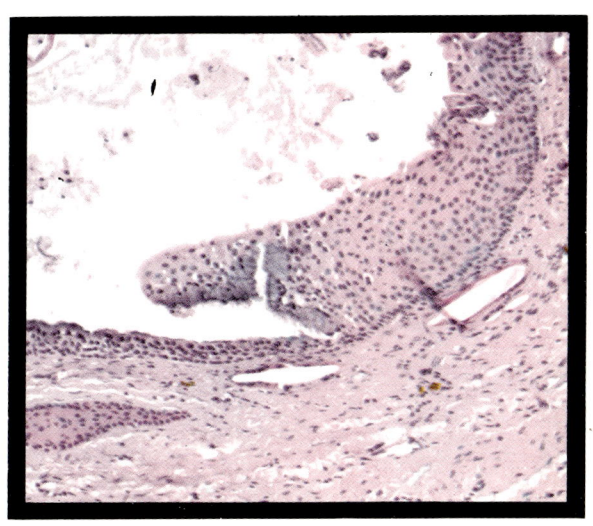

Globulomaxillary Cyst X 100

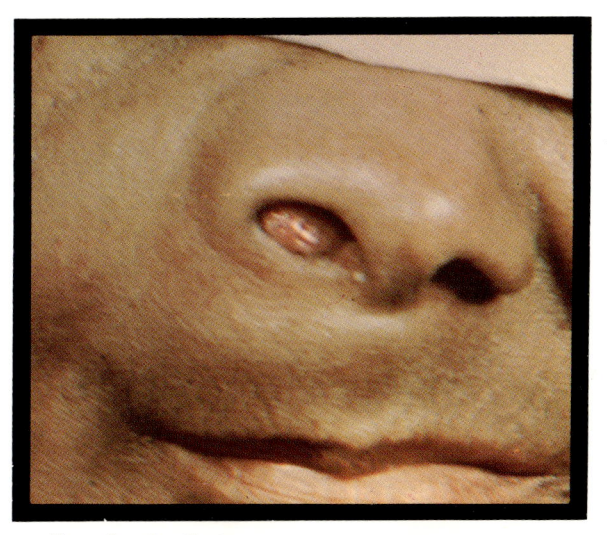

Nasoalveolar Cyst

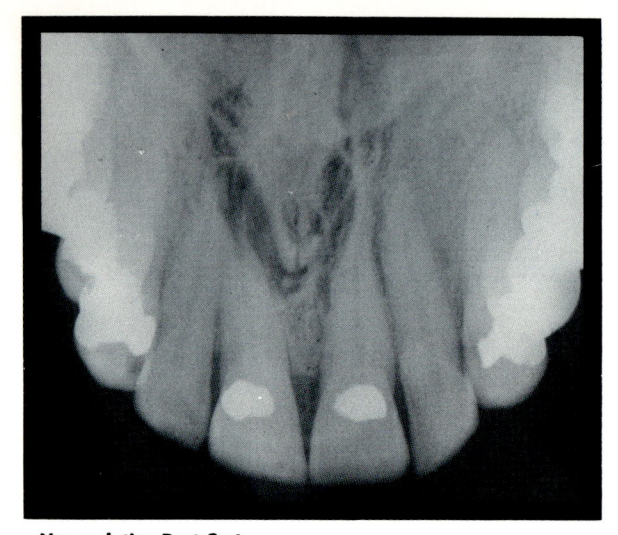

Nasopalatine Duct Cyst

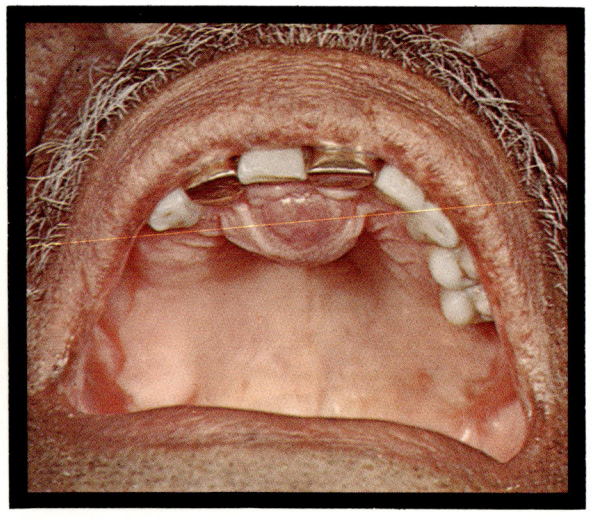

Nasopalatine Duct Cyst

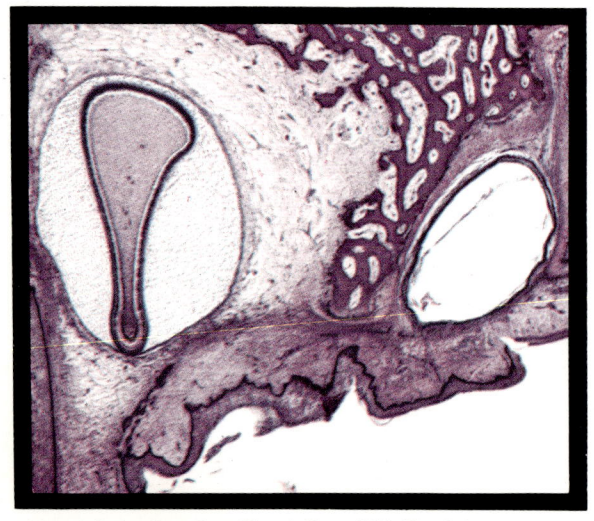

Nasopalatine Duct Cyst, Human Fetus (5½ Months)   X 25

NASOPALATINE DUCT CYST

After the palatine processes unite, as shown on page 28, and meet with the premaxilla anteriorly, there is still communication between the oral and nasal cavities by 2 epithelial-lined tubes, the nasopalatine ducts. These structures are located immediately to each side of the midline above the area that later will be the palatine papilla. In lower animals they are primordia of a pair of accessory olfactory organs, but in man they serve no useful purpose and ordinarily obliterate. If any portion of these ducts persists, the remaining epithelium may be the source of a nasopalatine duct (incisive canal) cyst.

(Top) The cyst is represented by the circular radiolucent area in the incisive canal region. The pulps of anterior teeth in this patient tested vital. A nasopalatine duct cyst may be located to one side of the midline if its origin is epithelial debris from only one of the ducts.

(Center) The marked swelling, as seen in the region of the palatine papilla, is caused by a nasopalatine duct cyst that was both intra- and extra-osseous. The nasopalatine duct cyst may be lined by pseudostratified ciliated columnar epithelium, stratified squamous epithelium or a modification of both. Mucous glands, hyaline cartilage, large vessels and nerves may be found in the cell wall. Inflammatory cells are infrequent.

(Bottom) A sagittal section through a human fetus of 5-1/2 months, taken from a region just to one side of the midline. At the upper left is a developing deciduous central incisor. The large, oval clear space at the far right is a nasopalatine duct cyst lined by stratified squamous epithelium. It lies near the incisive canal, which can be traced from the upper portion of the cyst to the upper right-hand corner of the photomicrograph. Below the cyst, extending into the oral cavity, is a mushroomlike protuberance, which is the palatine papilla. Nasopalatine duct cysts developing in this structure are sometimes designated as cysts of the palatine papilla.

DENTIGEROUS CYST

The dentigerous cyst develops about the crown of an unerupted tooth after amelogenesis is completed. It may involve the entire crown (central type) or only a portion of it (lateral type). The dentigerous cyst usually develops outside the ameloblastic layer. It may arise between the ameloblastic layer and either the stratum intermedium or the outer enamel epithelium or from cells proliferating from the odontogenic epithelium or from remnants of the dental lamina. In such instances it is lined entirely by epithelium. It is possible that a dentigerous cyst may result from fluid accumulating between the ameloblasts and the enamel, in which case the odontogenic epithelium lines the outer portions of the cyst with enamel centrally. The term dentigerous cyst is sometimes applied to cysts which develop about odontomas.

Both dentigerous and primordial cysts (p. 33) are sometimes classified as follicular cysts. The term eruption cyst is used for a dentigerous cyst in a superficial position over the crown of a tooth and manifested clinically by a bulging of the overlying mucosa. It may contain some blood and be mistaken, upon cursory examination, for a hemangioma.

(Top) Central dentigerous cyst occupying most of the ramus. Note that the involved 3rd molar is depressed inferiorly. All lesions appearing radiographically as dentigerous cysts should be examined histologically to rule out ameloblastoma. (See pp. 146-149.)

(Center) Radiograph of a lateral dentigerous cyst, involving only the distal portion of the crown. This should not be confused with a lateral periodontal cyst, which does not involve the crown. (See p. 32.)

(Bottom) Decalcified section of the cyst illustrated in the top picture. The keratin-filled cyst cavity (1) is lined by compressed stratified squamous epithelium (2). Just above the area formerly occupied by the enamel (5) is a blue line of columnar cells, the inner enamel epithelium. Between this line and the outer enamel epithelium (3) the stellate reticulum has degenerated, forming a microcyst. The main cyst at (1), however, probably developed from remnants of the dental lamina such as those seen at (4).

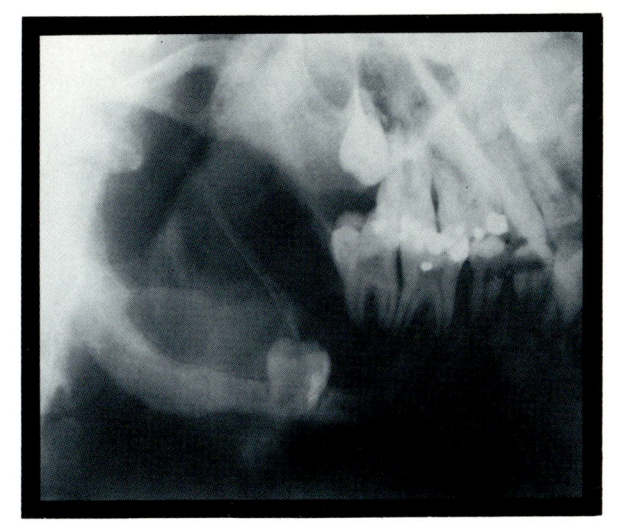

Central Dentigerous Cyst

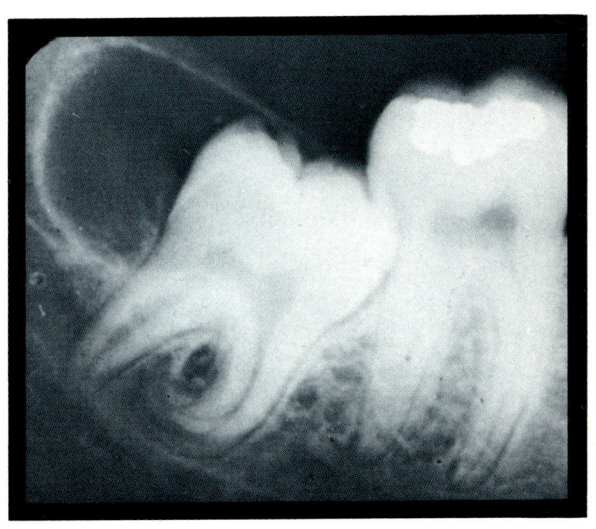

Lateral Dentigerous Cyst

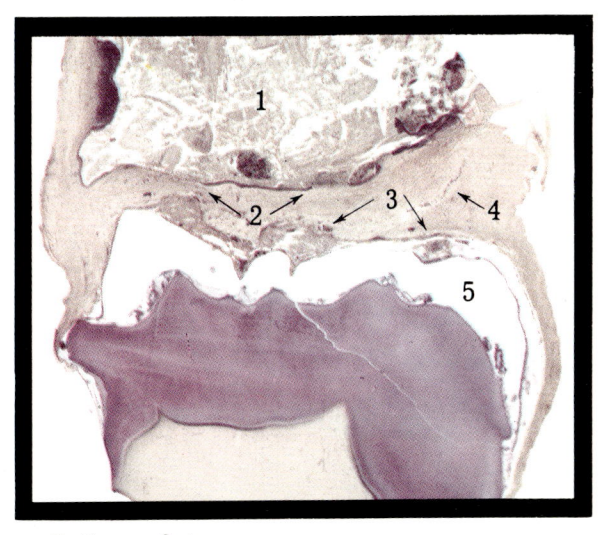

Dentigerous Cyst

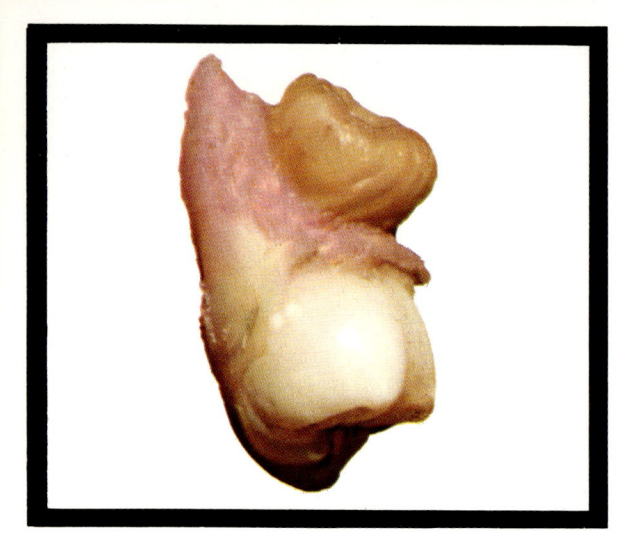

32 *Developmental Disturbances*

LATERAL PERIODONTAL CYST

A lateral periodontal cyst (lateral radicular cyst) occurs along the side of a tooth root. Its epithelial lining is derived from epithelial rests of Malassez, which are found in all periodontal membranes. It differs from a lateral dentigerous cyst in that the latter involves some portion of the crown and develops from epithelium of the enamel organ.

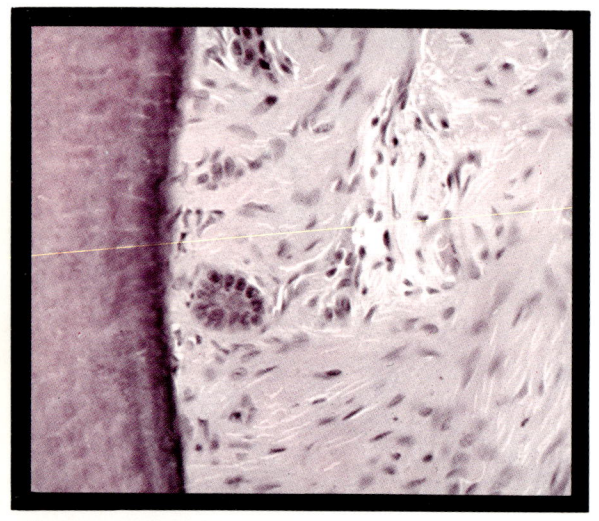

(Top) A large periodontal cyst on a molar tooth, located halfway between the apex and the cemento-enamel junction. Before extraction this tooth responded normally to vitality tests.

(Center) Photomicrograph showing a lateral root surface with attached periodontal membrane. At the far left is root dentin, bordered by cementum. The rest of the illustration consists of periodontal membrane. In this structure are 2 groups of epithelial cells, one at the top of the picture and the other in the central portion. The cells in the latter group are arranged in palisade fashion. These 2 groups of cells are remains of Hertwig's sheath, the source of epithelium for periodontal cysts. Inflammation in the periodontal membrane may cause these rests to proliferate, which will eventually lead to cyst formation. Lateral periodontal cysts occur most frequently on the roots of partially erupted vital mandibular 3rd molars as sequelae of chronic pericoronal inflammation. This type of cyst may also develop from extension of pulpal inflammation in a tooth with a lateral accessory pulp canal. Occasionally, remnants of Hertwig's sheath may proliferate to form a lateral periodontal cyst without any apparent cause.

(Bottom) This is a photomicrograph taken from a section of the tooth illustrated at the top of this page. In the lower left corner a portion of the pulp cavity can be seen. To the right of this area there is dentin, then a thin line of cementum, and finally a mass of fibrous connective tissue containing inflammatory cells. In this connective tissue is a cyst cavity lined by dark-blue-staining stratified squamous epithelium. There was no evidence of pulpal inflammation.

Lateral Periodontal Cyst

Remnants of Hertwig's Sheath   X 220

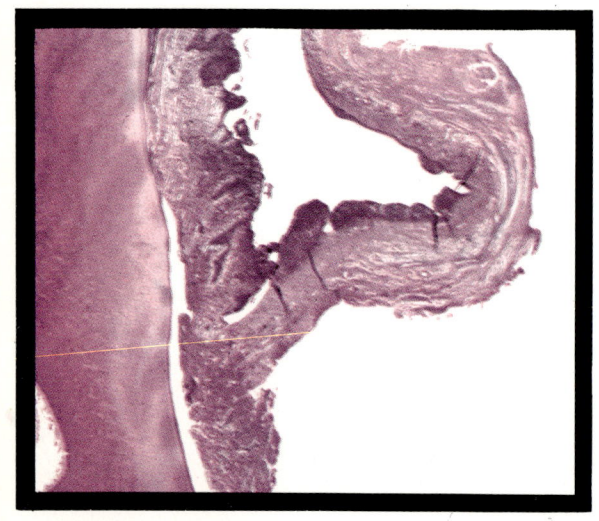

Lateral Periodontal Cyst   X 12

Developmental Disturbances

PRIMORDIAL CYST

The primordial cyst develops because of cystic degeneration of the bud, cap or early bell stage of an enamel organ. Because this metamorphosis occurs before the enamel organ has initiated induction of enamel or dentin, and tooth tissue has not yet been formed, this cyst always arises in place of, rather than in relationship to, a tooth. It is the least common of odontogenic cysts, occurring most often in the mandibular 3rd molar region. Examination and history demonstrate its presence in place of one of the 3rd molars. This cyst formerly was classified as a follicular cyst because of its origin within the dental follicle.

(Top) Radiograph of the 3rd molar region of a 13-year-old boy shows a radiolucent area in place of a calcifying 3rd molar. The other 3rd molars were present. Histologic examination of the surgical specimen revealed findings compatible with clinical diagnosis of primordial cyst.

(Center) At this stage of tooth development, or even earlier (see p. 14), the stellate reticulum may degenerate as a result of trauma, infection or some other factor. As the cells of the stellate reticulum liquefy, the remaining inner and outer enamel epithelia form a sac. This fluid-filled sac, with its connective tissue capsule, is the primordial cyst. Tooth development cannot proceed, but the cyst may enlarge slowly.

(Bottom) The cyst cavity (clear area at top) is lined for the most part with compressed stratified squamous epithelium. The lining at the right, however, somewhat resembles odontogenic epithelium. In this case the connective tissue cyst wall is conspicuously devoid of any inflammatory elements. Ordinarily, a primordial cyst cannot be distinguished histologically from other types of cysts seen in the jaw. To determine that a cyst is of the primordial variety, it is necessary that the histologic findings be supplemented by the clinical history and the radiologic examination.

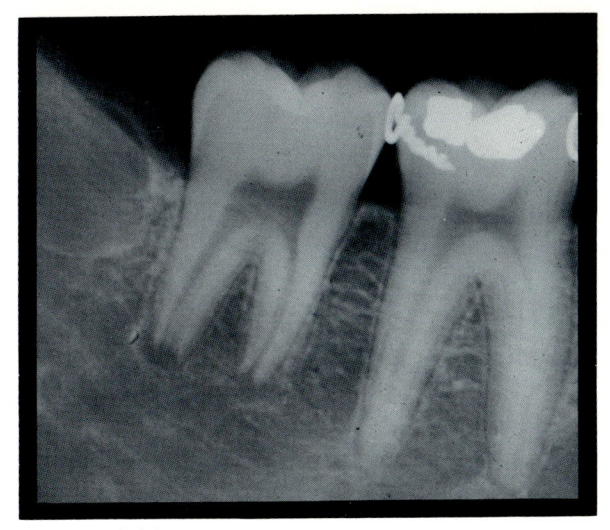

Primordial Cyst

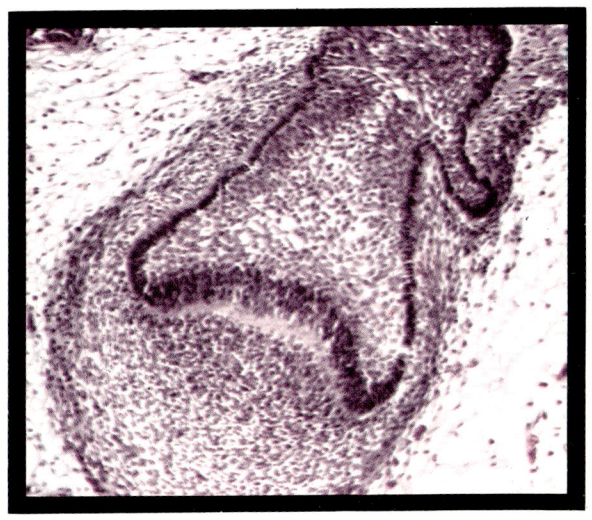

Developing Tooth   X 150

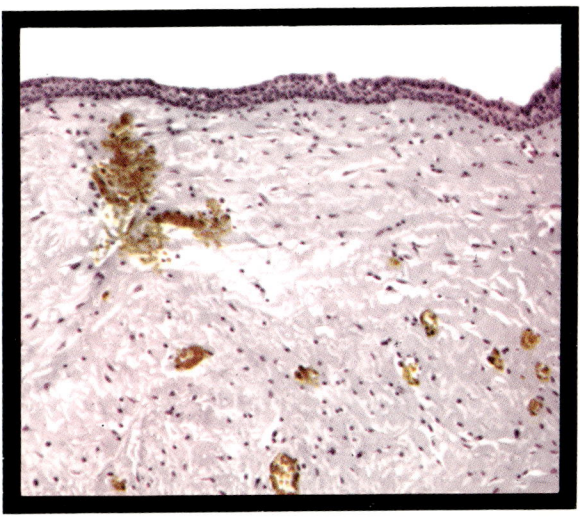

Primordial Cyst   X 90

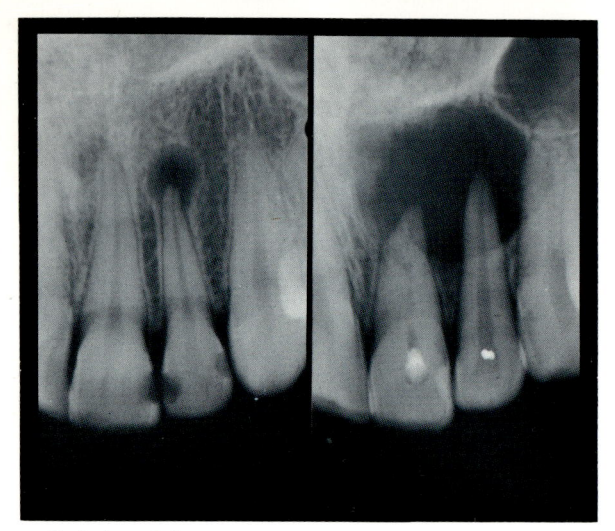

Periodontal Cysts

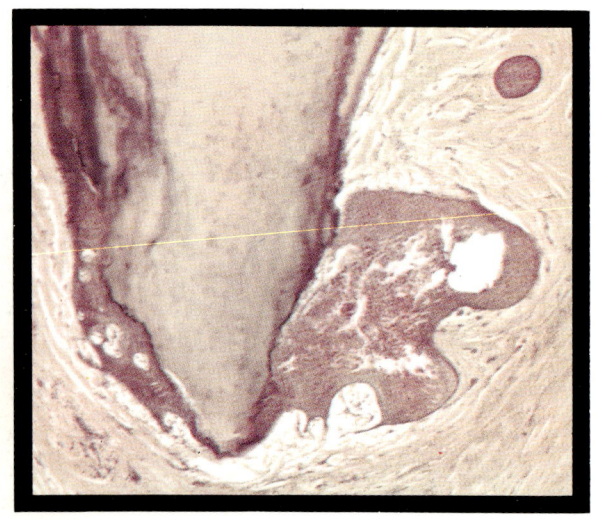

Proliferating Epithelial Debris   X 30

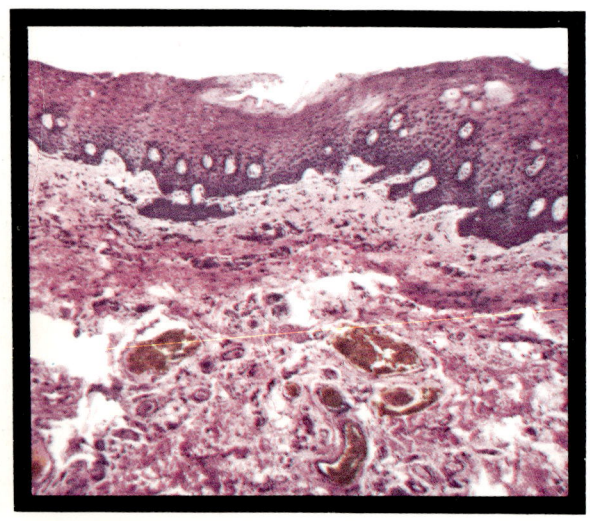

Periodontal Cyst   X 100

PERIODONTAL CYST

Periapical periodontal (radicular, root end, dental root) cysts are developmental in origin, since they form from residues of odontogenic epithelium, but the inciting cause is inflammation (p. 73). Usually there is a history of carious exposure of the pulp with ensuing pulpitis, which leads eventually to a chronic productive inflammatory process in the periapical tissue. The epithelial cells remaining from Hertwig's sheath (p. 16), present in all periodontal membranes, are stimulated to proliferate by the periapical inflammation. These epithelial cells, not having a blood supply of their own but being dependent on vessels in adjacent connective tissue, may multiply to such an extent that the central cells are so distant from their source of nutrition that they die and liquefy, thus forming a cyst. Another method of formation is the epithelization of the border of an abscess cavity related to the inherent urge of epithelium to cover a surface. Also epithelium may proliferate and enclave connective tissue, as suggested at the lower border of the epithelium in the center illustration.

(Top) Two periodontal cysts at the apices of anterior teeth. Radiographically an apical periodontal cyst cannot be differentiated definitely from a granuloma, even though the radiolucent area is surrounded by a line of increased density. Large circular well-demarcated areas of decreased density, however, are usually cysts.

(Center) This photomicrograph shows a marked proliferation of epithelium around the apical third of a tooth. It is evident that a cyst is beginning to form near the apex of the root, at right, because of the central degeneration of the epithelial mass.

(Bottom) A section from a periodontal cyst which was associated with the apex of a pulpless tooth. The cyst cavity (clear area at top) is lined by stratified squamous epithelium. In the fibrous connective tissue wall are dilated blood vessels and a few inflammatory cells. In other areas inflammatory cells were more abundant and the epithelium markedly hyperplastic. Clinical and radiographic evidence are necessary to validate the histologic diagnosis.

Periodontal Cyst (Cont.)

(Top) Periapical periodontal cyst on the lingual root of a maxillary 1st molar. The boundary of this cyst is sharply demarcated, and it is radiographically superimposed over the floor of the maxillary sinus due to the angle of exposure. The radiopacity of the border of the cyst is due to reactions of the bone to the slowly enlarging cyst. More rapid expansion would produce resorption without compensatory bone formation, with loss of sharp radiopaque boundary. Cysts in the maxillary sinus region are often unrecognized because of confusing their borders with those of the sinus or because they entirely fill the sinus cavity with common boundaries.

(Center) A residual cyst of the maxillary 1st molar region approximating the floor of the maxillary sinus. This type of cyst may develop from a periapical granuloma that contained epithelial remnants which were left behind when the associated tooth was extracted, or it could have been formed before removal of the tooth. Similar radiologic appearance could be produced by a primordial cyst (p. 33). In such a case the 1st molar would not have been formed. This must be determined from the history. A similar cyst could be residual after a larger cyst had been treated by marsupialization (Partsch procedure) at the time of extraction, with closure of the external opening and incomplete filling in of the epithelial-lined bone cavity. Residual cysts may also be derived from incompletely removed dentigerous cysts. Since this is possible, thorough histological study is indicated to rule out the possibility of ameloblastoma.

(Bottom) A mandibular molar with a cyst attached to its distal root. The entire root projects into the cystic cavity. If radiographs had not been available at the time of extraction, the tooth might have been removed and the cyst could have been left in the jaw. Epithelium might have closed the extraction wound, and the cyst could have continued its expansile growth. Such a cyst, either attached to the root, as in this case, or as a residual cyst as conjectured, may become of such large size as to occupy the entire body and ramus of a side of the mandible.

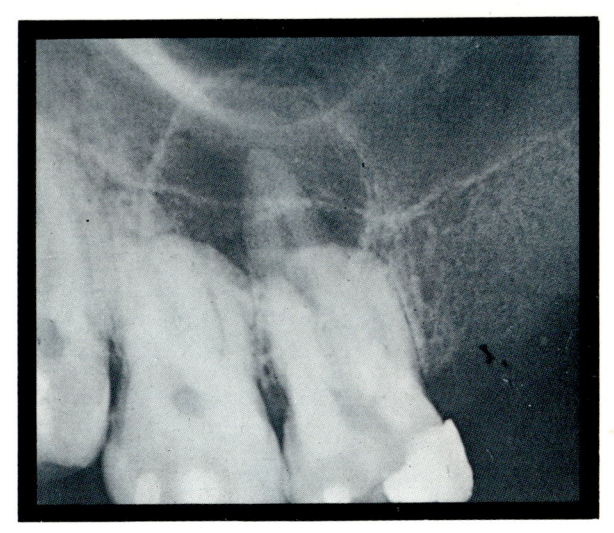

Periodontal Cyst

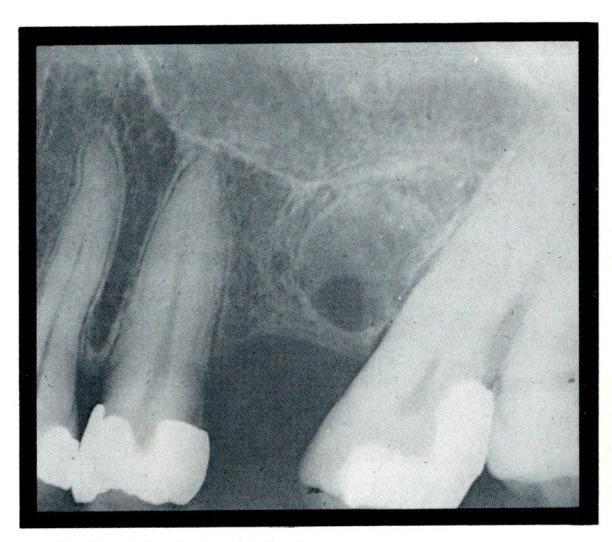

Residual Periodontal Cyst

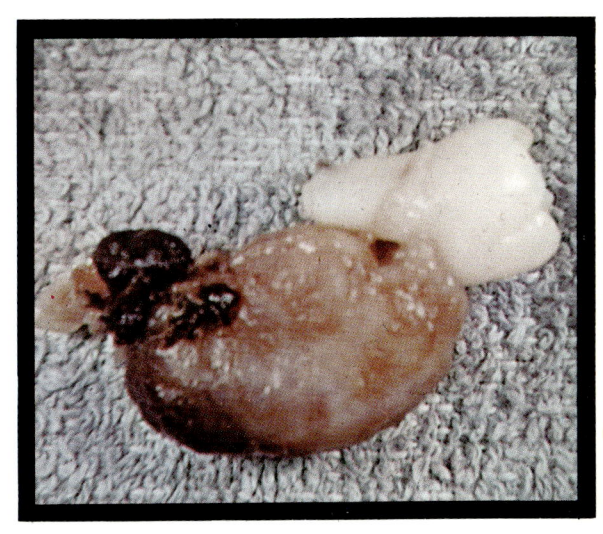

Periodontal Cyst

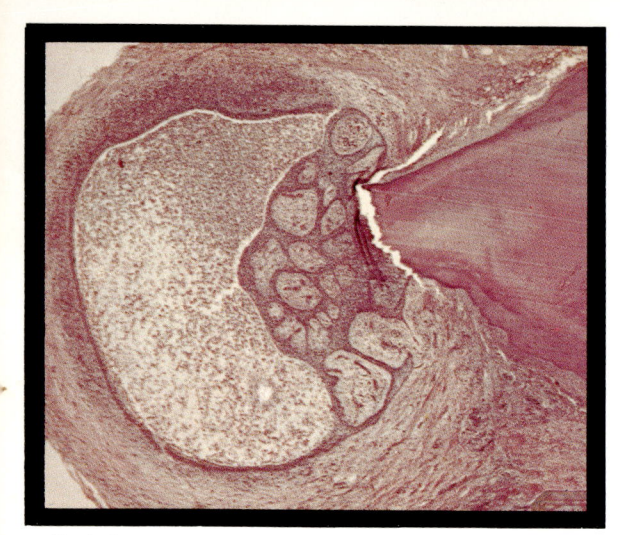

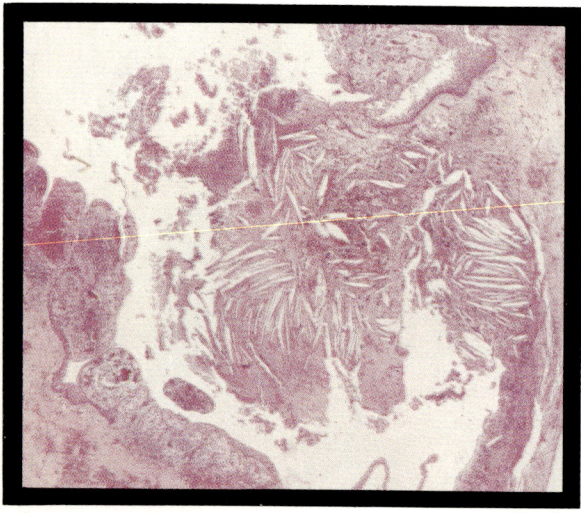

Periodontal Cyst (Cont.)

(Top) Low-power view of a periodontal cyst attached to the apex of a root. The connective tissue wall of the cyst is continuous with the periodontal membrane. The epithelium that lines the cyst is squamous and arose from epithelial debris of Malassez (epithelial rests). It closely approximates the root in the region of the apical foramen. Epithelial rests are present in all dental granulomas, and for this reason all are potential cysts. In the region of the apex the epithelium shows proliferative changes, as is indicated by the reticular pattern. The cyst cavity is filled with tissue debris and fluid. In many instances cholesterol crystals are present in such cystic cavities and may give an oily "glare" to the cystic contents, grossly.

(Center) A portion of a cyst wall in which there is destruction of part of the epithelial lining which is replaced by granulation tissue surrounding masses of cholesterol crystals. There is also epithelial proliferation with small epithelial islands in the granulation tissue. The cyst contents included abundant cholesterol crystals, as indicated by the numerous lenticular-shaped clefts. At times there is epithelial degeneration in cysts that permits the contents to contact connective tissue and initiate an inflammatory response. The cyst may fill with exudate, sometimes purulent, and the cyst is said to be "infected" even though no microorganisms are present. The reaction is to the toxic products of tissue degradation. The inflammatory change may be attended by pain which calls attention to the presence of the cyst.

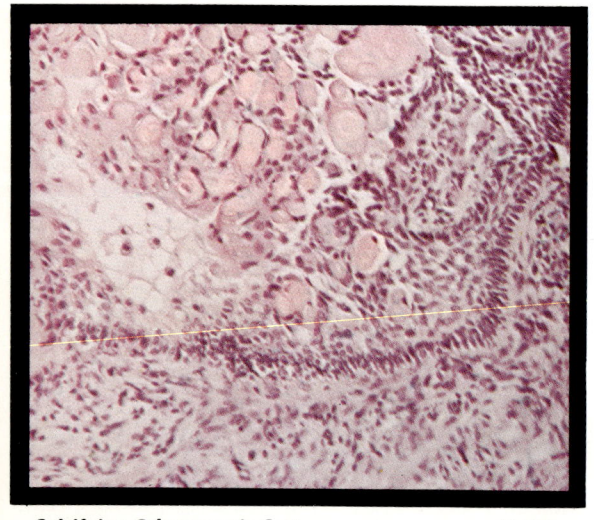

CALCIFYING ODONTOGENIC CYST

(Bottom) Photomicrograph of calcifying (and keratinizing) odontogenic cyst. These cysts are lined by squamous epithelium which forms masses of keratin in which large "ghost" epithelial cells are trapped. The degenerated ghost cells undergo calcification. Odontogenic type epithelium is in evidence. The cyst may be either intra- or extra-osseous. Radiographically the lesions are radiolucent with radiopaque flecks which vary with the degree of intracystic calcification. It is believed that the lesion, although cystic, is related to the epithelial odontogenic tumors. There is some tendency to recurrence after surgical treatment.

Developmental Disturbances

GEMINATION AND FUSION

Geminated teeth are formed by the splitting of a single tooth germ. The 2 resulting components may be approximately equal in size, or 1 may be rudimentary in size and form. While the term gemination may be applied properly to the formation of twin teeth that are separate entities, usually it is reserved for those instances of maldevelopment in which only partial cleavage of the tooth germ has occurred. Geminated teeth usually have a single root and a common pulp canal. Clinically, the normal number of teeth can be accounted for in the dentition, counting the bifid tooth as 1.

(Top) Gemination in which the double tooth developed from the formative organ of the maxillary right lateral incisor. The upper dentition consists of a normal number of teeth, the presence of an unerupted cuspid being revealed by radiologic examination. Clinical evidence of this fact is also apparent from the bulge above the edentulous area.

(Center) Fused teeth result from the union of 2 adjacent tooth germs. The 2 teeth may be united for their entire length or joined only by their crowns or their roots. The fusion must involve the dentin, for when 2 teeth are connected only by cementum, the condition is termed concrescence (p. 42).

Examples of complete fusion in mandibular anterior teeth are shown. In these 2 cases, as in most instances, there are separate pulp canals. Usually fusion may be differentiated from gemination by the appearance of a more definite separation between the 2 components, and by the fact that the number of individual teeth in the arch is reduced by 1, counting the anomaly as a single unit. Of course, this latter criterion will not apply if a supernumerary tooth is involved in the fusion. Gemination and fusion occur most frequently in mandibular deciduous incisor teeth.

(Bottom) Fusion between a supernumerary tooth *(left)* and a portion of a mixed complex odontoma. Near the incisal edge of the tooth the dentin of the 2 components is continuous. Sections at a deeper level revealed a pulp canal in the supernumerary tooth.

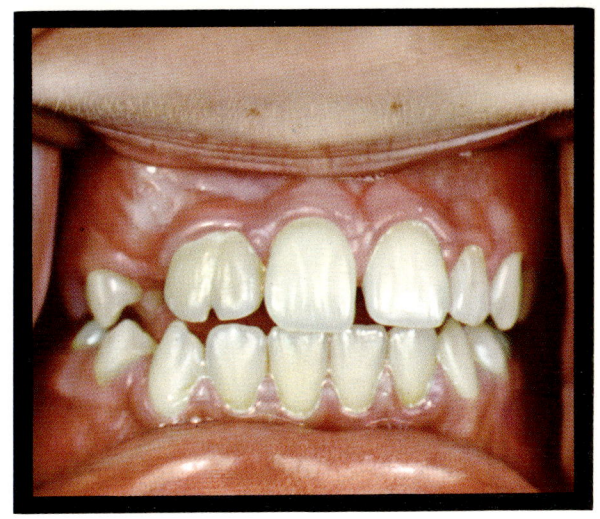

Gemination

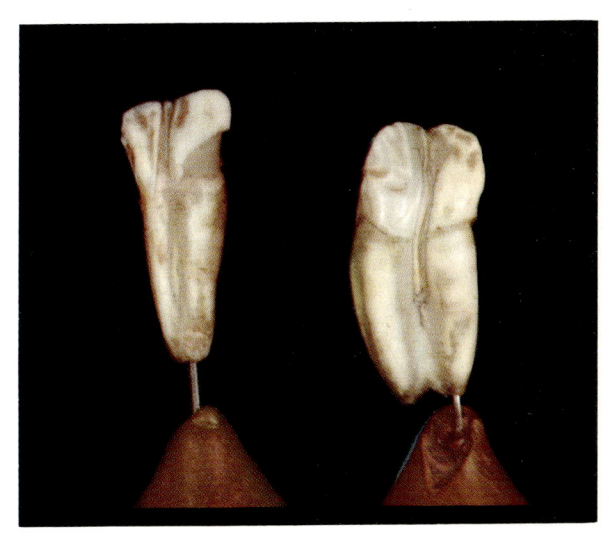

Fusion

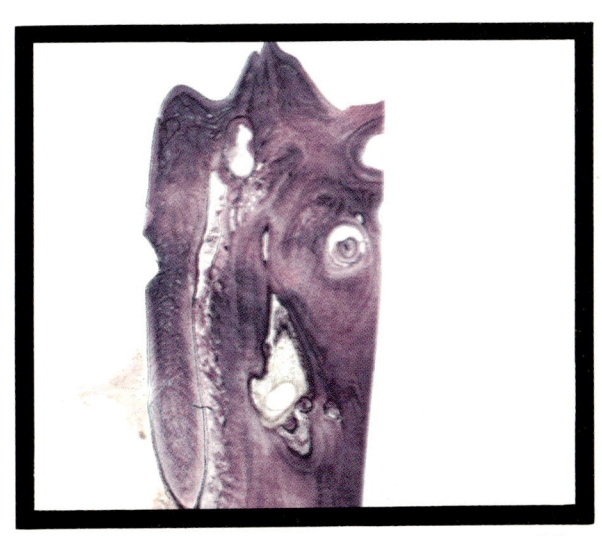

Fusion

X 5

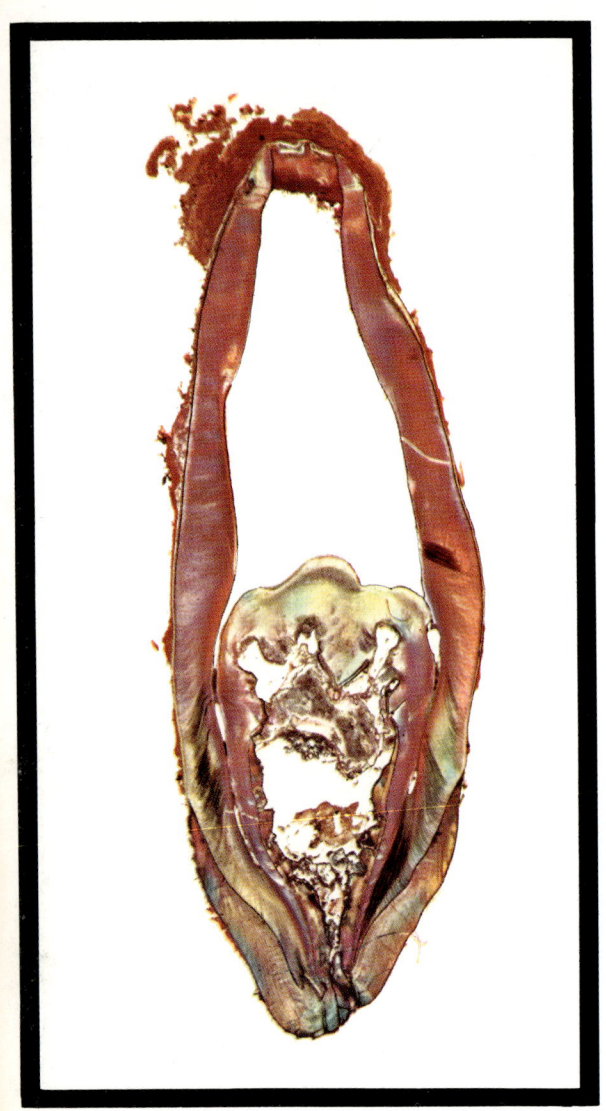

Dens Invaginatus — X 6

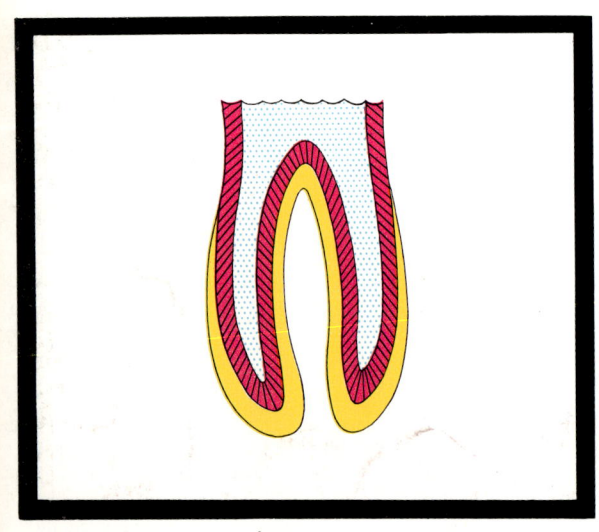

Schematic Dens Invaginatus

DENS INVAGINATUS

(Dens in Dente)

This anomaly appears radiographically (p. 39, *top*) as a "tooth within a tooth." Actually it is formed by the retarded growth of a portion of a single tooth germ or by the proliferation of a segment of the odontogenic epithelium into the dentinal papilla. Also known as dens in dente or gestant anomaly, it usually involves a maxillary lateral incisor. A communication exists between the oral cavity and the enamel-lined inner cavity which can be considered as an extremely deep pit. Debris and bacteria may accumulate in this inner cavity and caries usually develops unnoticed. For this reason pulpitis and periapical inflammation are commonly associated with dens invaginatus. This anomaly may be discovered in routine radiographic examinations or because pain occurs in an apparently intact tooth.

(Top) A ground section of a dens invaginatus in a maxillary lateral incisor photographed in polarized light. Near the tip of the cusp, in the lower part of the picture, a small opening into the inner cavity may be seen. At midcrown the structures may be observed from the surface to the center on either side in the following order: enamel, dentin, thin slitlike space occupied by pulp, dentin, enamel, central cavity space. A similar anomaly occurring in the roots may present a central cavity lined by cementum rather than enamel.

(Bottom) This diagram depicts how a tooth germ might enfold to form a dens invaginatus. The positions of the enamel (yellow), dentin (red) and pulp (dotted) are indicated. The coronal tips of enamel will more closely approximate each other, as seen above, leaving the inner space almost closed off from the oral cavity. During development part of the dental sac occupies this central cavity and, for this reason, cementum or bone may be found here. Upon eruption the dental sac, having no blood supply, necrotizes. Fine canals have been reported communicating between invaginated cavity and the pulp, accounting for pulpal involvement even in the absence of caries.

Developmental Disturbances

Dens Invaginatus (Cont.)

(Top) Radiographs of dens invaginatus in a molar tooth *(left)* and in a maxillary incisor *(right)*. In the right-hand specimen a thin radiolucent line begins at the incisal edge and leads into a central cavity which is bordered by radiopaque material which appears to have the same density as enamel. On either side of the "inner tooth" is a radiolucent space which represents the pulp chamber. Because of pulpal and periapical involvement most examples of dens in dente will be accompanied by periapical radiolucencies.

SEGMENTED ROOT

(Center) Radiographs of a tooth in which there was a disturbance in root formation causing it to be formed in 2 segments. Some factor, probably trauma, caused intrusion of the developing tooth which separated the epithelial diaphragm from the formed root. Proliferation of Hertwig's sheath continued root formation while the persistent epithelial diaphragm caused separation of the 2 portions of the root, resulting in the segmentation. This anomaly may have developed in much the same manner as do accessory pulp canals, except that the defective activity of Hertwig's sheath occurred around the whole circumference of the tooth.

DWARFED ROOTS

(Bottom) Three maxillary incisor teeth with normal-sized crowns and short, stubby roots. In addition to the hypoplastic roots, such teeth usually have an exaggerated labial contour with the incisal edge in a lingual position to the long axis of the tooth. When dwarfed roots of this kind occur, they are frequently found in pairs of teeth and may exist in several members of the same family. It is evident that these short-rooted teeth may be lost early due to passive eruption, and earlier still if there is periodontal disease. Underdeveloped teeth of this type should not be confused with normally formed teeth in which there has been apical resorption. Undersized roots of a different form are sometimes seen in disturbances in odontogenesis (pp. 51, 52, 63).

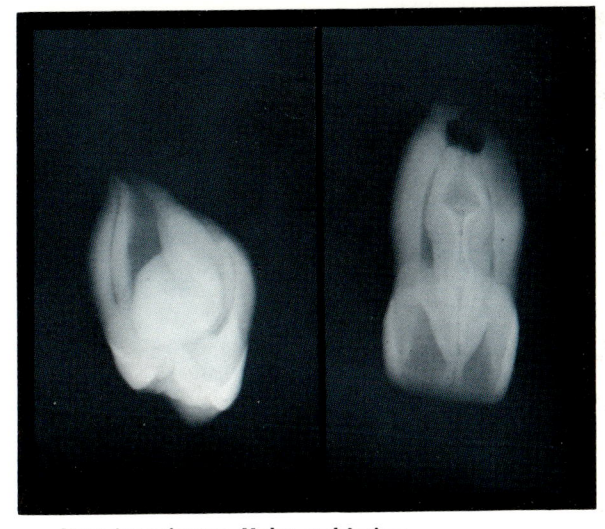

Dens Invaginatus, Molar and Incisor

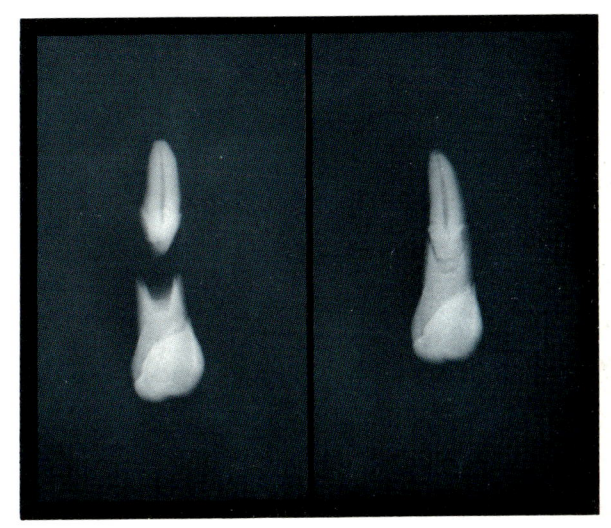

Segmented Root

Dwarfed Roots

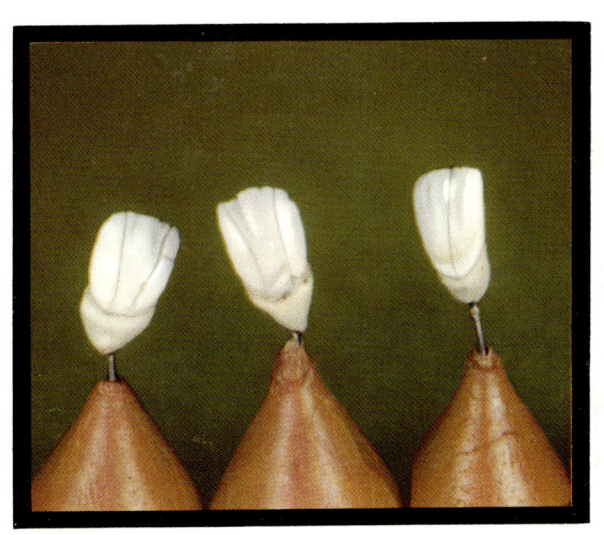

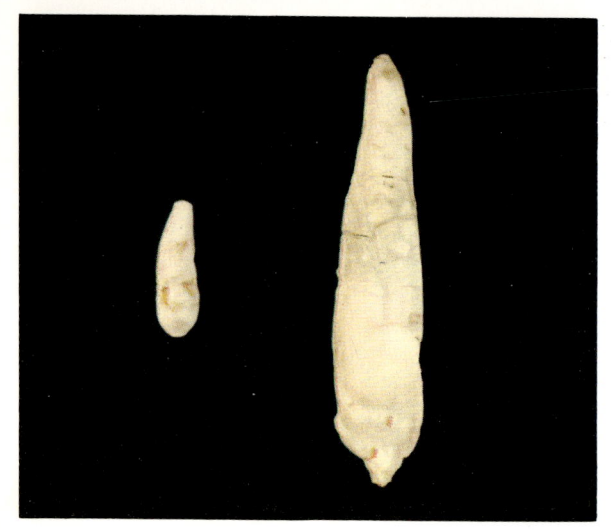

40 Developmental Disturbances

Microdontia and Macrodontia

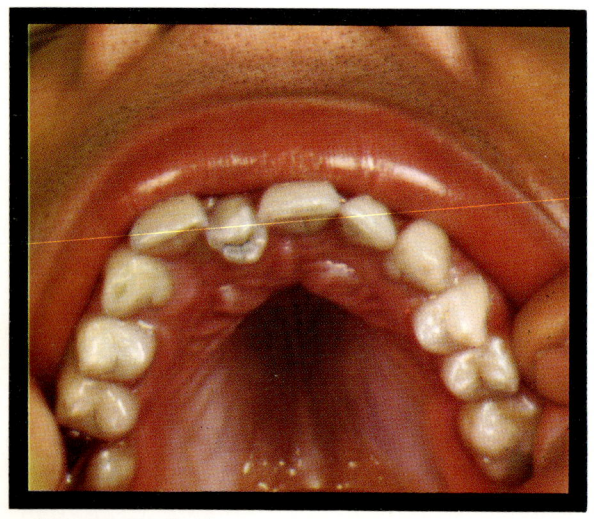

MICRODONTIA AND MACRODONTIA

(Dwarfism and Gigantism)

(Top) Examples of a very small tooth (microdontia, dwarfism) and a very large tooth (macrodontia, megalodontia, gigantism). Such variations in size may occur in single teeth, a few teeth, or all teeth of a given dentition. When all teeth are large or small, but proportionate to the general constitution, they may be considered as normal. Gigantism of individual teeth is most frequent in the incisor or cuspid region, while 3rd molars and maxillary lateral incisors are the teeth most frequently dwarfed. The maxillary lateral incisors may be peg-shaped. Both large and small teeth tend to occur in pairs and often follow a genetic pattern although other factors may be active (p. 63, *center*).

SUPERNUMERARY TEETH

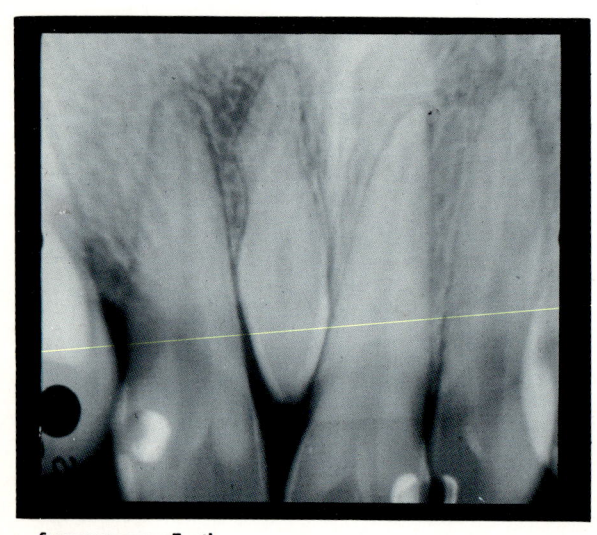

(Center) A supernumerary tooth with the crown form of a premolar has displaced the maxillary right central incisor and prevented the eruption of the right lateral. Supernumerary teeth, in addition to interfering with normal eruption, may be situated between the roots of adjacent teeth, causing a diastema; they may erupt into the buccal or lingual embrasures and also may occur outside of the normal line of the dental arch. These extra teeth are observed most frequently in the maxillary incisor and the 3rd molar regions. They are produced as a result of accessory tooth buds differentiating from the dental lamina. Even when erupted, supernumerary teeth are often unobserved or overlooked.

Supernumerary Tooth

(Bottom) A radiograph showing a median diastema caused by an unerupted supernumerary tooth. The term mesiodens is sometimes applied to a tooth in this location because it is mesial to the 2 central incisors. Teeth that occur distally to 3rd molars are designated as distomolars, while those appearing laterally may be called paramolars. Among the explanations proposed for the appearance of supernumerary teeth in the incisor and the premolar regions is reversion to the typical mammalian formula of 6 incisors and 8 premolars in either jaw.

Supernumerary Tooth

ECTODERMAL DYSPLASIA

This hereditary disease of faulty ectodermal development is characterized by a few or many of the following abnormalities: lack of sweat and sebaceous glands; smooth, atrophic skin; total or partial anodontia; defective hair, nail and iris formation; atrophic rhinitis; deficiency of lacrimal, pharyngeal, conjunctival and salivary glands; prominent forehead; saddle-type nose; thick lips; and dysphonia. In the anhidrotic type (lack of sweat glands), the inability to perspire greatly interferes with the well-being of the individual because the heat-regulating mechanism cannot keep the body at the proper temperature.

(Top) A 5-year-old boy exhibiting manifestations of ectodermal dysplasia. He has very fine, sparse, silken hair and scant eyebrows and eyelashes; frontal eminences are quite prominent; and the nose is depressed at the root. The skin is smooth and glossy, and the lips are thick. Abnormality was first suspected at 8 months, when teeth had not yet appeared. Shortly thereafter, with the advent of warm weather, the child felt hot, showed signs of distress, and had an unusual thirst. When he was placed in an air-conditioned room, these symptoms disappeared.

(Center) Intra-oral view of the above patient wearing complete artificial dentures, the lower one being slightly dislodged by the cheek retractor. Radiographs did not reveal tooth buds of either the primary or the permanent dentition. At the corners of the nose the dryness and thinness of the skin are well demonstrated. This patient has neither rhinitis nor a deficiency in salivary flow but does have a constant rough quality of voice.

(Bottom) Another case of ectodermal dysplasia, characterized by hypotrichosis, anhidrosis, photophobia and partial anodontia. Mild partial anodontia (congenital absence of 1 or 2 pairs of teeth) is a relatively common defect in the general population and is not usually associated with ectodermal dysplasia. When all or most of the teeth are missing, however, the syndrome should be suspected.

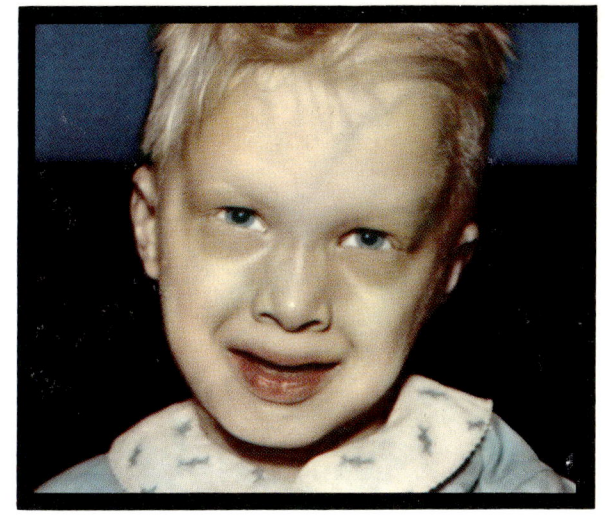

Ectodermal Dysplasia

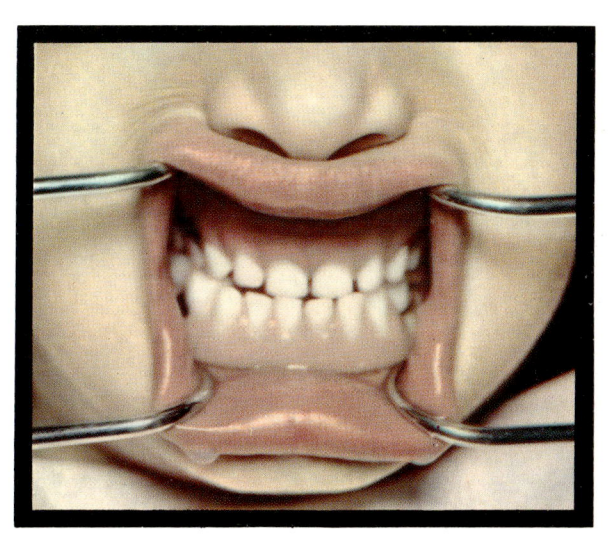

Complete Anodontia

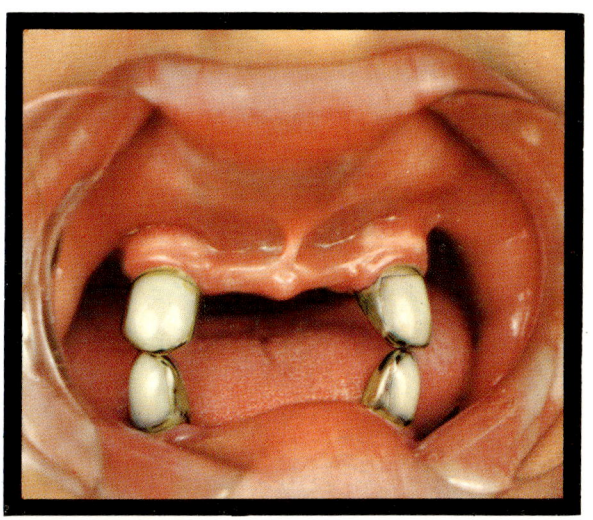

Partial Anodontia

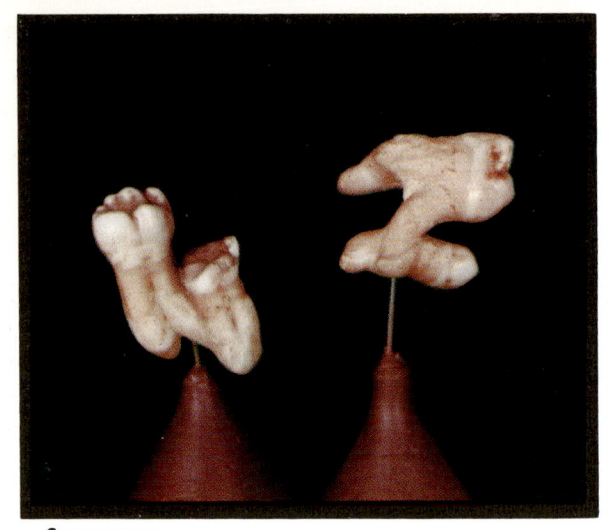

Developmental Disturbances

Concrescence

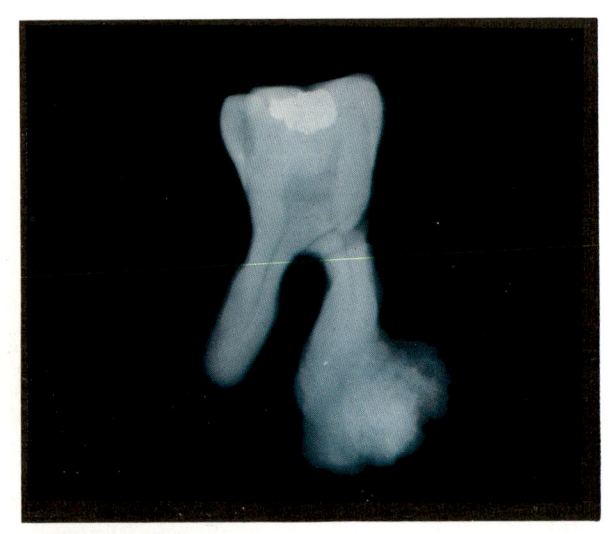

Hypercementosis

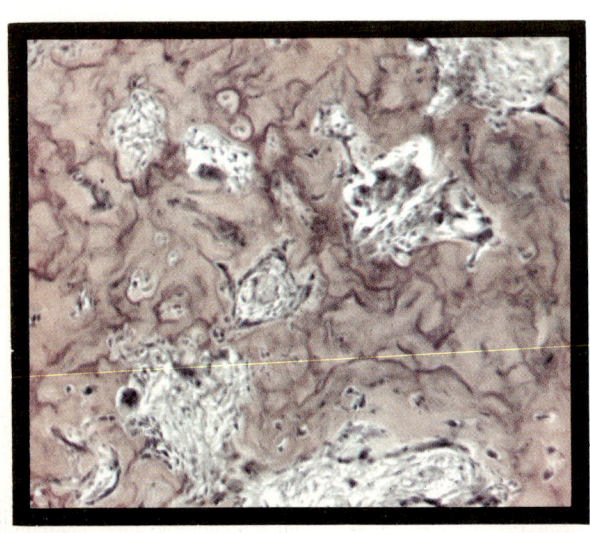

Cementoma   X 90

CONCRESCENCE

The term concrescence denotes the cemental union of 2 fully formed teeth which originally were separate entities. Two factors are essential for this condition: (1) excessive deposition of cementum and (2) close approximation of the roots of adjacent teeth. The process is similar to that which occurs when a fractured root is repaired (p. 60). Concrescence differs from fusion in that the union in the latter is between 2 developing teeth (tooth germs), with a resulting coalescence of their respective dentins (p. 37). Concrescence is observed most frequently in the maxillary molar region.

(Top) Two examples of concrescence. In the one on the left, the root of a 2nd molar is joined by cementum to the root of a 3rd molar which was completely unerupted. At right, a partially erupted supernumerary tooth and a 1st molar are united.

HYPERCEMENTOSIS

The formation of excessive cementum on the root (hypercementosis) may be due to trauma, local (p. 62) or general (p. 134) metabolic dysfunction, periapical inflammation or a defect in development. In the latter case there is an inherent tendency toward generalized extensive production of cementum probably due to inadequate inhibiting factor rather than to excessive cementoblastic stimulation. Unlike cementoma formation (p. 62), developmental hypercementosis is not preceded by bone resorption.

(Center) Radiograph of an extracted tooth showing extreme hypercementosis. Obviously, if another tooth root had been very close to it, concrescence would have resulted.

(Bottom) The microscopic structure of an area of the cementoma seen above. The cementum is trabecular in pattern. At the periphery of the "marrow" spaces several cementoclasts (large cells) can be seen. This differs from the usual pattern of bone in that the cement lines are irregular, and the lacunae are scarce and haphazardly arranged. Sometimes, however, it is impossible to distinguish cementum from bone histologically. Cementum is modified bone attached to and part of the tooth.

Developmental Disturbances

ENAMEL PEARLS

Enamel pearls (nodulous anomalies, enamel drops, enamelomas) are small masses of enamel found apically to the amelocemental junction. They occur most frequently at the bifurcation of molar roots and may appear in radiographs as round radiopacities. Their presence is of clinical significance only when gingival recession or periodontal disease involves the bifurcation or root surface supporting the enamel pearl. These anomalies are formed when a portion of Hertwig's sheath remains in contact with the dentin and is stimulated to differentiate into functional ameloblasts.

(Top) The left molar with fused roots has an enamel pearl on the lateral root surface and hypercementosis at the root apex. The right molar (maxillary) has a large pearl in the bifurcation area.

(Center) A photomicrograph of an enamel pearl in the bifurcation of a mandibular molar tooth. Delicate pale-blue-stained enamel matrix lies in a baylike depression of the purple stained dentin. Remnants of the amelogenic tissue appear below this enamel pearl. Only the organic matrix material is seen in this decalcified specimen. The inorganic salts have been removed by acid.

DILACERATION

Dilaceration, technically, refers to distortion of the root or crown caused by a tearing during tooth development with a resultant crease at the point of distortion and a very sharp bend. Through usage the term is now used for any severe angulation with distortion of the roots such as that seen in mandibular 3rd molars distorted by lack of space for development. The roots of all posterior teeth tend to have a distal inclination, but the term dilaceration should be used only for sharp distortions.

(Bottom) A dilacerated tooth which may have resulted from an injury to the tooth germ *(left)*, and one which may have occurred because of insufficient space in which to develop *(right)*.

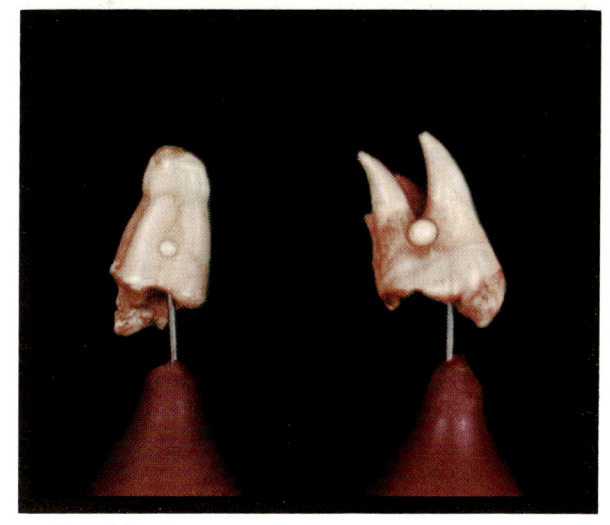

Enamel Pearls

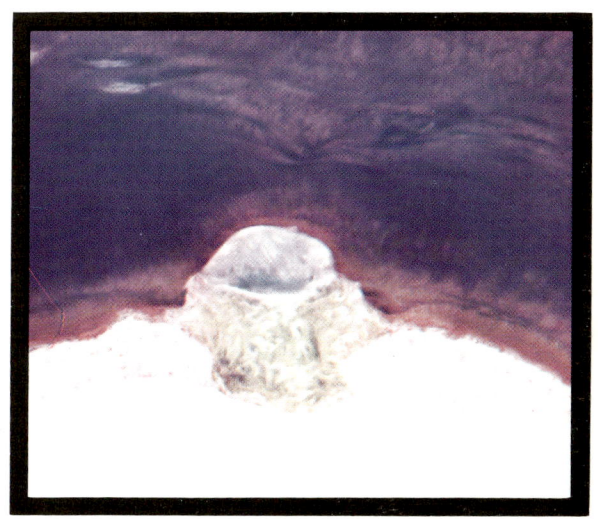

Enamel Pearl   X 100

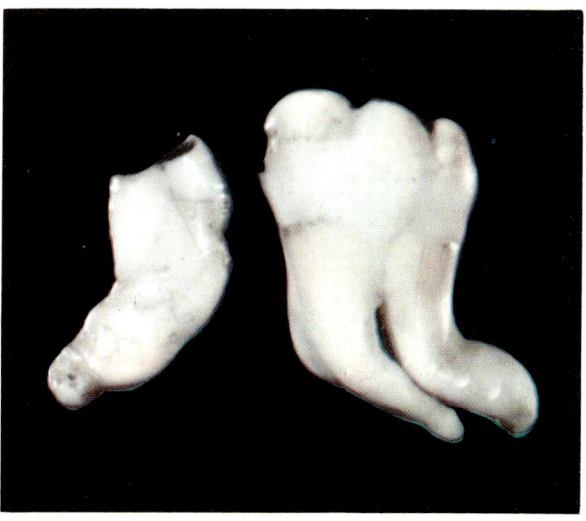

Dilaceration

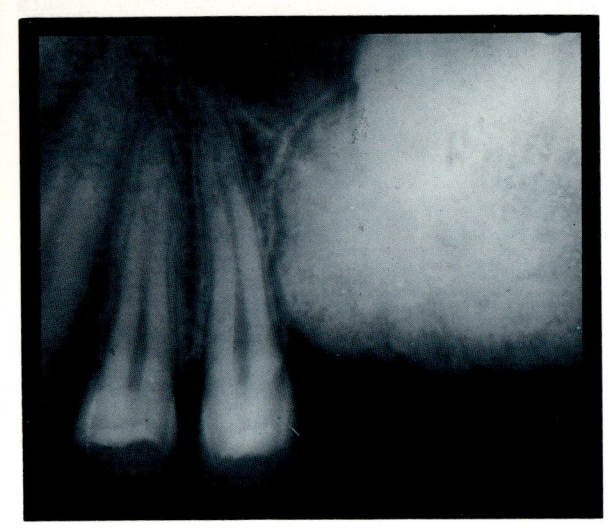

Complex Composite Odontome

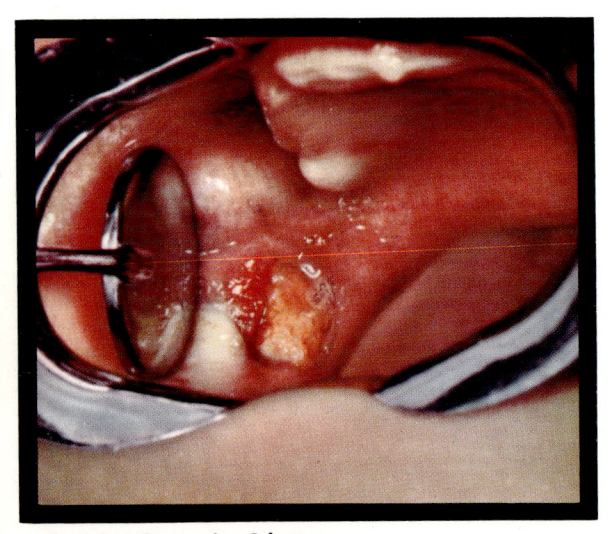

Complex Composite Odontome

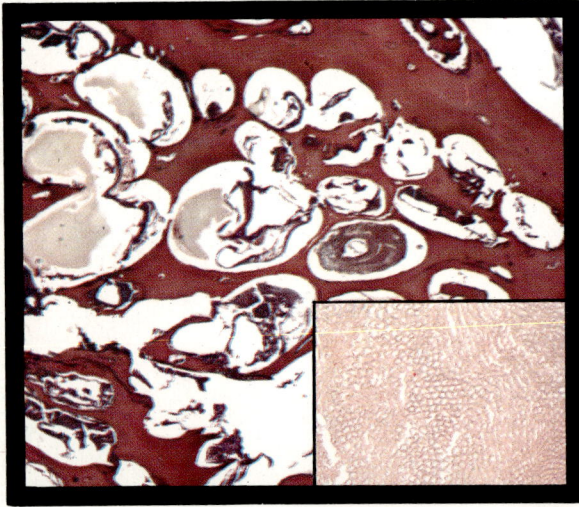

X 20   Complex Composite Odontome   X 180

ODONTOME

(Odontoma)

An odontome, or more specifically a composite (mixed) odontome, is a tumorous anomaly of calcified dental tissues involving both ectodermal (enamel) and mesodermal (dentin, cementum, pulp) structures. Two types of composite odontomes are recognized: (1) the complex type, which consists of a single mass of dentin, cementum and enamel in abnormal relation; and (2) the compound type, consisting of several small masses in which the anatomic relation of the dental tissues is such that the structures formed by these tissues are more or less recognizable as rudimentary teeth. Occasionally, features of both types are evident in a single case. In that event the designation of the lesion should be determined by its most predominant characteristic, or it may be referred to as a complex-compound composite odontome. Because these lesions are limited in growth, they are not true neoplasms, as the older term odontoma would imply, but are defects of development.

(Top) Radiograph of part of a large complex composite odontome in the maxillary molar region. The radiopaque mass surrounded by a radiolucent line is fairly diagnostic of the anomaly. This defect of development may arise from regular or supernumerary tooth buds.

(Center) Illustration of an exposed complex composite odontome in the mandibular 3rd molar region of a 65-year-old woman, depicting the gross characteristics of this type of odontome. The emergence of such anomalies is rare. In this patient, its exposure may be attributed to bone resorption in an edentulous area associated with a denture that had been worn for many years.

(Bottom) A photomicrograph from a section of the complex composite odontome shown at the top of this page. The dental tissues are arranged haphazardly and are not in the form of a tooth. The dense portion composing the bulk of the section is a mixture of dentin and cementum. The various-sized circular areas were filled with enamel, but because of decalcification, only remnants of the enamel matrix are now present. The inset shows the enamel pattern from one of these areas at higher magnification.

Odontome (Cont.)

(Top) A compound composite odontome that apparently has prevented the eruption of the permanent bicuspid. It is composed of numerous small radiopaque masses having the same density as tooth structure. One can be fairly certain of the diagnosis from a radiograph, but histologic examination should be made because occasionally it may reveal that the lesion is a neoplasm (odontoameloblastoma, p. 149) rather than a simple anomaly.

(Center) Components of a compound composite odontome. The denticles found in these anomalies may vary in size, number and configuration. Some of them duplicate specific tooth forms, while others are amorphous masses. As many as 200 such denticles have been observed in a single lesion.

(Bottom) A photomicrograph of a small compound composite anomaly that developed extraosseously. Clinically, this lesion, which was located between the maxillary lateral and central incisors, appeared to be a fibroid epulis. Only upon sectioning was the odontome discovered. The patient, when a small child, received a severe injury in this region, which may account for the misplaced odontogenic epithelium from which the anomaly developed. Near the upper border of the illustration is surface epithelium of the oral cavity (dark blue). Next is a mass of dense fibrous connective tissue staining a reddish color. In the midst of the connective tissue near the lower border, blue-staining dentin and cementum appear. The partially clear area contains fragments of enamel matrix.

The following entities, classified as odontomes or odontomas by some authors, are not to be confused with the anomalies discussed on this and the preceding page: simple soft odontoma (odontogenic fibroma, p. 149); mixed soft odontoma (fibroameloblastoma, p. 149); simple calcified odontoma (cementoma, p. 62); cementoblastoma, dentinoma, geminated odontome (gemination, p. 37); dilated composite odontome (a type of dens invaginatus, p. 38).

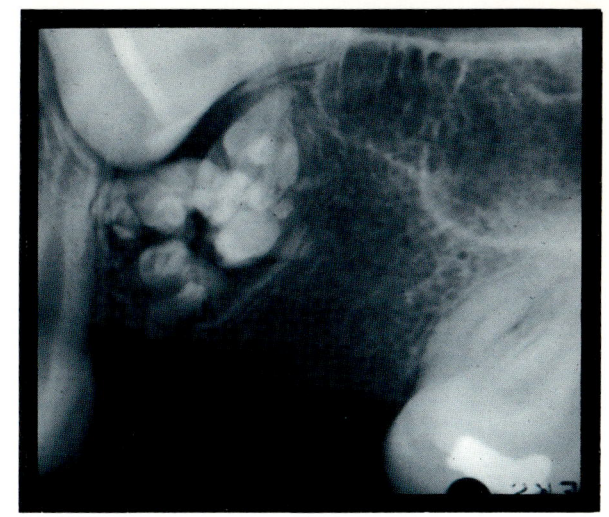

Compound Composite Odontome

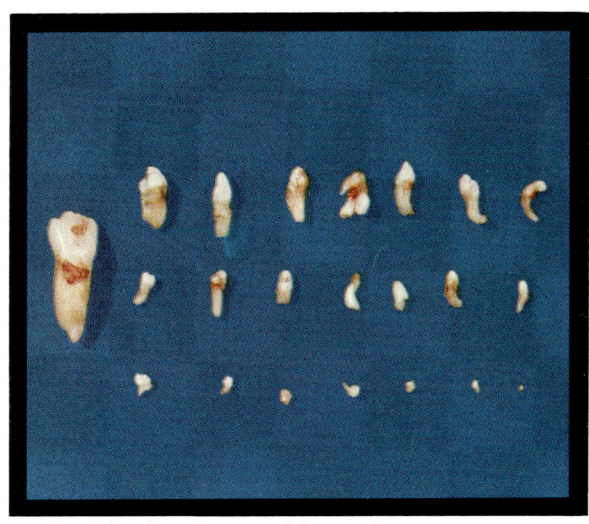

Denticles from Compound Composite Odontome

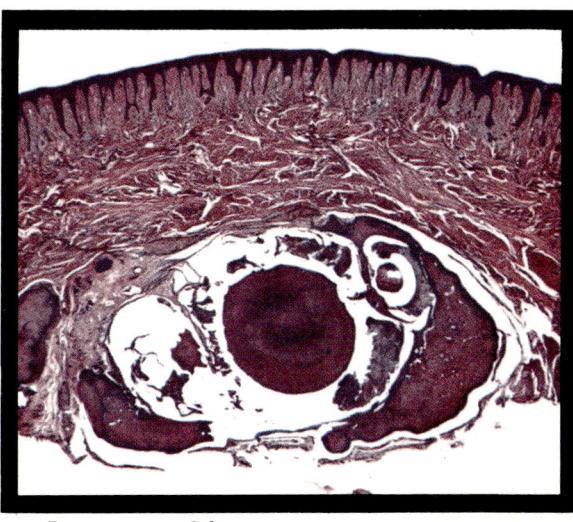

Extra-osseous Odontome

X 14

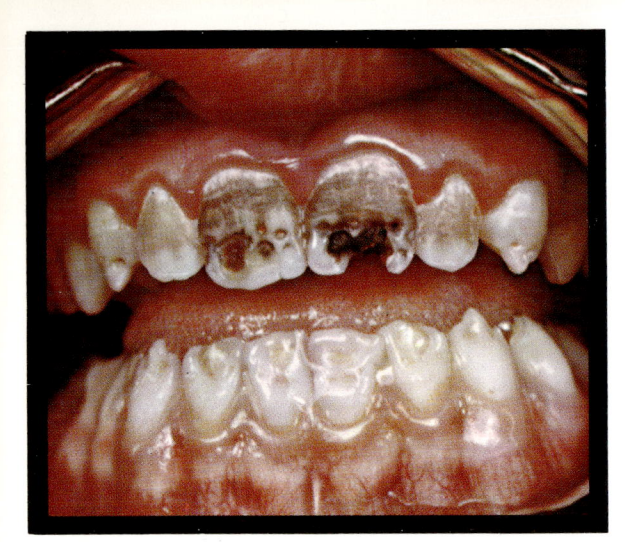

Enamel Hypoplasia

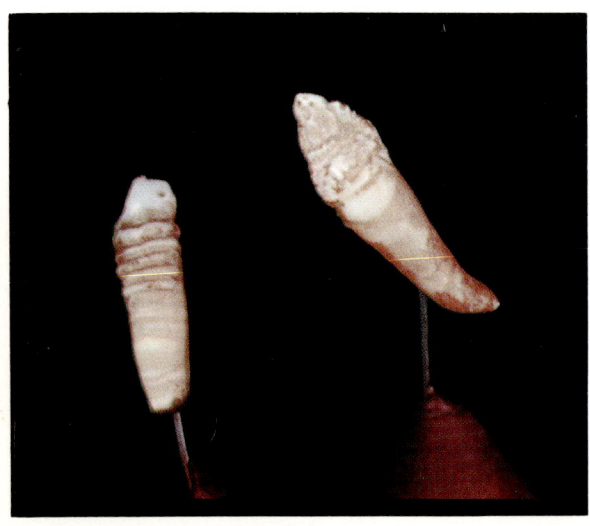

Intermittent Enamel Hypoplasia

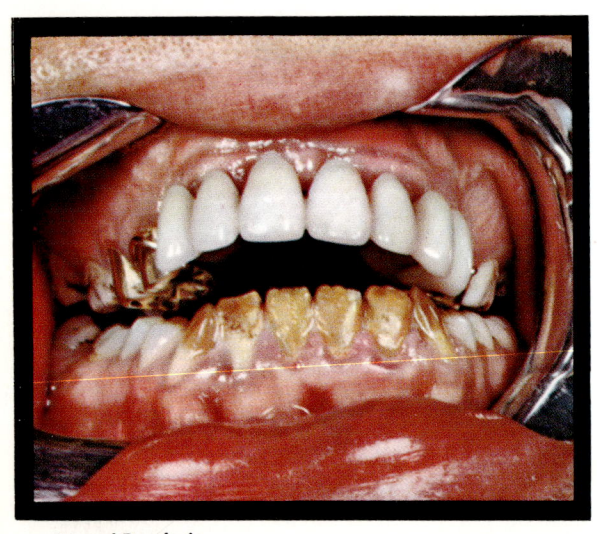

Enamel Dysplasia

ENAMEL DYSPLASIA

Enamel dysplasia is a broad term including two types of abnormal enamel development: enamel hypoplasia and enamel hypocalcification. Enamel hypoplasia may be produced by any disturbance of sufficient severity to interfere with ameloblastic function during formation of enamel matrix (apposition of enamel). Enamel hypocalcification may be caused by any factor which inhibits enamel maturation (the calcification of enamel). Local, systemic or hereditary disturbances may be etiologic factors in either type. Local factors such as periapical inflammation or trauma to a deciduous tooth may cause either hypoplasia or hypocalcification of the permanent successor. Nutritional deficiencies (particularly of vitamins A and D), endocrine dysfunction and generalized infection during odontogenesis are among the systemic causes. An excessive amount of fluorides in the drinking water during odontogenesis is the most frequent cause of hypocalcification. The term amelogenesis imperfecta is applied to hereditary types of enamel dysplasia.

(Top) Severe hypoplasia with pits and grooves at different levels on different teeth. The defects occur in the enamel that was being formed at the time of the disturbance. An exanthematous fever is often considered as the specific systemic factor responsible for this form of hypoplasia, but investigation will often reveal that the time of interruption of amelogenesis does not correspond to the time period of the disease.

(Center) Two teeth showing enamel hypoplasia of rhythmic character. The multiple zones of defective enamel resulted from intermittent interference with the appositional stage of amelogenesis.

(Bottom) Almost total aplasia of enamel in the lower incisors and cuspids. There is a small amount of enamel near the gingiva on the lower right cuspid and a sharp ridge demarcating its border. These teeth do not show attrition because of the open bite. The maxillary anterior teeth, now replaced by a partial denture, were affected similarly.

Enamel Dysplasia (Cont.)

(Top) This example of enamel dysplasia is designated as amelogenesis imperfecta, since the abnormality was exhibited by several members of the family as a dominant nonsex-linked Mendelian trait. Two brothers of the patient, similarly affected, also showed minor dysplastic defects of other ectodermal structures. This patient presents abnormal enamel development ranging from a complete absence of enamel formation to a deposition of enamel matrix that failed to become fully matured. Failure of enamel formation is apparent on the maxillary lateral incisors, which look as if they had been prepared for jacket crowns. Soft, immature enamel, although abraded from most of the teeth, is still present on the maxillary left central. At the neck of the maxillary right central is a very thin layer of smooth, shiny, hard, mature enamel through which is reflected the underlying dentin. If all the teeth were of this consistency and appearance, the abnormality might be further classified as hereditary brown hypoplasia. (Also see p. 49, *bottom*.)

(Center) Photomicrograph of a developing tooth from a 43-day-old infant born 3 months prematurely. The diagonal clear space in the center is an artefact separating the enamel organ *(right)* from the previously formed blue-staining enamel matrix. To the right of the artefact, partially surrounding a globule of abnormal enamel matrix, is a proliferation of poorly differentiated cells. This proliferation of odontogenic epithelium is apparently a reparative procedure—an attempt to replace degenerated ameloblasts. The cells in this zone are probably nonfunctional, and the area would have been represented clinically as a pit or groove.

(Bottom) In this photomicrograph from the same patient, the V-shaped clear space is artefact. Proceeding to the right from the artefact is first a reddish band of normal enamel matrix, next a vacuolated area, and then a row of ameloblasts. It is believed that the foamy enamel matrix (vacuolated area), caused by some disturbance to the ameloblasts, would have been reflected in the clinical appearance of the tooth as a hypoplastic defect.

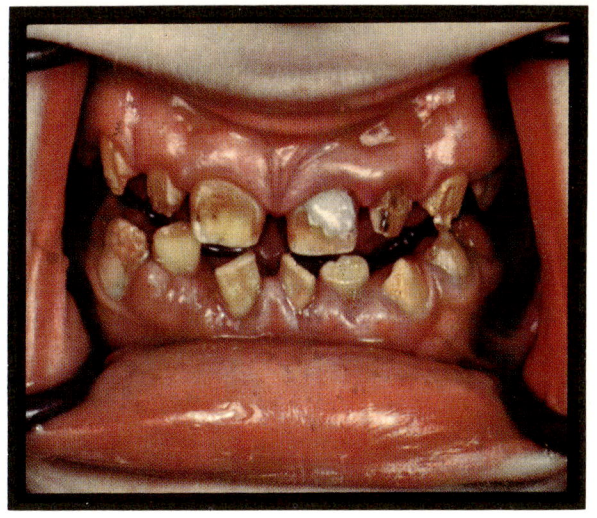

Amelogenesis Imperfecta

Enamel Hypoplasia X 100

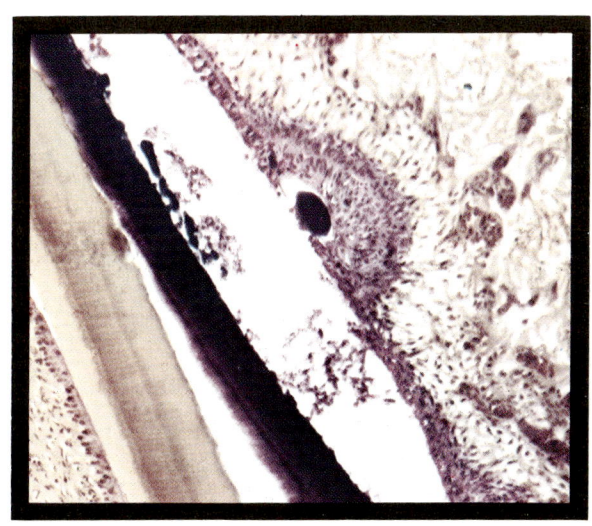

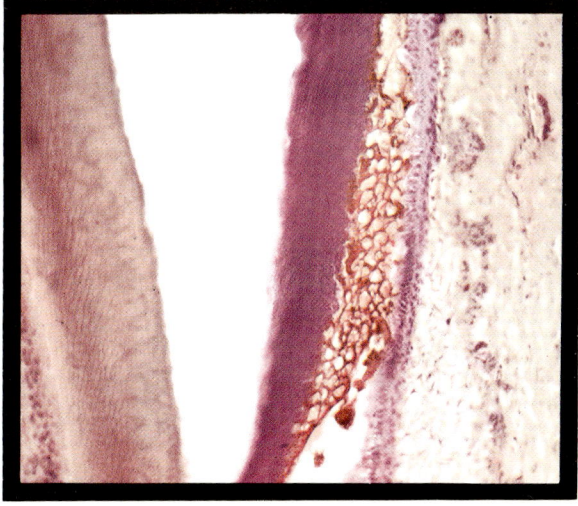

Enamel Hypoplasia X 100

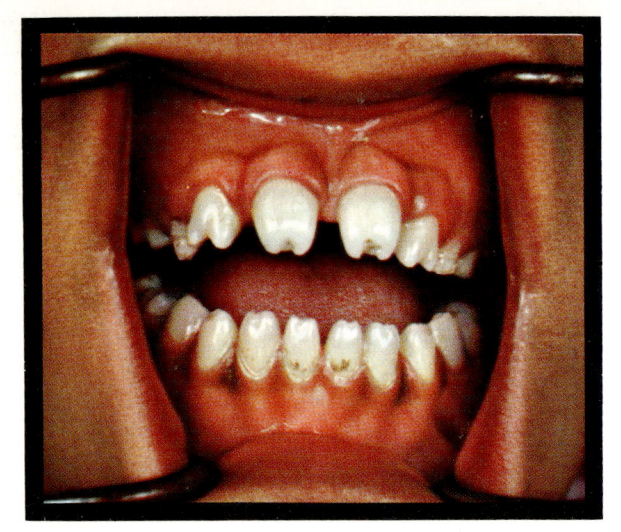

Hutchinson's Incisors

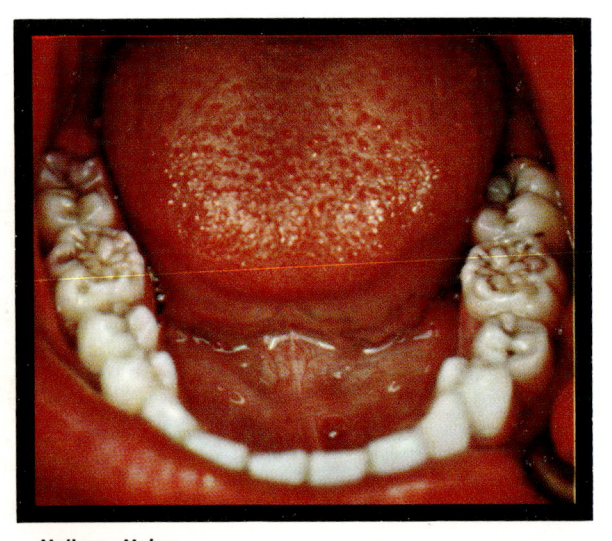

Mulberry Molars

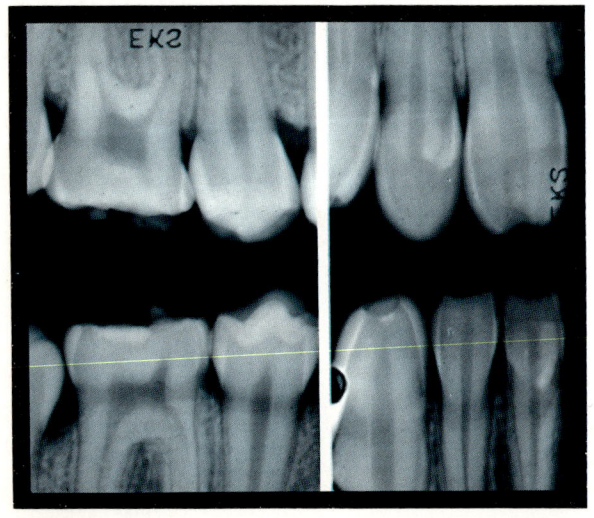

Mulberry Molars   **Hutchinson's Incisors**

Enamel Dysplasia (Cont.)

Enamel hypoplasia of both dentitions may result from prenatal syphilis. In the permanent teeth this specific infection also interferes with morphodifferentiation and dentinogenesis. The enamel organ may be directly invaded by *Treponema pallidum*, or may be secondarily affected by inflammatory processes in the surrounding tissues. The spirochete does not enter the fetal circulation until after the 16th week, and its effect on tooth development does not extend beyond early infancy; therefore, only those stages of odontogenesis that occur during this period can be affected. Since morphodifferentiation of the deciduous teeth has already been completed by the 16th week, their size and shape cannot be altered, but enamel apposition may be disturbed and result in hypoplastic defects that, although caused by syphilis, are not especially pathognomonic of the disease. The permanent teeth (12 anteriors and 4 first molars) are so distinctively affected, when involved, that clinically they can be consistently recognized.

(Top) Typical Hutchinson's incisors in a patient with prenatal syphilis. They are notched, screwdriver-shaped teeth with rounded incisal angles. Although faulty matrix formation often accentuates the notch, the abnormal contour is mainly due to alteration in the ameloblastic layer at the time of morphodifferentiation. Hutchinson considered such teeth, keratitis, and nerve deafness as a triad characteristic of congenital syphilis.

(Center) One of the types of 1st molars seen in this disease. Hypoplasia of the enamel, along with the altered shape, gives the occlusal surface a mulberrylike appearance. A variation characterized by a clinched appearance of the crown is known as the bud molar. Attrition of both these types may result in a flat-surfaced tooth with exposed dentin.

(Bottom) Bitewing radiographs showing the characteristic notching and converging lateral borders of the anterior teeth and the marked hypoplasia of the enamel on the occlusal surfaces of the 1st molars. Diagnosis of congenital syphilis should not be based on dental defects alone. (See pp. 114, 115.)

Enamel Dysplasia (Cont.)

(Top) A mild case of mottled enamel (endemic dental fluorosis), which is an acquired form of enamel hypocalcification caused by the consumption of water having an excessive amount of fluorine. To cause mottling, the water must contain more than one part per million of the element and be consumed during the tooth-development period. The fluorine, unless in extremely high concentration, does not injure the ameloblasts sufficiently to interfere with enamel apposition, but the matrix formed by such ameloblasts does not mature completely. When decalcified microscopic sections are made of mature enamel, which is acid-soluble, only a scant amount of matrix may be seen. When teeth with mottled enamel are likewise prepared, a considerable amount of enamel matrix is apparent in the brown areas. Because this hypocalcified enamel is high in organic content, it is relatively acid-resistant and appears microscopically not unlike young enamel matrix of a developing tooth, depicted at the top of page 6. When teeth of this type originally erupt, there are cloudy, opaque areas, but these porous regions gradually absorb extrinsic material and assume a yellow or brown color.

(Center) The single chalky-white opaque spot in the left maxillary central incisor is an example of focal hypomaturation (nonendemic mottling) of enamel. When the surface was removed in preparing this tooth for an acrylic crown, the underlying enamel in this region was found to be soft. The groove above the area of hypocalcification reflects a disturbance in matrix formation. Not all white spots are examples of hypomaturation. Some may be due to altered matrix apposition, which changes the index of refraction. Other white areas, especially if generalized, may be caused by lack of pigment. Decalcification in the early phases of dental caries may produce a similar-appearing white spot.

(Bottom) An example of severe amelogenesis imperfecta. The enamel on the lower anterior teeth is nearly normal, but the remaining teeth show varying degrees of enamel aplasia and hypomaturation. This patient's 2 sisters were affected likewise. (Also see p. 47.)

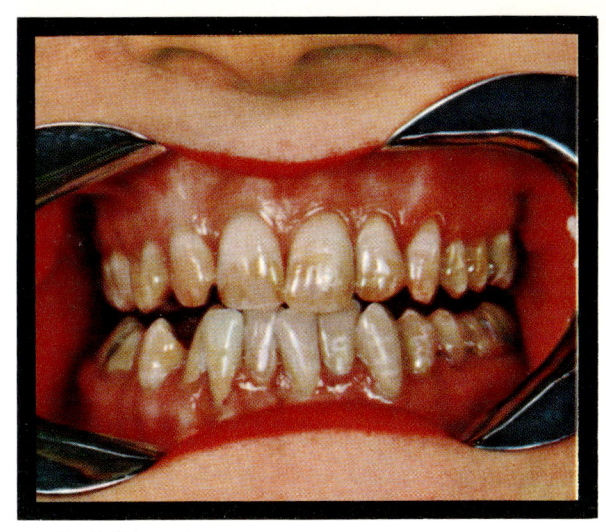

Mottled Enamel

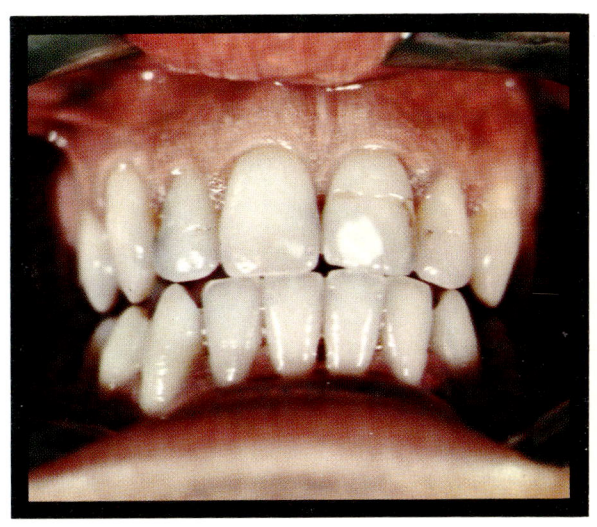

Focal Hypomaturation

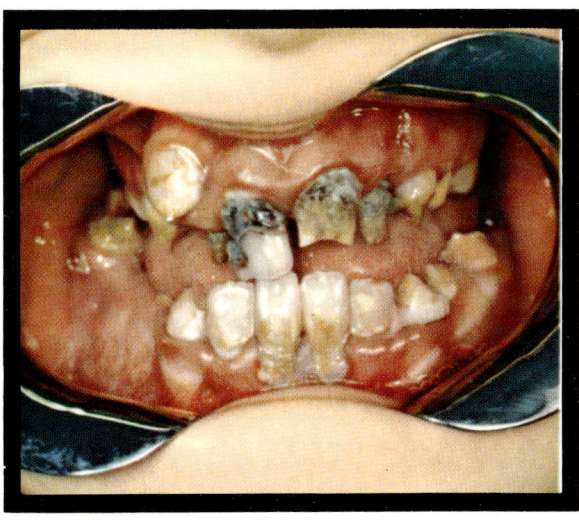

Amelogenesis Imperfecta

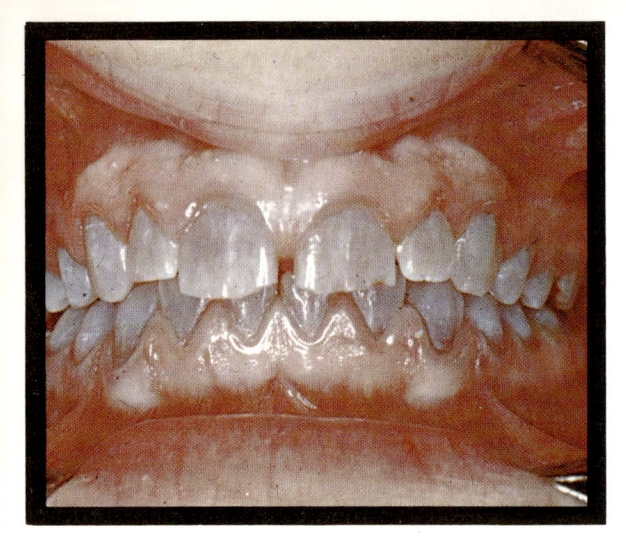

Dentinogenesis Imperfecta

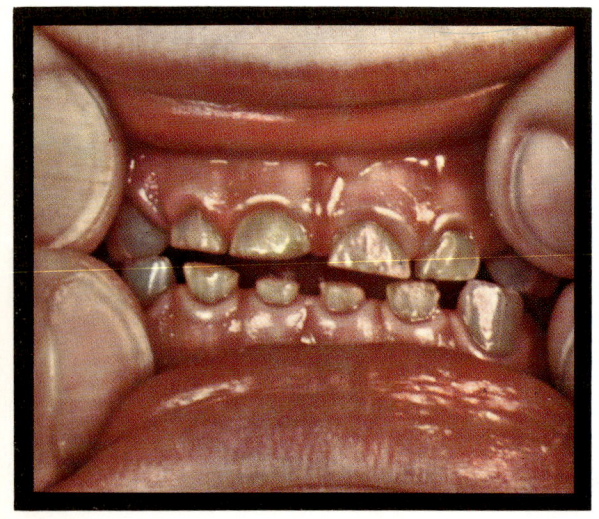

Dentinogenesis Imperfecta, Severe Attrition

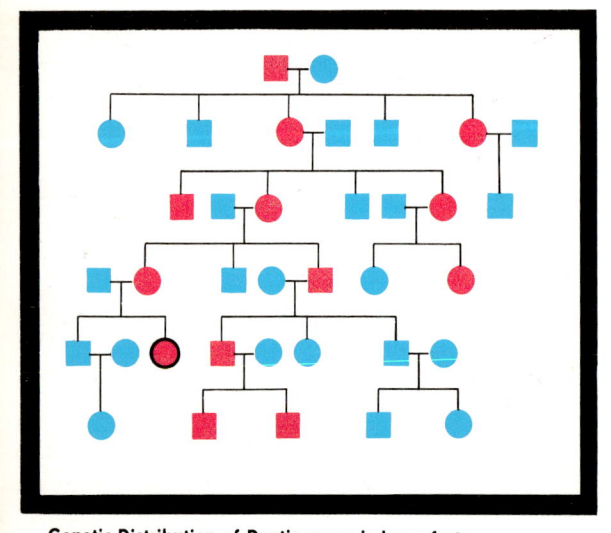

Genetic Distribution of Dentinogenesis Imperfecta

DEFECTS OF DENTIN FORMATION

Dentinogenesis Imperfecta

(Hereditary Opalescent Dentin)

This anomaly of imperfect formation of dentin is characterized by a peculiar tooth color, severe attrition and rapid obliteration of pulp chambers and root canals. The tooth color may be bluish-brown, violet or amber with an iridescence in certain lights. Enamel tends to chip or shear away from the dentin. Histologically, chemically and physically, the enamel is normal. The dentin, however, is very atypical. Dentinal tubules are few in number but of a large diameter; they are arranged haphazardly and sometimes appear at right angles to the normal direction. The dentin is poorly calcifed, and occasionally cellular inclusions are seen. Opalescent dentin is softer and has a greater water and organic content than normal dentin. Dentinogenesis imperfecta occurs in both the deciduous and permanent dentitions of the same patient.

(Top) Dentinogenesis imperfecta in a young patient with attrition of the maxillary incisor which would be excessive for normal teeth at this age. The teeth are opalescent with a violet hue. Almost complete obliteration of the pulp chambers and root canals was demonstrated radiographically.

(Center) Dentinogenesis imperfecta in a young patient showing severe attrition as contrasted with the patient above. Here the incisor teeth appear purplish-brown and the cuspids more of a violet color. Probably these variations in color are due to different dentin compositions and, in part, to the angle at which light strikes the enamel surfaces. The excessive wear followed the chipping of enamel from the functional surfaces. The radiographic appearance in this case was typical for dentinogenesis imperfecta (see p. 50, *top*).

(Bottom) Genetic pattern of dentinogenesis imperfecta in a family. The red symbols indicate individuals with hereditary opalescent dentin, the squares being males and the circles females. The patient in whom the disease was first observed is shown by a black-ringed circle. Dentinogenesis imperfecta is not sex-linked and is a dominant genetic disease that, when present in one parent, is transmitted by chance to approximately half of the offspring.

Dentinogenesis Imperfecta (Cont.)

The genetic disturbance of the mesenchyme in this disease results in abnormal dentin formation. Not only are the tubules sparse and irregular but the calcification is somewhat incomplete. The dentino-enamel junction usually is smoother than that in normal teeth. As the pulp chambers and root canals are rapidly filled with calcified, but irregular, dentin, they are soon obliterated radiographically. This is important diagnostically.

These teeth appear to be highly caries-resistant. The sensitivity of the teeth is usually low or negative, but occasionally they give normal responses to pulp tests. Because of their relatively thin roots, they may be prone to root fracture, although they have been successfully treated by jacket and full-veneer crowns.

(Top) These radiographs are of the same patient, those on the right at 7 years of age and those on the left at 17 years. Upper right shows obliteration of incisal pulp chambers and obliteration of root canals almost as fast as they form. The lower right illustrates involvement of both dentitions with severe attrition of deciduous molars and obliteration of pulp chambers in deciduous and permanent teeth. The upper left demonstrates complete obliteration of pulp chambers and heavy incisal wear. The lower left shows obliteration of pulp chambers, but a pulp canal may be visualized in distal root of 2nd molar. Because of excessive wear the 1st molar was lost, and the 2nd molar required a crown.

(Center) Low magnification *(left)* shows normal thin layer of cementum (at top), relatively normal outer layer of dentin and irregularly formed dentin below. The blue lines in the center are due to matrix failure and compression of many dentinal fibers. Under higher power *(right)* the irregular pattern is evident. Tubules of normal size and arrangement are seen at the center. Nodular areas show cross sections of large tubules, irregular tubules and atubular matrix.

(Bottom) Blue sclera may be seen alone or with dentinogenesis imperfecta. Either, neither or both may occur with osteogenesis imperfecta (p. 53). The blue color is due to the dark choroid showing through a thin sclera.

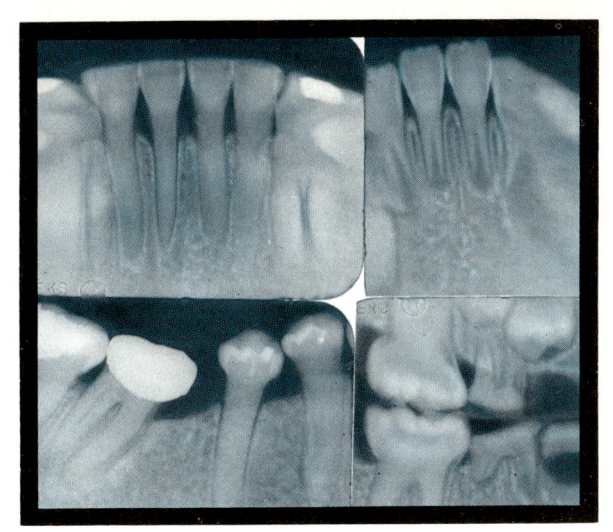

Dentinogenesis Imperfecta

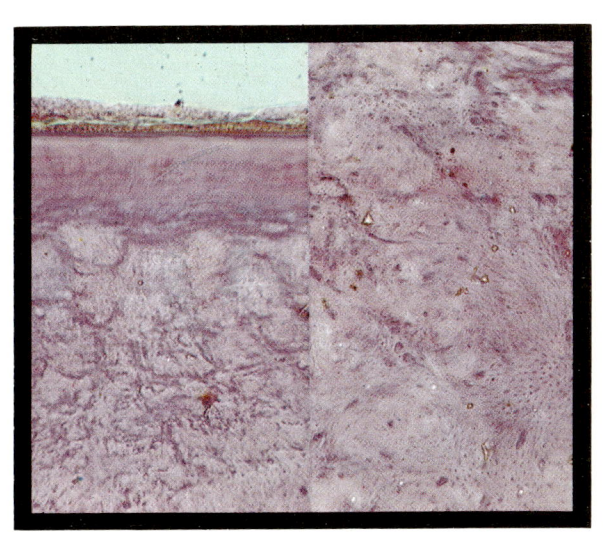

Dentinogenesis Imperfecta   left, X 50; right, X 150

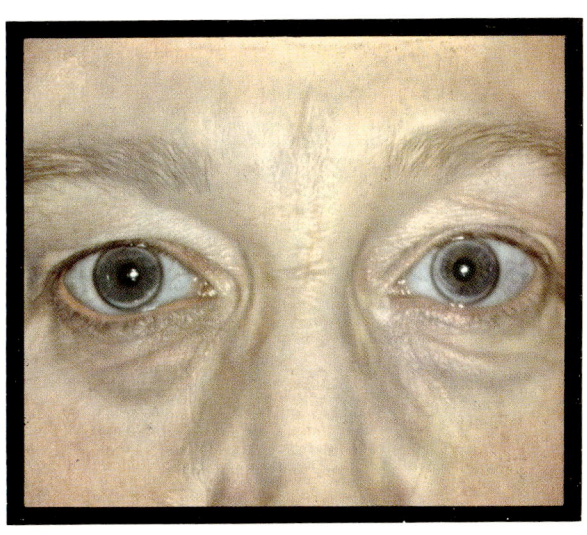

Blue Sclerae

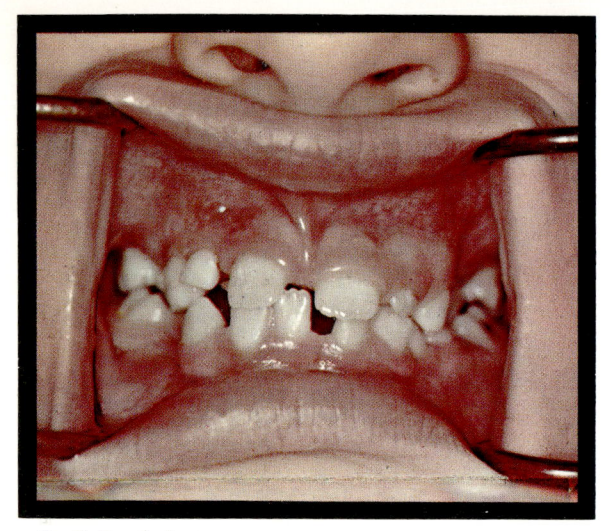

Developmental Disturbances

Dentin Dysplasia

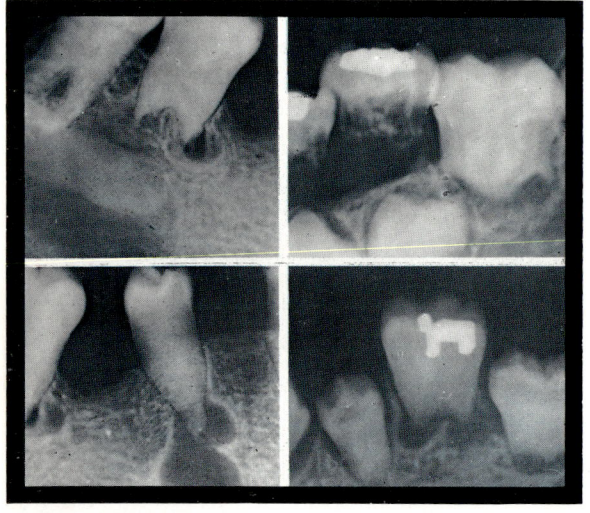

Dentin dysplasia is a form of mesodermal dysplasia now generally considered to be an entity distinct from dentinogenesis imperfecta. It differs from the latter in that the teeth are of normal color; there is no tendency for the enamel to chip off and no rapid attrition; and there is altered, retarded, and/or deficient root formation with radiolucent areas at the apices of some teeth. It is similar to dentinogenesis imperfecta because of early obliteration of pulp chambers and root canals by atypical dentin.

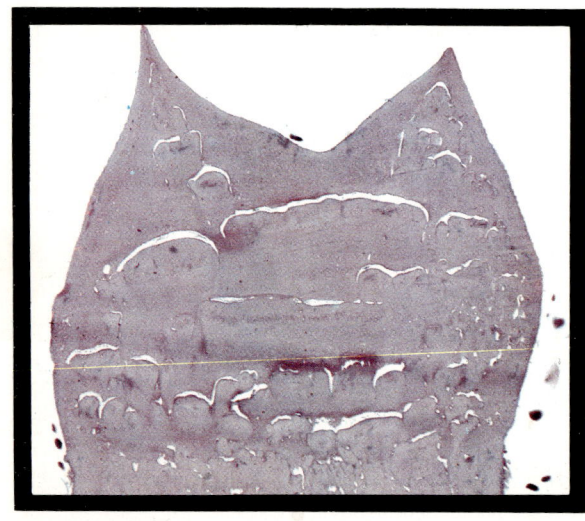

(Top) Clinical picture of dentin dysplasia. The teeth are of normal color with no attrition. Looseness, malposition and early loss of teeth may be attributed to retarded root formation and lack of supporting bone.

(Center) Radiographs of patient in top picture are on the right. They show normally shaped crowns, obliteration of pulp chambers, retarded root formation and apical radiolucencies. The radiographs on the left (from another patient) show sharply defined periapical radiolucencies, absence of pulp chambers and canals, and roots that are better formed but still defective. Sometimes horizontal radiolucencies are seen in the tooth crowns. The apical areas are fibrous but may become inflamed via periodontal pockets, especially on short-rooted teeth, and may develop into abscesses, granulomas or cysts.

(Bottom) In the decalcified section (without enamel) the only normal dentin is on the periphery. The remainder, which nearly obliterates the pulp chamber, is quite bizarre. Numerous horizontal crescent-shaped clear areas are evident. At higher magnification it is observed that dentin, with large tubules, curves around nodules of atubular dentin. The apical ends of the nodules are poorly defined, and tubular dentin appears to stream out of them. The cause of this pattern is not known, but it has been conjectured that the nodules are denticles.

Dentin Dysplasia

Dentin Dysplasia

Dentin Dysplasia   X 32

Developmental Disturbances

ODONTODYSPLASIA

(Top) This peculiar form of odontogenic dysplasia may involve one or several teeth. The teeth have a ghostlike appearance and have been termed "shell teeth." Both dentin and enamel are affected, the dentin being sparse and poorly formed and the enamel thin and rough. Histologic studies suggest that a violent local metabolic disturbance occurred at about 6 years of age. One or several teeth may be involved.

OSTEOGENESIS IMPERFECTA

Osteogenesis imperfecta and dentinogenesis imperfecta are manifestations of mesenchymal dysplasia that are definitely familial and genetically dominant. Osteogenesis imperfecta (brittle bones) may be associated with blue sclera, otosclerosis and/or dentinogenesis imperfecta. While osteogenesis imperfecta usually is divided into 2 types—congenital (prenatal) and tarda (postnatal)—they may simply represent variations in time and severity of clinical manifestations. In the early form the child is stillborn or dies in early infancy. The late form may appear in infancy or even as late as early adult life. Multiple fractures, associated with failure of osteoblastic function, abnormal osteoblastic function or reduction in osteoblasts are noted. Osteogenesis imperfecta and dentinogenesis imperfecta may occur concomitantly or independently in any single family. An affected individual may show one or both conditions.

(Center) Dentinogenesis imperfecta (hereditary) opalescent dentin in a 14-year-old female with osteogenesis imperfecta. The teeth have the usual dark, purplish-brown color, and the root canals and pulp chambers were practically obliterated as viewed in radiographs. This girl had already suffered multiple fractures with resultant deformity.

(Bottom) Osteogenesis imperfecta has resulted in over 20 fractures of the legs of this 14-year-old girl. Improper healing had led to angulation and bowing with marked deformity. Her teeth were opalescent in color, the enamel had chipped from the dentin on several of them, there was abnormal attrition, and the pulp chambers and root canals were practically obliterated. The scleras were blue. This patient had severe osteogenesis imperfecta tarda and severe dentinogenesis imperfecta.

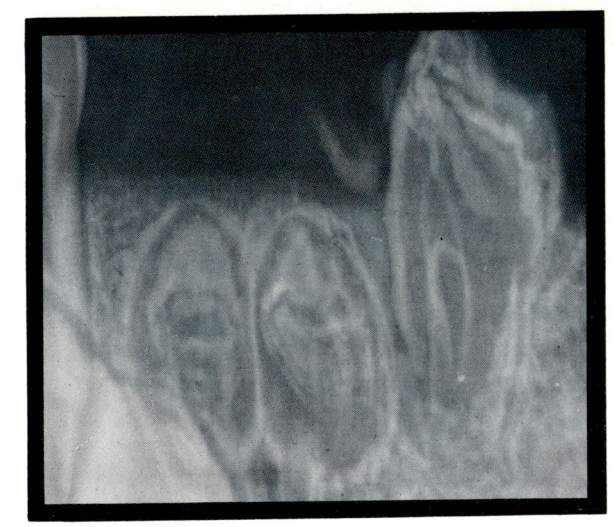

Odontodysplasia

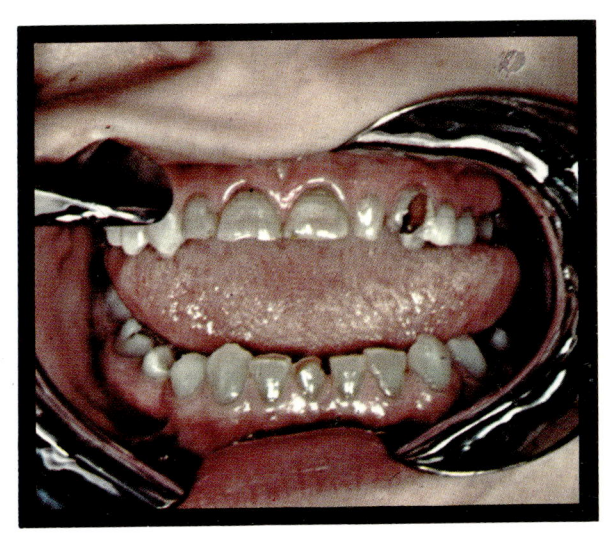

Dentinogenesis Imperfecta

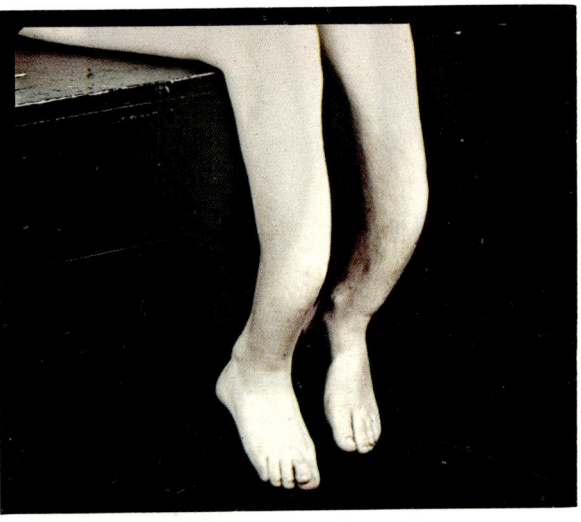

Osteogenesis Imperfecta, Repeated Fractures

54 *Developmental Disturbances*

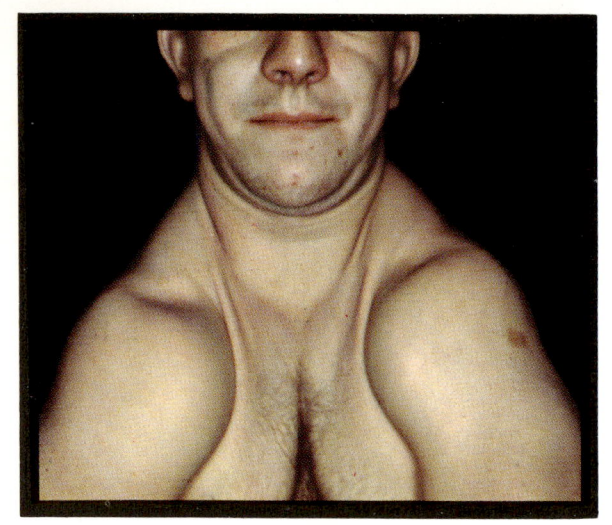

Cleidocranial Dysostosis, Excessive Shoulder Mobility

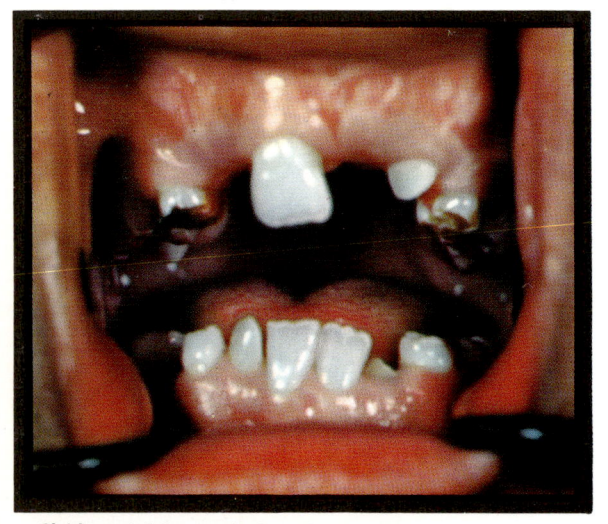

Cleidocranial Dysostosis, Retarded Eruption

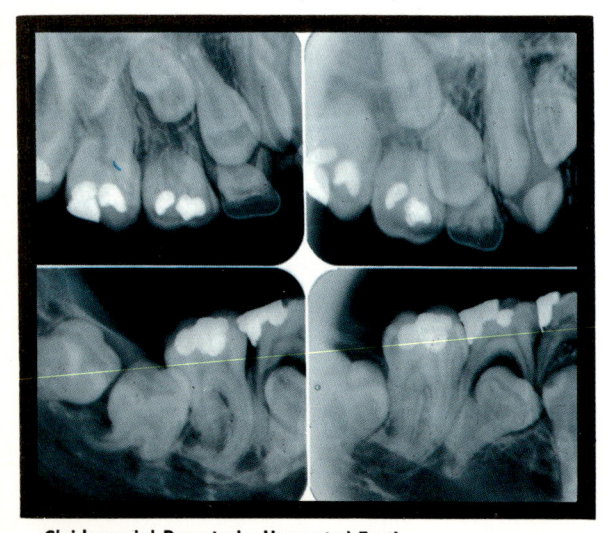

Cleidocranial Dysostosis, Unerupted Teeth

CLEIDOCRANIAL DYSOSTOSIS

This hereditary developmental disturbance is characterized primarily by defective ossification of the clavicles and bones of the skull that are not preformed in cartilage. The aplasia or hypoplasia of the clavicles enables the patient to move his shoulders forward to such an extent that he may be able to touch them together in front of the sternum. There may be a retarded closure of the fontanels and an exaggerated development of the transverse diameter of the skull. The root of the nose may be broad, the bridge depressed, and the accessory sinuses may be missing or small. Because there is usually some underdevelopment of the long bones, these individuals are frequently of relatively short stature. This disease is often associated with failure of shedding and eruption of teeth, the presence of numerous unerupted supernumerary teeth, and underdevelopment of the maxilla. This last abnormality gives a prognathic effect to the mandible. Mentality is not affected.

(Top) Cleidocranial dysostosis (Marie and Sainton's disease) in a 24-year-old male, showing the characteristic excessive mobility of the shoulders. Radiographic examination revealed defective development of the skull, clavicles and cervical spine, as well as the presence of numerous unerupted permanent and supernumerary teeth. The patient is short, stocky and broad-shouldered. The nose is broad, and the maxilla underdeveloped.

(Center) Another case of a 21-year-old male in which only a few of the permanent teeth have erupted. This should not be confused with craniofacial dysostosis, which is characterized by more serious defects.

(Bottom) Radiographs of the patient shown in the previous picture, illustrating dilaceration and failure of exfoliation and eruption. Extraction of deciduous teeth usually does not aid the eruption of the permanent ones. When a prosthesis is contemplated, it is acceptable practice to leave the numerous deeply unerupted teeth in place if it appears that their removal would result in an excessive bone loss. In all cases of multiple unerupted teeth the clavicles should be examined radiographically.

3
Diseases of the Teeth and Supporting Structures

INTRODUCTION

Diseases of the teeth and supporting structures may be classified according to etiology, but for purposes of discussion it is much easier and more convenient to divide them according to the tissues involved, as follows: (1) diseases of the calcified portions of the teeth, (2) diseases of the pulp and their sequelae, and (3) diseases of the periodontium.

The calcified portions of the teeth may be worn away by the abrasive action of numerous foreign substances or by abnormal masticatory forces. Noncarious loss of tooth substance may also be due to erosion. Teeth may be stained extrinsically by such substances as chromogenic bacteria, food, drugs and tobacco, or intrinsically during development by circulating pigments. A "pink tooth" may result from internal resorption of the dentin. Resorption of the apical portion of a permanent tooth root may be caused by improper tooth movement, endocrine imbalance, Paget's disease, neoplasia, inflammation or may be idiopathic.

Dental caries remains the most common and important disease process affecting the hard structures of the teeth. The disease is related to the composition, form and position of the teeth; to certain characteristics of the saliva and to the diet, in particular the carbohydrates and possibly the phosphates. It is generally agreed that the lesions of caries begin with decalcification and that acidogenic bacteria in the dentobacterial plaque are essential to the process. Proteolytic bacteria may play some role. Although dental caries is initiated by bacterial action, it is not an infection in the usual sense, for the tissue is not invaded by bacteria or their toxins, and the tissues that are injured (enamel and dentin) are incapable of inflammatory response.

The pulp has great recuperative powers and will recover from injuries provided that the causative agent is not too pronounced or long-acting. This tissue protects itself by the formation of secondary dentin in response to abrasion, erosion, attrition, cavity preparation and dental caries. Under certain conditions it will heal even when exposed. The pulp and periodontal membrane have the ability to repair a root fracture.

When the pulp is severely injured by thermal changes, trauma, microorganisms or chemical agents, the resulting pulpitis may not be resolved. If such is the case, inflammation of the periapical tissues will eventually occur if proper endodontic therapy is not instituted. Injury of the tissue in the periapical region by irritants emanating from the pulp canal may result in formation of a so-called dental granuloma (chronic periapical productive periodontitis). A granuloma may in time form a periodontal (radicular, periapical) cyst. A localized collection of pus (abscess) at the periapex may also be a sequela of pulpitis. Pus from a periapical abscess may burrow through the bone to the gingiva, forming a parulis (gingival abscess, "gum boil"). This gingival lesion may rupture, and a draining sinus may develop. Periapical infections may sometimes spread and involve the various fascial spaces of the head and neck.

Diseases of the periodontium are in general inflammatory. Gingivitis is usually initiated by local irritation but may be modified by systemic factors. Most types of gingivitis are infections. Occasionally blastomatoid enlargements occur from long-standing irritation of the gingiva. Periodontitis is always preceded by gingivitis and occasionally also by degenerative changes in the periodontal membrane (periodontosis). Trauma from occlusion and systemic factors may contribute to periodontal disease, but per se they do not initiate periodontitis.

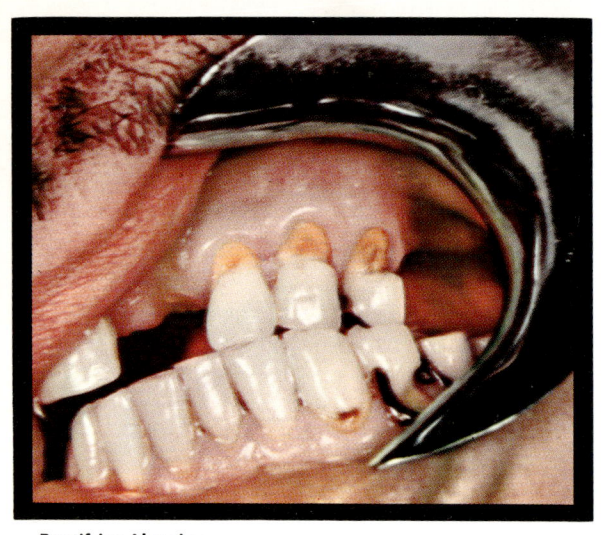

Dentifrice Abrasion

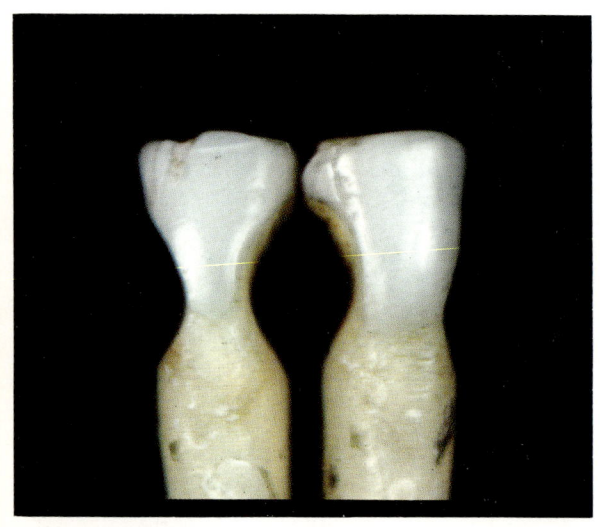

Toothpick Abrasion

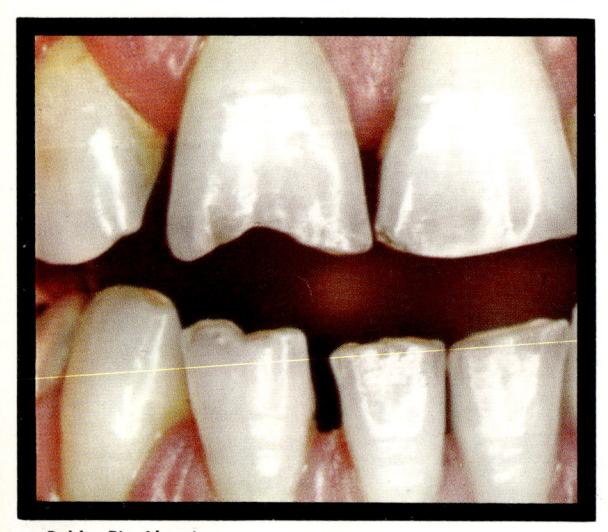

Bobby-Pin Abrasion

ABRASION

The term abrasion is commonly used to designate defects in tooth tissues resulting from the abrasive action of substances other than food. Abnormal tooth wear may result from improper oral hygiene procedures, from holding objects with the teeth, and from chewing on various foreign substances.

(Top) Sharp wedge-shaped defects on the maxillary left lateral, cuspid and 1st bicuspid teeth, caused by the abrasive action of a dentifrice. Less severe dentifrice abrasion of this type may be observed frequently on the root surfaces in adults in whom gingival recession has exposed the cementum. While overzealous and improper brushing contributes to this form of abrasion, toothbrush bristles alone will not cause the defects. If enamel is involved, it is only by undermining, for modern dentifrices are not abrasive enough to wear away enamel. The cuspids are involved more frequently than any other teeth, owing to their prominence. The defects may be more marked on the left side of the mouth in right-handed people, and vice versa.

(Center) The misuse of toothpicks, dental floss and dental tape may cause abnormal tooth wear. The substantial loss of tooth substance seen in the illustration was caused by the pernicious habit of rotating a toothpick between the lower central incisor teeth. Strenuously polishing the teeth with dental floss or tape apical to the cemento-enamel junction may result in the notching of the root surfaces. This notching is more likely to occur when the floss or tape is used in conjunction with a dentifrice.

(Bottom) The notches in the incisal edges of the maxillary right central and mandibular right lateral were produced by repeatedly using these teeth to open bobby pins. Similar defects, though of lesser magnitude, may be produced by thread biting. Continually holding tacks, nails, pins, or other hard substances in the teeth may also result in abnormal incisal wear. Large notches involving several teeth are sometimes observed in individuals who habitually hold a pipe in one location, especially if the stem is made of clay.

Diseases of the Teeth and Supporting Structures

Abrasion (Cont.)

(Top) Excessive wearing of the crowns of teeth is observed most frequently in habitual tobacco chewers. The greatest amount of damage is usually seen in the lingual cusps of the maxillary teeth and the buccal cusps of the mandibular teeth. The pattern of wear, however, may vary with the habits of the patient. In some instances the abrasion may be limited to one side, and in others the entire dental arch may be involved. The loss of tooth substance in tobacco chewers is also accompanied by staining of the exposed dentin. At times the teeth may be worn to the gingival margin without exposure of dental pulps. This is possible because the pulp responds with progressive formation of secondary (reparative) dentin.

(Center) Marked abrasion of the anterior teeth resulting from the chewing of betel nuts. Ordinarily these teeth are stained a dark mahogany red, but in the case illustrated prophylaxis was given so that the pattern of wear could be better demonstrated. The so-called betel nut is the fruit of the areca palm. It is commonly chewed for medicinal purposes by natives of southern India, Ceylon, Malaya, Thailand, Formosa, Guam, the Philippines and several of the small South Pacific islands. The amount of abnormal tooth wear associated with the use of the nut depends partly on the manner in which it is prepared for chewing. It may be chewed with or without the husk, but is often cut into pieces and each piece wrapped in a leaf of the betel vine with a small amount of ground sea shells or powdered coral.

(Bottom) Severe abrasion in a sand blaster. Fine particles of sand suspended in dust entered this patient's mouth during inspiration and resulted in the excessive wearing away of the occlusal and incisal tooth surfaces when the individual brought his teeth together into occlusion. The presence of the abrasive material in the mouth probably caused the patient to grit his teeth subconsciously, thus increasing the wear. The sharp edges of enamel resulting from occlusal and incisal abrasion from any cause may irritate the lingual, buccal and labial mucosa and should be eliminated either by careful rounding or by restorative procedures.

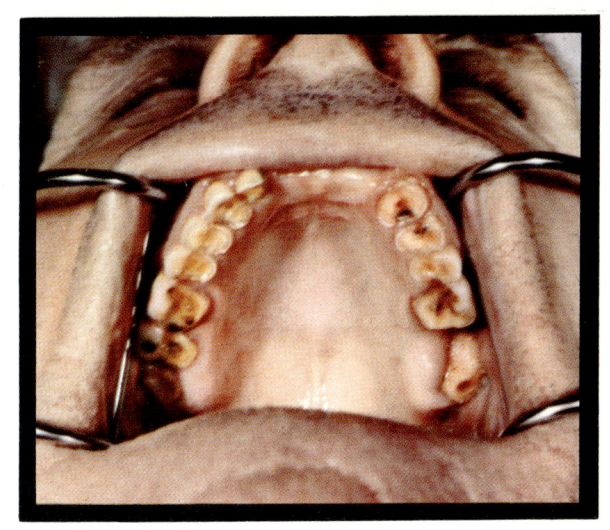

Tobacco Abrasion

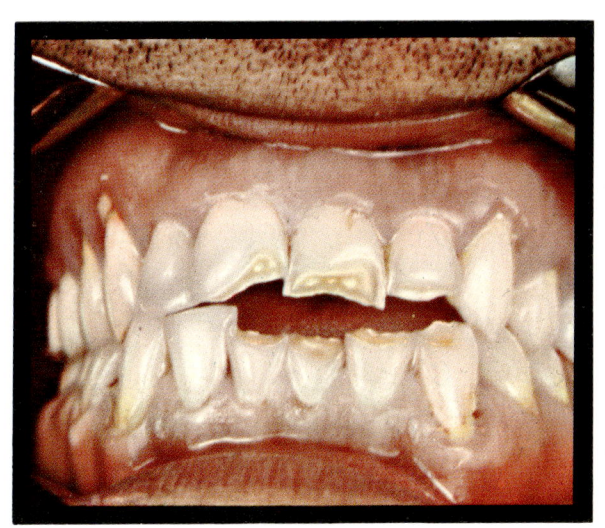

Betel-Nut Abrasion

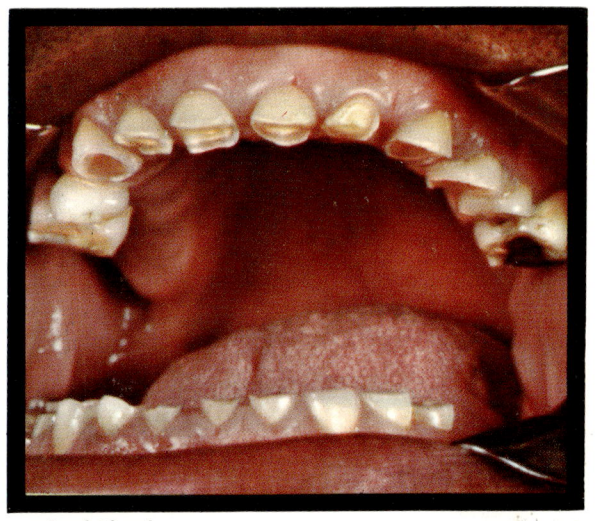

Sand Abrasion

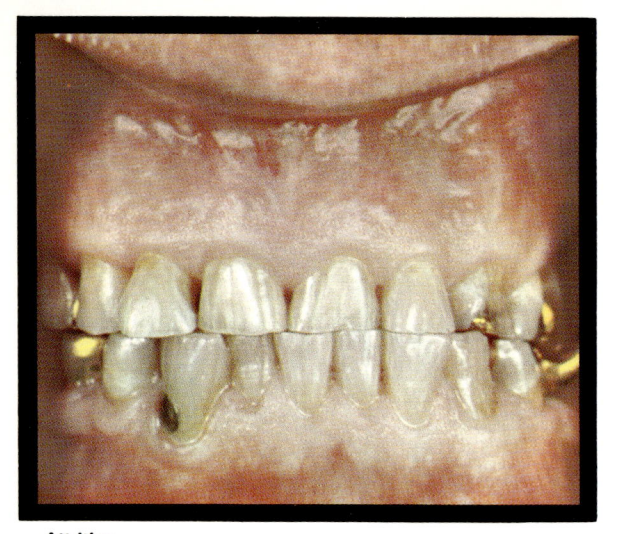

Attrition

Acid Erosion

Idiopathic Erosion

58 *Diseases of the Teeth and Supporting Structures*

ATTRITION

(Top) Attrition and abrasion are not synonymous. Attrition is the physiologic wearing away of the teeth during mastication, while abrasion refers to any other type of mechanical wear. Attrition always involves functional surfaces and may be excessive due to bruxism (night grinding), gritty food, premature contacts (centric or excentric) or abnormal tooth structures (pp. 50, 51 and 53). Excessive wear at contact points may occur in conjunction with excessive and incisal attrition resulting in accentuation of the physiologic mesial drift of the teeth. The pulp is protected from exposure in severe cases by the formation of secondary (reparative) dentin.

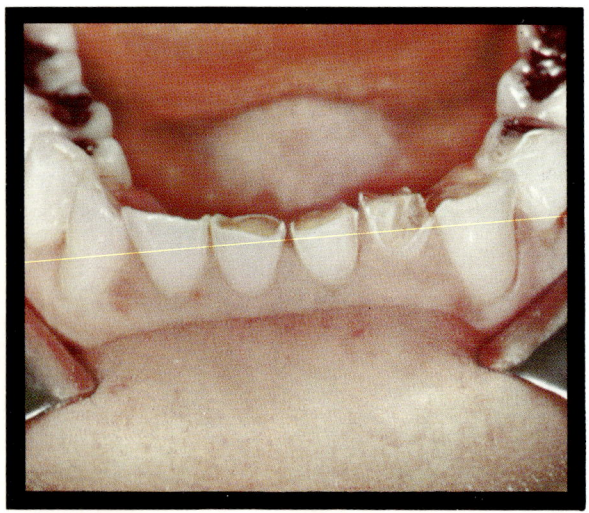

EROSION

(Center) The use of acid in the treatment of gastric disease and the repeated regurgitation of gastric contents may result in acid erosion of the teeth. Although the saliva tends to buffer the acid, the concentration may be too high in certain areas for neutralization to occur. The acid may cause the decalcification of enamel in the regions it first touches, as seen here in a patient who took dilute hydrochloric acid from a glass tumbler. The deleterious effect of this type of therapy may be alleviated by immediate use of baking soda as a mouthwash. Once the dentin has been exposed by acid action, it may wear down rapidly, and the enamel may chip even after the acid is eliminated. People who habitually use lemons may exhibit acid erosion — usually on the labial surfaces of the anterior teeth if they suck on the fruit, and on the lingual surfaces if they chew it.

(Bottom) Noncarious dissolution of labial and buccal enamel of unknown cause is commonly classified as idiopathic erosion. The lesions observed in this type of erosion are frequently saucer-shaped but may also be flattened, wedge-shaped or very irregular. They are differentiated from dentifrice abrasion because they originate in the enamel rather than on the root surface. After the dentin is exposed, however, these lesions may be deepened as a result of dentifrice abrasion.

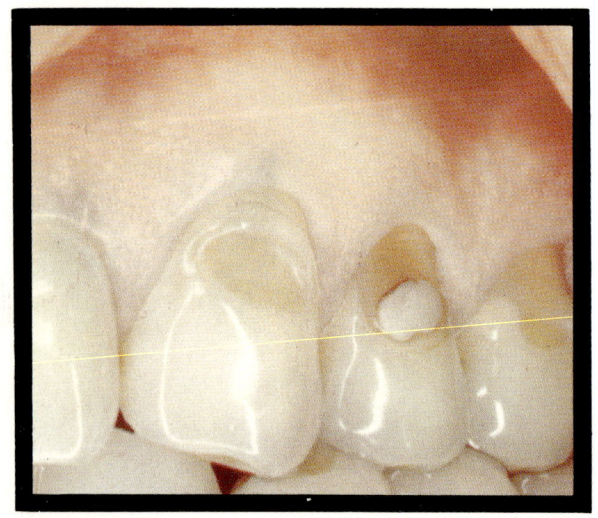

STAINS

Those stains which come from within the tooth are called intrinsic stains. The most common example is discoloration of the crown by blood pigments that enter the dentinal tubules after pulpal injury. During tooth development generalized intrinsic staining may result from pigments associated with systemic disease or from medications. More frequently, stains are caused by the accumulation of material on the tooth surface. These are extrinsic stains, and the color depends on the substance responsible; e.g., tobacco, drugs, foods, microorganisms, and blood from the gingival crevice. Extrinsic stains may be associated with soft deposits or with calculus.

(Top) This 4-year-old child shows dark-greenish-blue intrinsic pigmentation of the deciduous teeth. The child became jaundiced shortly after birth as the result of erythroblastosis fetalis. The greenish-yellow skin color was intense during the first 10 weeks of life; by the 27th week the icterus had completely disappeared. Circulating pigments caused staining of the dental tissues that were developing during the first 3 months of life. The pigmentation is primarily in the dentin. Intrinsic staining also may occur in congenital porphyria (red-brown) or with tetracyclines (yellow-brown).

(Center) Tetracyclines administered during tooth development are incorporated into dentin and enamel. The teeth fluoresce in ultraviolet light. The ground section shown is a deciduous incisor from a 5-1/2-year-old girl who received oxytetracycline intermittently for 4 to 7 days at a time between the 5th and 15th month of life. In ultraviolet light the tetracycline-affected bands have a brilliant yellow color.

(Bottom) Brown pellicle is found on the teeth of some individuals who do not use an abrasive-containing dentifrice. The pellicle may vary in thickness and coloration. This brown-stained, structureless film may be readily removed and its recurrence prevented by appropriate oral hygiene procedures. In this case the pellicle varies from very heavy on the upper centrals to mild on lower right cuspid. Children with poor oral hygiene may show green stain with a similar distribution.

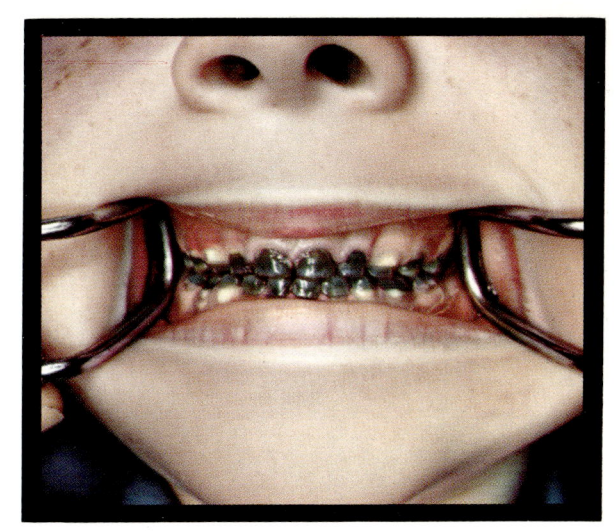

Intrinsic Stain, Bilirubin

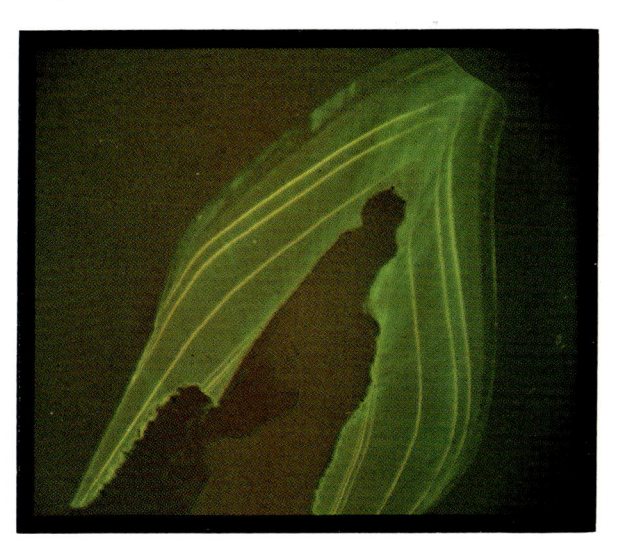

Tetracycline Fluorescence, Ground Section

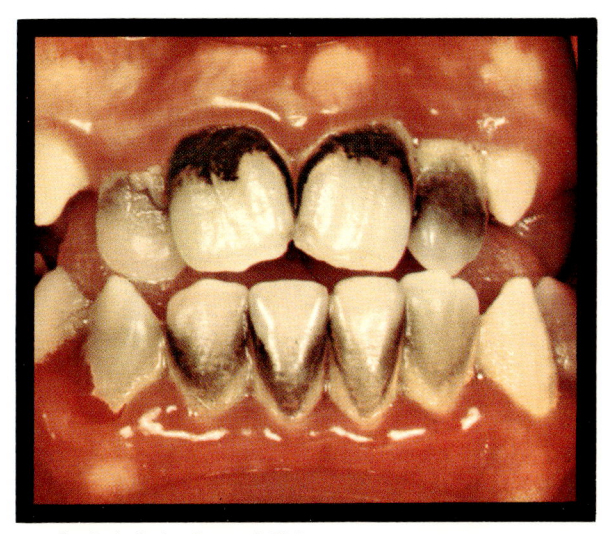

Extrinsic Stain, Brown Pellicle

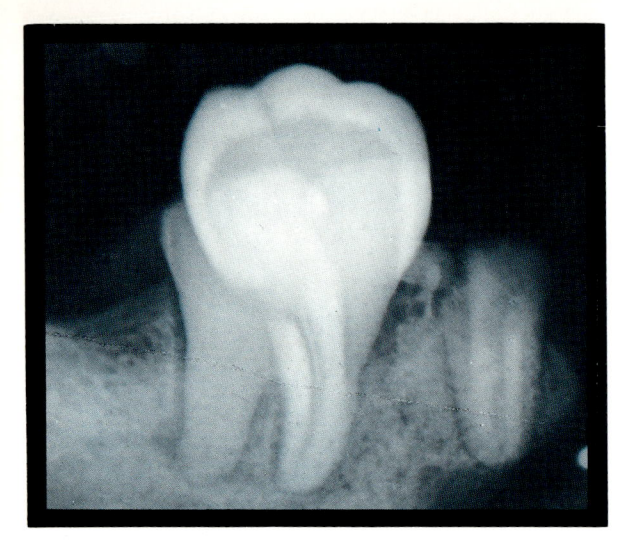

Fractured Molar Tooth

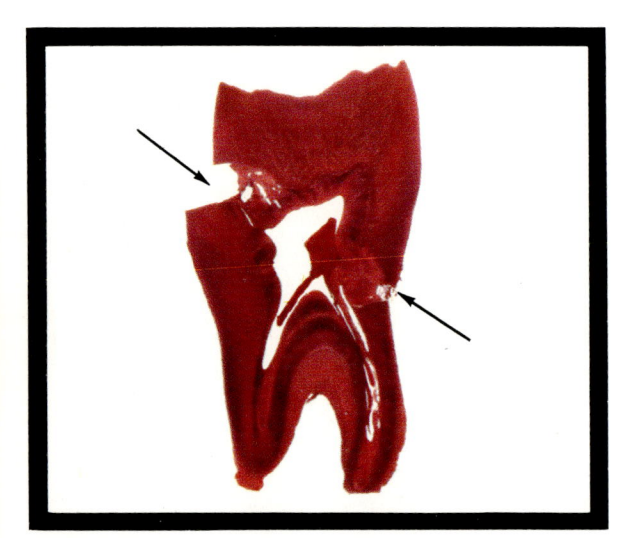

Healed Fracture   X 3

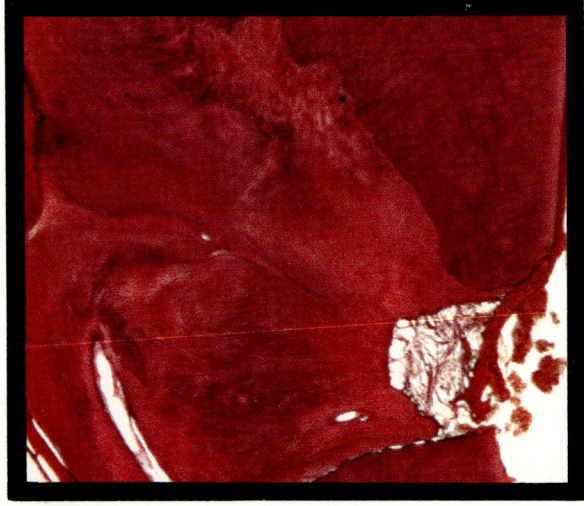

Fracture Area   X 40

60 *Diseases of the Teeth and Supporting Structures*

ROOT FRACTURES

Root fractures are not common, but because of their possibility, periapical radiographs should always be taken following traumatic incidents. When the fracture line is apical to the epithelial attachment, healing frequently occurs, especially if the crown segment is immobilized. A fractured root heals in somewhat the same manner as an osseous fracture. There is an ingrowth of vascular fibrous connective tissue from the pulp and periodontal membrane, and subsequently the dentin surfaces resorb. Later a bony type of material is deposited. This material varies with the case and may be tubular or atubular dentin, bone or cementum. In some instances the calcific continuity of the root is reestablished. In other cases a small amount of fibrous connective tissue may remain separating the tooth segments, and thus a fibrous union or pseudoarthrosis is the final result. Reducing the possibility of secondary infection by keeping the neck of the involved tooth clean, applying mild antiseptics to the gingival crevice, and using antibiotics systemically may aid materially in the successful healing of a fractured root.

(Top) This molar tooth was fractured by a rocket-shell fragment. Even though the 2 portions of the tooth are not properly aligned, healing occurred. The tooth was removed 14 months after injury in order to accommodate a prosthesis. At the time of removal this tooth reacted normally to pulp tests.

(Center) Low-power photomicrograph of the same tooth. The line of fracture is indicated by the arrows. The calcified material uniting the fractures is evident. Most of the pulp tissue was lost in the processing of the specimen.

(Bottom) A higher magnification of the healed area on the right side of the same tooth shows the bonelike structure of the repairing tissue contrasted with the blue-staining tubular dentin above and below. Small scalloped regions in the dentin indicate that some resorption preceded the process of osteoid formation. The small clear area at the right has not repaired completely. It is probable that some of the calcified material associated with the healing was formed by the pulp, and other portions by the periodontal membrane.

INTERNAL RESORPTION

In this disease (also termed "idiopathic resorption") the pulp tissue undergoes a metamorphosis, resulting in resorption of the dentin from the pulpal walls. The pulp cavity in such cases, rather than being occupied by loose, delicate connective tissue which is bordered by odontoblasts, is devoid of the latter cells and filled with very vascular granulation tissue. A history of trauma may sometimes be elicited, but in most instances no cause for this phenomenon can be determined. Radioactive material inhaled, ingested or injected may initiate internal resorption of dentin, and that possibility always should be considered. If the process of resorption reaches the enamel, a pink spot may be seen in the crown because the highly vascular granulation tissue shows through the translucent enamel. Internal resorption ceases at times, and bonelike tissue is deposited both in the resorbed areas and haphazardly throughout the pulp. Dentin resorption usually begins from the inside, although in some instances it is possibly initiated in the periodontal membrane. Technically, the latter type is classified as external resorption. In cases in which there is perforation of the root it is not always clear whether internal or external resorption has occurred.

(Top) Internal resorption as seen radiographically in a maxillary 2nd molar tooth. While most of the crown and a portion of the distal root are radiolucent, it is apparent that some osteoid formation has already occurred.

(Center) In this cross section of the tooth shown above, loss of purple-staining dentin from the pulpal wall is evident. It is also apparent that osteoid (red-stained) has replaced some of the lost dentin, and that trabeculae have developed in the pulp. The presence of the trabeculae probably accounts for the somewhat mottled appearance in the radiograph.

(Bottom) A higher magnification of one of the trabeculae extending from the pulpal wall shows tubular dentin surrounded by osteoid or osteodentin. A line of osteoblasts is seen in the baylike area along the upper left portion of the spicule. Inflammatory cells are apparent in the fibrous pulp tissue.

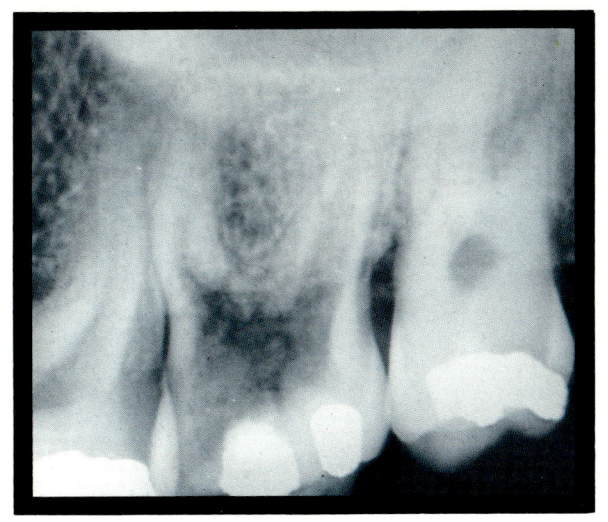

Internal Resorption, Second Molar

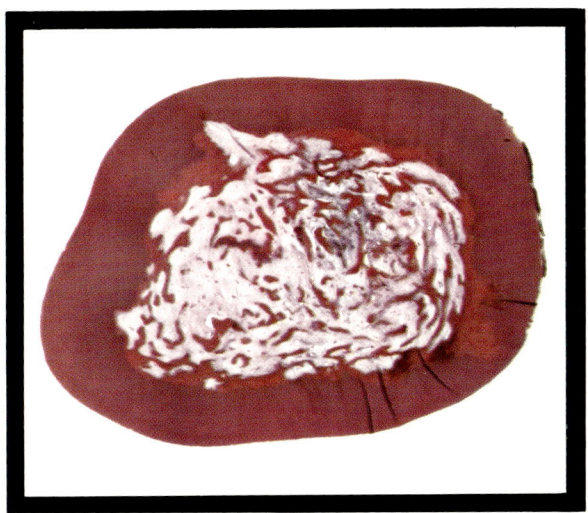

Internal Resorption, Cross Section   X 6

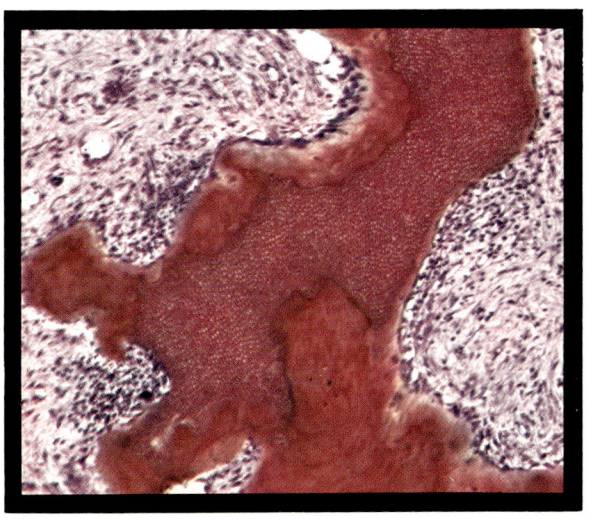

Internal Resorption, Same Specimen as Above   X 100

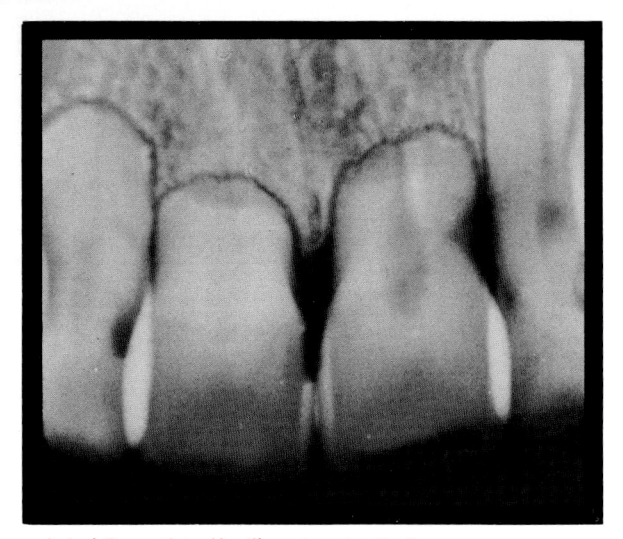

Apical Resorption, Maxillary Anterior Teeth

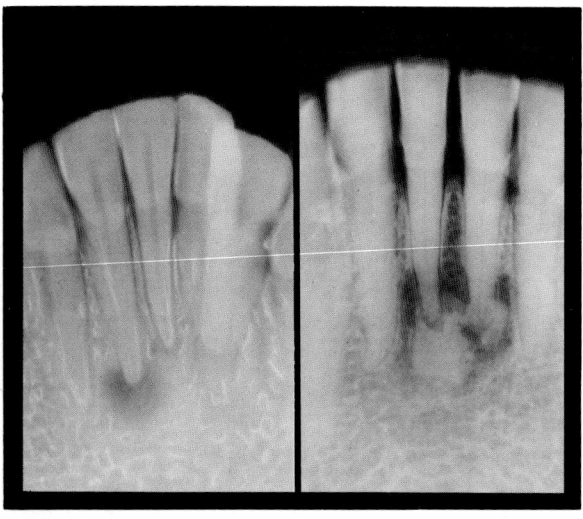

Cementomas, Early and Advanced Stages

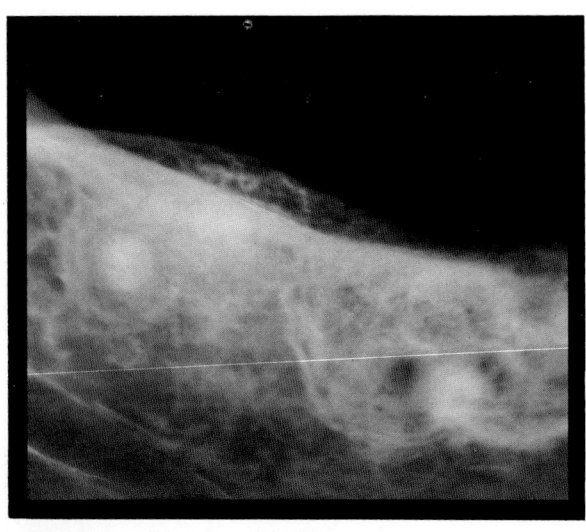

Cementomas, Edentulous Mandible

APICAL RESORPTION

(Top) Apical resorption may occur following orthodontic treatment, as a result of endocrine imbalance (particularly hypothyroidism), in association with Paget's disease, or no precise cause may be evident. In the normal individual receiving proper orthodontic therapy, no gross resorption should be expected. The patient's history is of great importance in determining the cause of any given resorption. Inflammation, especially suppurative, in the periapical region may cause root resorption, but the resorbed areas are not replaced by bone. Malignant neoplasm, either local or metastatic, may cause root resorption (pp. 153 and 168). Apical resorption should be differentiated from underdeveloped roots (pp. 39, 52, 63). Histological examination of teeth frequently reveals small areas of resorption not demonstrated radiographically.

CEMENTOMA

(Cementosis)

(Center) The so-called cementoma, which is nonneoplastic, usually develops over a period of years. Initially there is a resorption of bone about the apex of a tooth having a normal pulp *(left)*. Gradually the area of resorption is replaced by cementum or bone *(right)*. The cause of this localized disturbance in bone metabolism is not known, although incisal and occlusal trauma have been implicated as possible exciting factors. The first stage of a cementoma (also designated as a periapical fibroma) cannot be differentiated radiographically from bone resorption resulting from periapical inflammation. If the periapical radiolucency is the first stage of a cementoma, the associated tooth should be normal in color and in its response to vitality and percussion tests. Cementomas are frequently multiple and most often occur in the mandible, especially in association with the anterior teeth. In general, surgical intervention for either stage of this lesion is not indicated.

(Bottom) Radiopaque areas in an edentulous mandible which proved upon histologic examination to be composed of cementum. Since preextraction radiographs were not available in this case, it is not known whether these lesions existed prior to extraction or developed afterward. Similar-appearing radiopacities may be composed of sclerotic bone which has developed idiopathically or in association with Paget's disease.

RADIATION EFFECT, TEETH

Experimental studies and clinical evidence indicate that radiant energy may interfere with normal development of the teeth. Clinically, this energy usually is derived from a source being used in treatment of neoplastic disease. The effect of radiation on developing teeth depends on the dosage, given, the stage of tooth development, the proximity of the dental structures to the irradiated area, and the degree to which these structures are shielded. Contingent on the foregoing, there may be no interference with tooth development, or there may be failure of root formation, dwarfing of the crown or root, or complete absence of development. Fully developed teeth may undergo circumferential cervical destruction as an indirect result of extensive irradiation of the head-and-neck region.

(*Top*) This 12-year-old patient received x-ray irradiation for treatment of a hemangioma of the cheek at the time of development of the teeth. The skin of the face shows a characteristic "orange-peel" appearance over the field of direct irradiation. There is a failure of development of the left side of the face and jaws which is more apparent when the mouth is closed.

(*Center*) Radiograph of the left side of the maxilla in the same patient. The roots of the bicuspids and 1st molar have failed to form. The crown of the 2nd bicuspid is abnormally small.

(*Bottom*) Fully-developed erupted teeth seldom are affected by direct irradiation but sometimes become hypersensitive, and their pulps may degenerate. Heavy therapeutic doses of radiant energy directed in the region of the salivary glands may lead to their atrophy if they are not adequately shielded. The resultant xerostomia and qualitative changes in the saliva probably are the cause of rampant cervical destruction of the teeth in such patients. These rampant lesions of dental caries may lead to "amputation" of the crown. Extraction of teeth from jaws that have been heavily irradiated is contraindicated, so that extraction of teeth before irradiation generally is advised to prevent caries and the need for later removal (see p. 101).

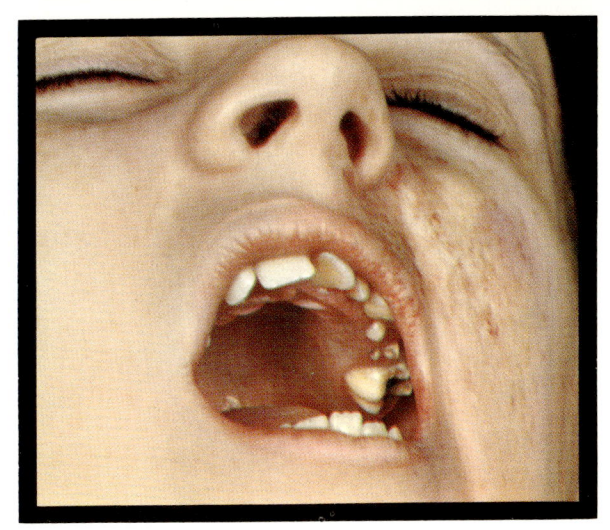

Radiation Effect—Skin, Bone and Teeth

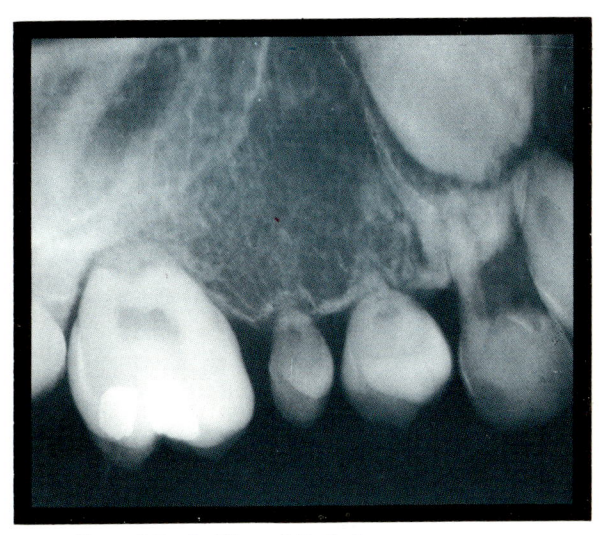

Malformed Teeth, Effect of Radiation

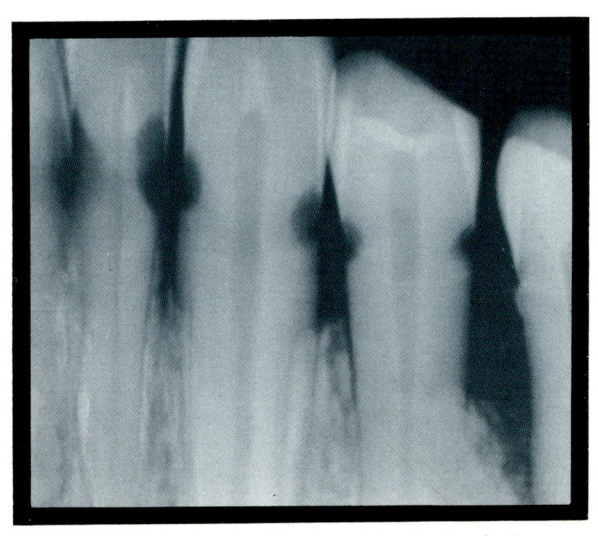

Cervical Destruction Resulting from Extensive Irradiation

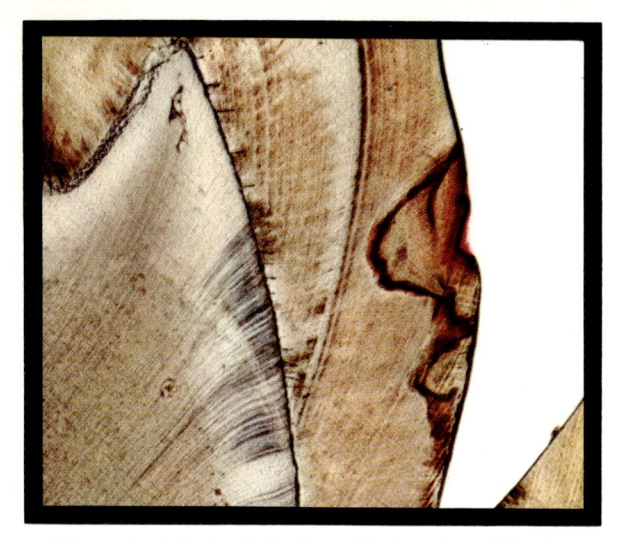

Interproximal Caries, Early Enamel Lesion, Ground Section

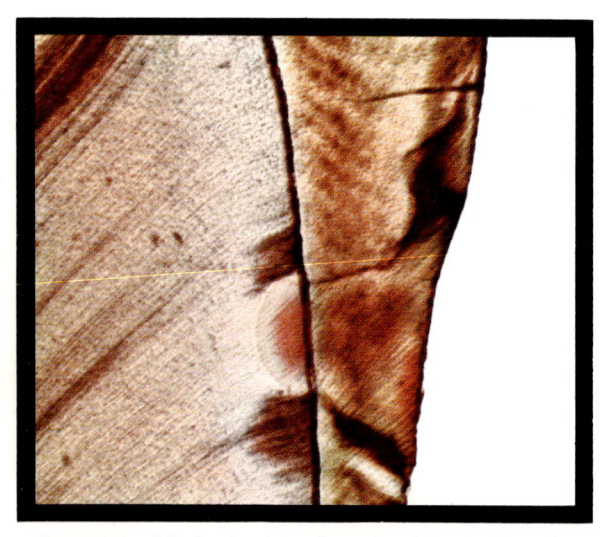

Interproximal Caries Involving Enamel and Dentin, Ground Section

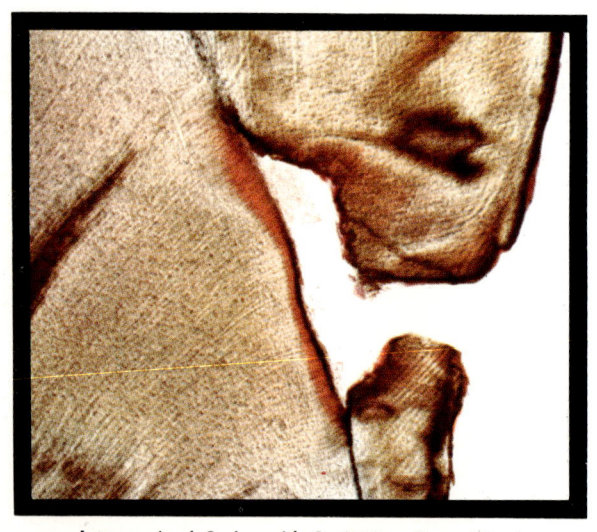

Interproximal Caries with Cavitation, Ground Section

DENTAL CARIES

Dental caries is initiated by decalcification beginning at the tooth surfaces. It is generally accepted that the decalcifying acids are produced in the dentobacterial plaques by the action of bacteria on carbohydrates. The dentobacterial plaques are found on protected areas of the teeth that are not kept clean by the action of the tongue, lips, cheeks, the food bolus, or oral hygiene. Carious lesions therefore most frequently occur in the occlusal fissures, interproximally or cervically. A few individuals are immune to caries regardless of their carbohydrate intake. These fortunate immunes seem to have some peculiar quality to their saliva that inhibits bacterial growth or metabolism. Optimal amounts of fluorides ingested in the water during tooth development will lower the incidence of dental caries.

(Top) The initial lesion of dental caries, clinically, is a white spot which may become stained. Histologically, the appearance of such a lesion, on the interproximal surfaces, is a cone-shaped region of decalcification with its broad base at the surface. In the section shown there are 2 such cone-shaped lesions extending toward the dentino-enamel junction. At one point along the surface some enamel has disintegrated. A sharp explorer might be expected to reveal this defect.

(Center) In this section the carious process has extended into the dentin, but there still is no cavitation. There is broad involvement of the enamel surface, and the apex of the cone of decalcification has reached the dentino-enamel junction. Here the process spreads laterally, and a cone of decalcification in the dentin is stained red. A surrounding halo of white suggests that the dentinal calcification has increased (sclerosis) as a defense against the advance of caries. Clinically, this lesion would be radiolucent.

(Bottom) This section shows frank cavitation, presumably due to disintegration of the decalcified enamel. The overhanging enamel could easily be fractured during mastication or by an operative hand instrument. The carious process is advancing within the dentin as indicated by the red-stained area and the reactive region beneath.

Diseases of the Teeth and Supporting Structures 65

Dental Caries (Cont.)

Dental caries, beginning in pits and fissures, presents a somewhat different pattern in its advance through the enamel from that of smooth-surface caries although the chemical and physical processes involved probably are identical. As the process of caries follows the direction of the enamel rods, it diverges from the enamel surface of the fissure or pit, spreading as it advances toward the dentin. This results in a cone-shaped lesion with its base toward or at the dentino-enamel junction. Even though there may be extensive destruction of the underlying enamel and dentin (*center*), the site of initiation of caries usually remains small, and the patient may be unaware of the lesion until pain is felt due to pulp involvement or until the roof of the enamel over the cavity collapses under masticatory forces. A small opening leading to a large carious lesion may be overlooked during a screening or cursory clinical examination. The elimination of very deep sulci by operative procedures prior to clinical evidence of caries is an acceptable procedure.

(Top) Caries is seen beginning in a fissure with decalcification extending from its sides and bottom. If this process had continued, a greater area would be involved at the dentino-enamel junction than at the surface as indicated by the width of the pale yellow lesion in the dentin.

(Center) When occlusal caries reaches the dentin, it usually spreads laterally as seen here. There may be separation of the enamel from the dentin and later fracture of the enamel "roof." The red-staining regions of enamel and dentin are zones of decalcification. The process of decalcification of enamel from the underlying dentin (red region above separation) is known as undermining, secondary or backward caries of the enamel. A zone of increased calcification (sclerosis) surrounds the red zone of decalcification in the dentin, but not in the enamel, which has no such defense mechanism.

(Bottom) In this section the caries is far-advanced, and the red-staining zone appears to have reached the pulpal wall. The process of cavitation has left overhanging enamel which could be fractured easily.

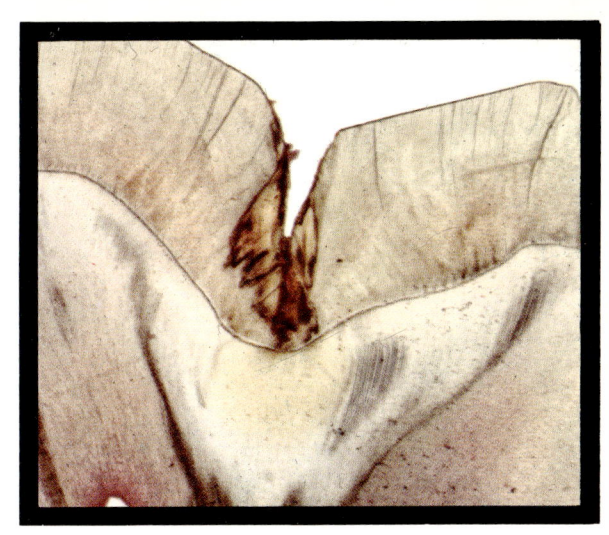

Fissural Caries, Ground Section

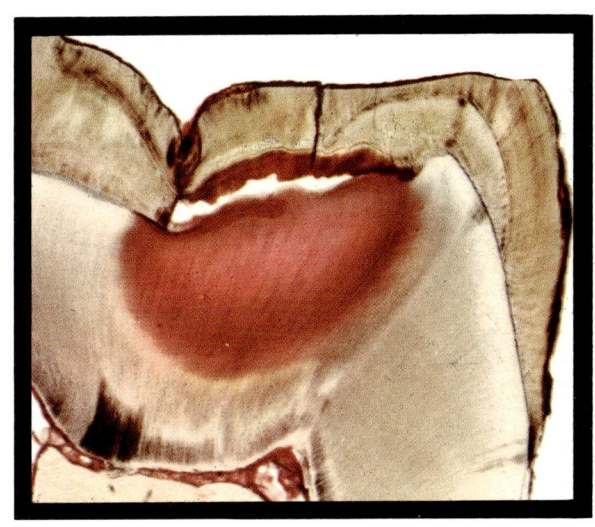

Fissural Caries with Marked Dentinal Involvement, Ground Section

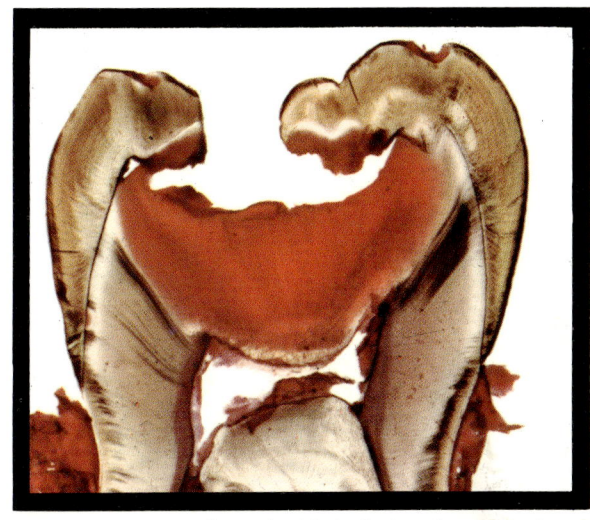

Fissural Caries, Advanced with Cavitation, Ground Section

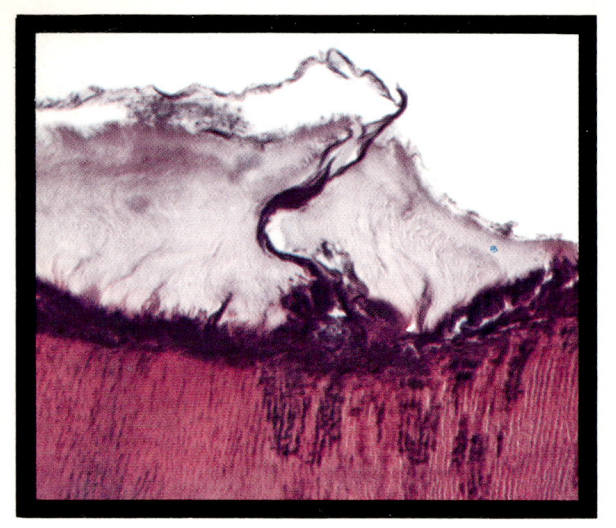

Enamel Lamella, Decalcified Section   X 200

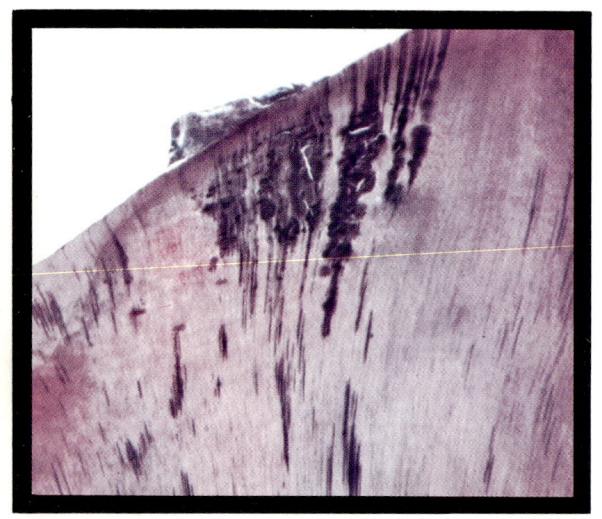

Dentinal Caries, Decalcified Section   X 35

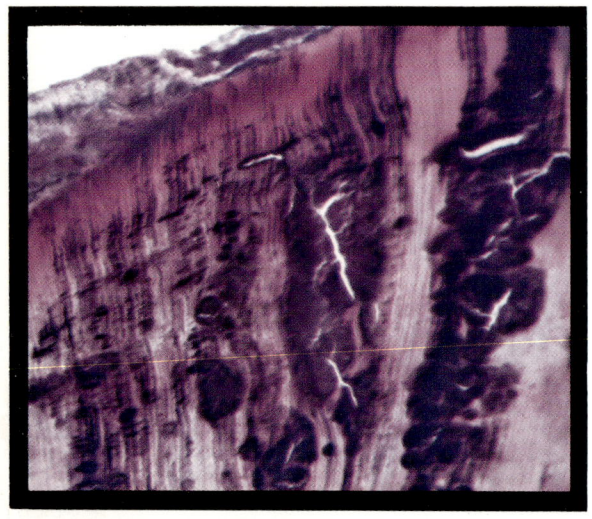

Dentinal Caries, Decalcified Section   X 150

Dental Caries (Cont.)

When sections are decalcified in the laboratory, all the enamel except the organic portion (matrix and lamellae) is lost, and even this portion is lost unless special technics are used. The dentin, having a greater organic content (about 30 per cent vs. 2 per cent), is well preserved after histologic preparation.

(Top) The light-lavender-staining material above is enamel matrix in a decalcified section. A lamella is seen as a darker-staining, curved structure extending through the matrix. The dark-staining granules in the red-stained dentin are microorganisms in dentinal tubules. One theory of caries suggests that the initial lesion of caries is caused by proteolysis of the lamellae, but the evidence favoring the decalcification theory is far more substantial.

(Center) Caries is seen in the dentin. A small dentobacterial plaque is present on the surface. The carious process follows the dentinal tubules. The inorganic portion of the dentin probably is first decalcified by bacterially produced acids. Because of its higher inorganic content the dentin is not extensively dissolved, and its morphology is not altered by the decalcification. When proteolytic activity is combined with or follows decalcification, the dentin is completely disintegrated. The dark streaks in the photomicrograph are enlarged tubules containing microorganisms. At various places along the bacteria-packed tubules beadlike enlargements are seen. These distentions (liquefaction foci) are assumed to occur from the pressure of bacterial growth after the dentinal matrix is softened by decalcification. They enlarge by proteolysis and coalescence.

(Bottom) A higher magnification of the specimen above shows details of the dentobacterial plaque at the surface with the raylike arrangement of some of its organisms. Filaments (actinomycetes), bacilli and cocci commonly make up this plaque that sometimes is erroneously called the mucin plaque. In the dentin the details of the microorganisms in the tubules and the liquefaction foci, with cracks where the entire dentinal substance has been lost, are apparent. The bacteria may extend into tubules in advance of the process of decalcification and may even infect the pulp while the dentin is intact.

Diseases of the Teeth and Supporting Structures 67

Dental Caries (Cont.)

(Top) This dentobacterial plaque is stained to show some of the microorganisms. Dentobacterial plaques are masses of different species of microorganisms. The filaments appear to form the basic structure, clinging tenaciously to the tooth surface. Many of the organisms of acidogenic nature in the plaque rapidly convert carbohydrate into acid. Other bacteria produce proteolytic enzymes that dissolve the organic materials of the tooth. Plaques are difficult to remove by ordinary oral hygienic procedures and reform rapidly after their removal.

(Center) In the left photomicrograph there is a plaque on the surface of the dentin, and bacteria have penetrated along the tubules. Foci of liquefaction are also apparent. The right photomicrograph shows microorganisms in enlarged dentinal tubules. A few are extending out into the lateral branches. The bacteria may progress along the tubules to the pulp or destroy the surrounding dentin by decalcification and proteolysis.

(Bottom) Colonies of lactobacilli are seen as small dots in a petri dish containing a selective culture medium. The larger white dots are colonies of yeast. The small inset shows lactobacilli under high magnification. A selective medium may be used to estimate the number of lactobacilli in a given amount of saliva. While recent studies indicate that the salivary lactobacillus count is not a reliable indicator of future caries activity in individuals, studies of lactobacilli in the saliva by this and other methods have yielded valuable information on the cause and possible methods to control caries. Germ-free-animal studies have firmly established the important role of microorganisms in the process of dental caries.

There are four generally accepted methods for control of dental caries: (1) cleaning teeth immediately after eating, (2) reducing the frequency of intake of carbohydrates, (3) fluoridation of water supplies and topical application of fluorides by approved technics, and (4) early restoration of carious lesions.

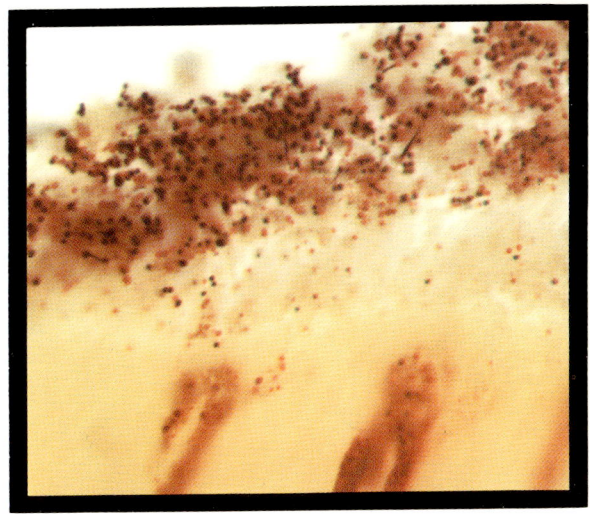

Dentobacterial Plaque, Brown and Brenn Stain, Decalcified Section X 918

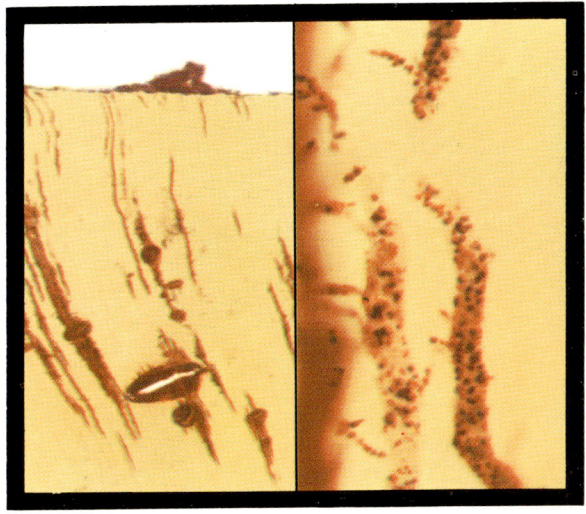

X 85 **Dentinal Caries** X 920
Brown and Brenn Stain, Decalcified Sections

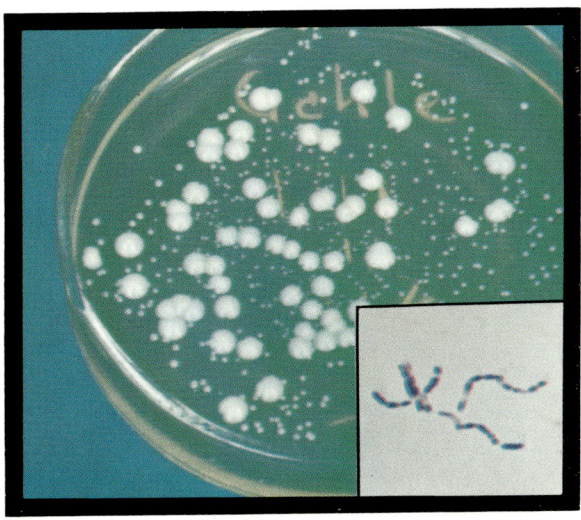

Lactobacillus Colonies **Lactobacilli** X 1080

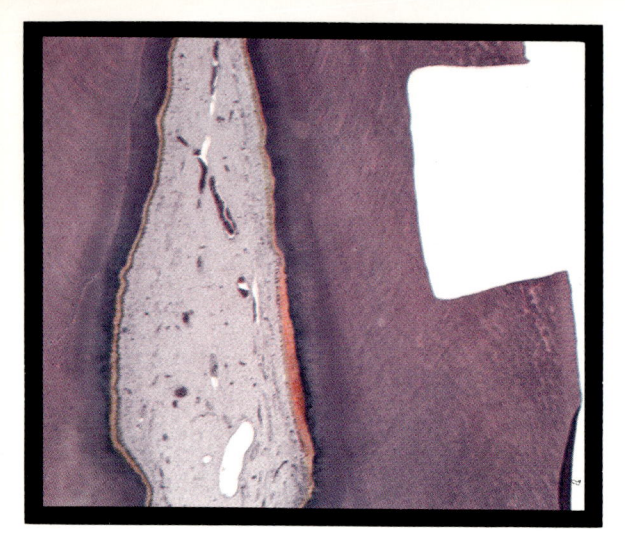

Secondary Dentin Beneath Cavity Preparation X 15

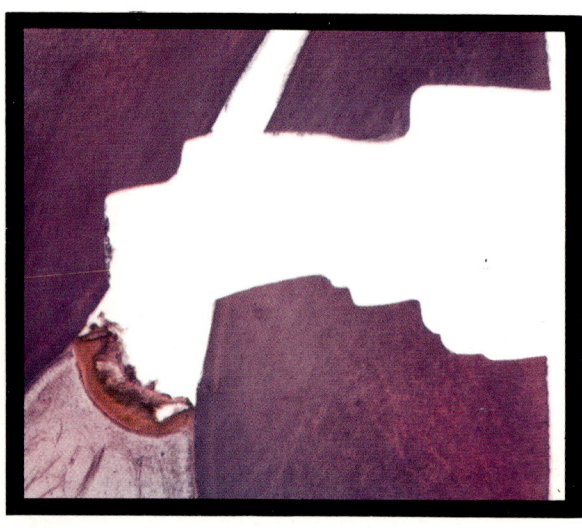

Pulp Healing, Bridge of Dentin in Region of Exposure X 20

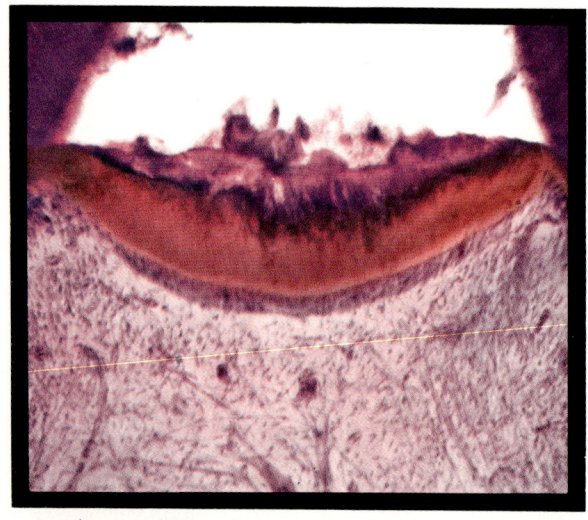

Pulp Healing, Bridge of Dentin, Normal Pulp X 100

SECONDARY DENTIN FORMATION

(Top) Secondary dentin as a protective layer is formed on the pulpal wall when odontoblastic processes are irritated. This reaction may occur as a result of dental caries, cavity preparation, abrasion, attrition or erosion. The cells of the pulp normally continue to produce dentin after tooth formation is considered to be complete, but stimulation of odontoblastic processes accelerates this dentin formation in the region of the involved odontoblasts. This is exemplified in the photomicrograph, which shows a cavity preparation at the right and a slight excess of red-staining secondary dentin along the pulpal wall. If the course of the dentinal tubules is traced from the axial cavity wall to the pulp, it will be seen that this secondary dentin has been formed at the pulpal ends of the cut tubules. Secondary dentin also may be termed reparative dentin.

PULP HEALING

Pulp capping has been practiced for many years, and claims have been made in favor of various drugs and technics for this procedure. For the most part these claims have been based on clinical evidence alone. However, it is common knowledge that necrosis of the pulp may occur, or a mild chronic inflammation exist, without symptoms. In general, the success of a pulp-capping operation should be based on histologic evidence. Therefore only those procedures should be used which have been proved by laboratory studies to be consistently followed by complete pulp healing.

(Center) Successful pulp capping in a human tooth. At lower left is normal pulp tissue which is covered by a bridge of dentin. In this case the pulp was deliberately exposed and the wound covered with a paste of calcium hydroxide and tap water. The tooth, which needed to be removed for orthodontic purposes, was extracted 10 weeks after the pulp-capping procedure.

(Bottom) Photomicrograph of another section from the tooth shown in the center picture. At the base of the newly formed tubular dentin is a row of well-differentiated odontoblasts. The underlying pulp is vital, quite cellular, and free of inflammatory elements.

Diseases of the Teeth and Supporting Structures

PULP CALCIFICATION

Calcifications in the pulp may appear as roughly circular areas (denticles, pulp stones, pulp nodules) or as diffuse, irregular deposits. Denticles may be attached to the wall of the pulp or may be free within the pulp cavity. True denticles are composed of tubular dentin, but most pulp stones are lamellar structures with few, if any, tubules. Diffuse areas of calcification are usually limited to the radicular portion of the pulp.

(Top) Radiopaque areas (pulp stones) are apparent in the coronal pulps of the maxillary 1st and 2nd molars. These denticles are distinct, but frequently they are only faintly discernible, and many pulp stones are found in histologic sections which could not be demonstrated radiographically. Some individuals show pulp stones in nearly every tooth. Referred pain is sometimes attributed to pressure of pulp stones on nerves, but removal of teeth with pulp stones and no other symptoms seldom eliminates neuralgic pain. Caution is important, and hasty decisions to extract such teeth as possible causes of pain should be avoided.

(Center) One large denticle and several small ones lying free in the coronal pulp of a molar tooth which was symptomless but was removed to accommodate a prosthetic appliance. None of these pulp stones is composed of tubular dentin. It is apparent that the largest one has been formed in concentric layers. No inflammatory cells are present, and, except for the calcific deposits, the pulp is normal. Pulpal calcifications are a common histologic finding and are probably present in about 80 per cent of adult teeth. Many of these denticles are quite small, however, and are not apparent radiographically.

(Bottom) The irregular, purplish-staining areas in the central portion of this photomicrograph are regions of diffuse calcification. Pulpal degeneration is evident by the lack of odontoblasts and the general character of the tissue. There is a tendency for calcium salts to be deposited in the pulp, as elsewhere in the body, in tissue which is necrotic or degenerating. Diffuse, linear, dystrophic calcification in the pulp is generally limited to the radicular portion and is observed most frequently in older individuals.

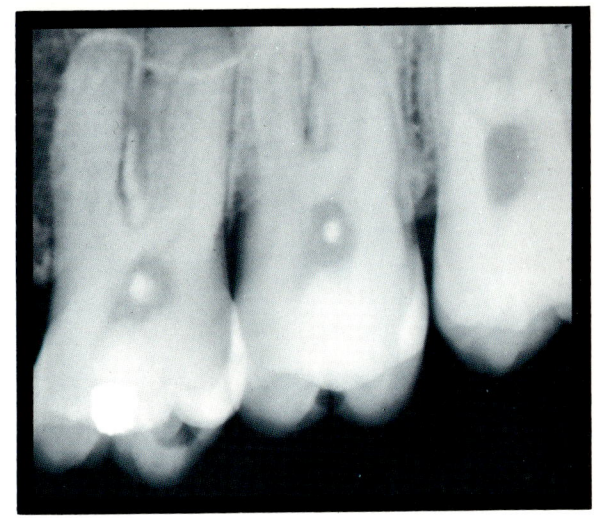

Denticles in Coronal Pulp of First and Second Molars

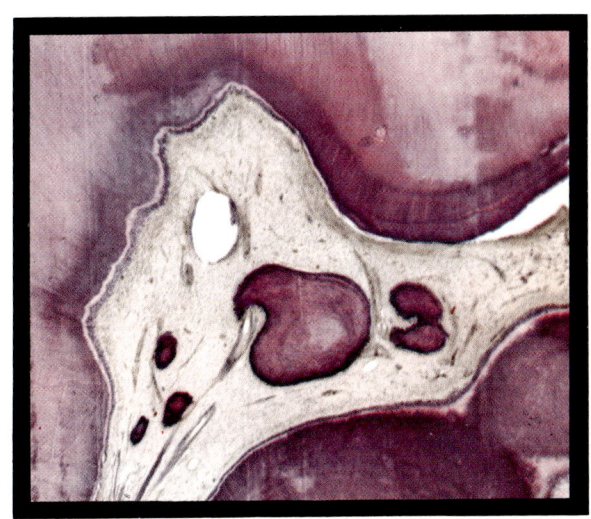

Denticles in Coronal Pulp of Molar Tooth   X 18

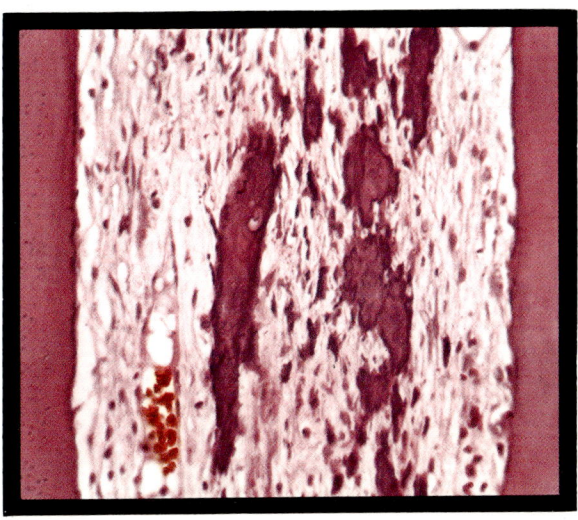

Linear Calcification in Radicular Pulp   X 200

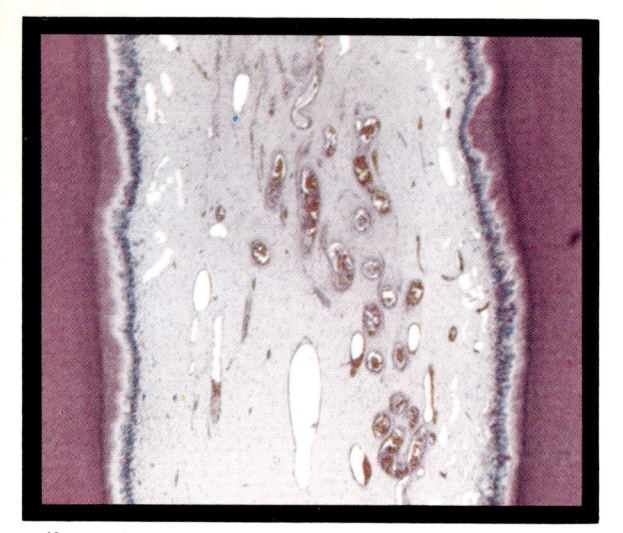

Hyperemia   X 40

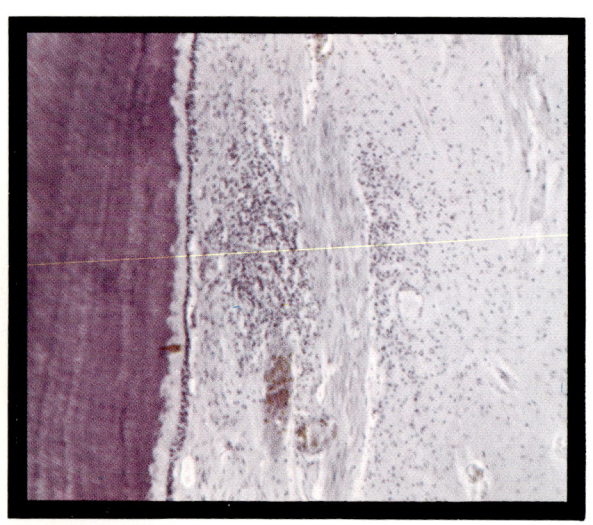

Mild Focal Pulpitis   X 98

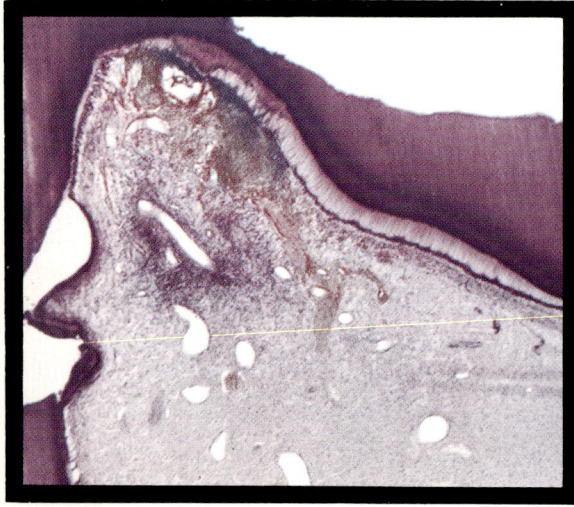

Advanced Partial Pulpitis   X 35

PULPITIS

(Top) Dilatation of capillaries and their engorgement with red blood cells (hyperemia or congestion), as shown in the radicular pulp of this tooth, may or may not be an early manifestation of inflammation. Noninflammatory hyperemia will occur if the venous outflow to the pulp is obstructed while there is no hindrance to the arterial flow. It may also result from minor irritations not of sufficient magnitude to cause inflammation. In noninflammatory hyperemia there is an increase in intercellular fluid because the fluid cannot return to the vessels due to increased venous pressure. This type of hyperemia is reversible, provided that the causative factor is soon eliminated.

The hyperemia occurring in an early phase of inflammation is followed quickly by the exudation of the fluid and cellular elements of the blood. This exudate is of a higher specific gravity than the transudate of noninflammatory edema. Exudation occurs as the result of vasodilation, increased permeability of vessel walls, and elevation of capillary pressure. It is believed that certain factors liberated by injured cells are responsible for initiating some of the vascular changes as well as directly attracting the polymorphonuclear leukocytes to the area of injury.

(Center) A small focus of lymphocytes and plasma cells is seen in the vicinity of nerve tissue. Pulpitis, like inflammation in other tissues, is a response of the pulp to an irritant that is intense enough to injure cells. Pulpal cells may be injured or killed by microorganisms, by toxic subtances, by excessive thermal change and by trauma. Occasionally, pulpitis occurs secondarily by extension of periodontal inflammation or as a result of bacteremia.

(Bottom) A large occlusal carious area in a molar tooth is apparent at the top of the photomicrograph. In relation to this area, at the periphery of the pulp, is a thick layer of predentin. Numerous capillaries in the pulp are dilated, and in the pulpal horn there is extensive hemorrhage and a marked influx of inflammatory cells.

Diseases of the Teeth and Supporting Structures

Pulpitis (Cont.)

(Top) Histologic examination of this tooth, which was removed after the patient experienced 12 hours of excruciating pain, reveals a large occlusal defect, below which are several layers of secondary dentin. In the coronal portion of the pulp is a distinctly localized mass of inflammatory cells. It is composed mainly of dead and disintegrating polymorphonuclear neutrophils. The necrotic tissue in this area is beginning to liquefy. Histologically this abscess (localized collection of pus) is acute, for there is no evidence of fibrosis at its periphery.

(Center) In this instance the suppurative exudate is not localized, and the entire pulp is involved. The photomicrograph shows only a small area of the pulp in one of the roots. It is apparent that the pulp tissue is necrotic, and that much of it is liquefied. The inflammatory cells present are mainly polymorphonuclear neutrophils.

(Bottom) A large portion of the coronal pulp is exposed and presents an ulcerated surface. In the necrotic area there are polymorphonuclear neutrophils, fibrin, and colonies of microorganisms. A bandlike bluish line, running the whole length of the defect, separates the viable from the nonviable tissue. This line is due to a peculiar diffusion of chromatin from dead cells. Below the necrotic area is an extensive infiltration of inflammatory cells which involves most of the coronal pulp.

Interest in pulpal reactions has been stimulated since the introduction of operative procedures involving high-speed instruments. The studies of several investigators suggest that the pulp has greater recuperative powers than was formerly recognized, but all warn that every effort should be made to minimize operative trauma to the pulp by using an effective fluid coolant with high-speed instruments. However, with severe injury the pulp may not recover because its recuperative powers are limited by lack of room for swelling, and because it has no collateral blood supply.

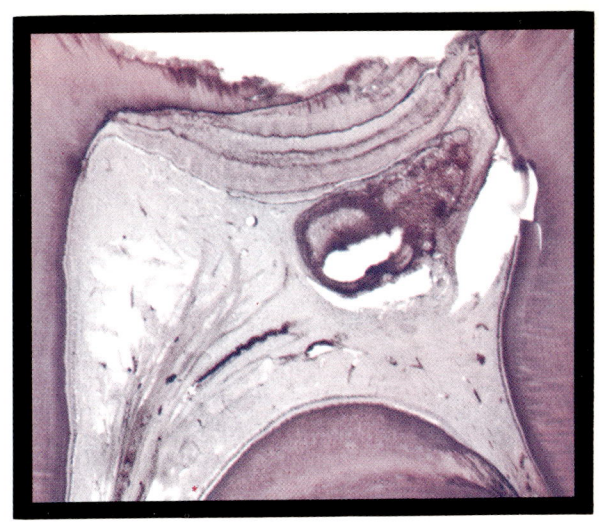

Acute Pulpal Abscess   X 22

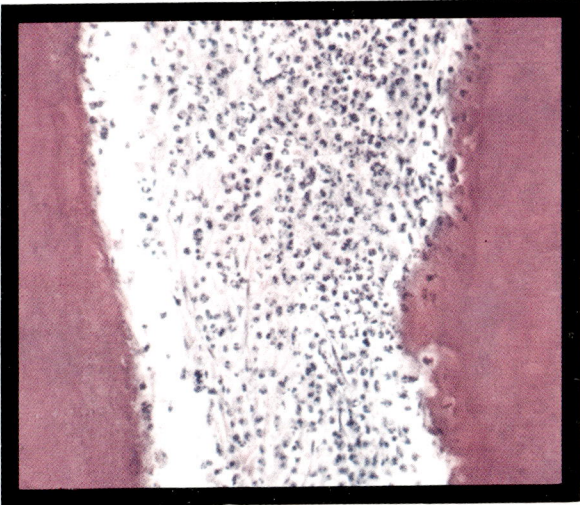

Total Suppurative Pulpitis   X 190

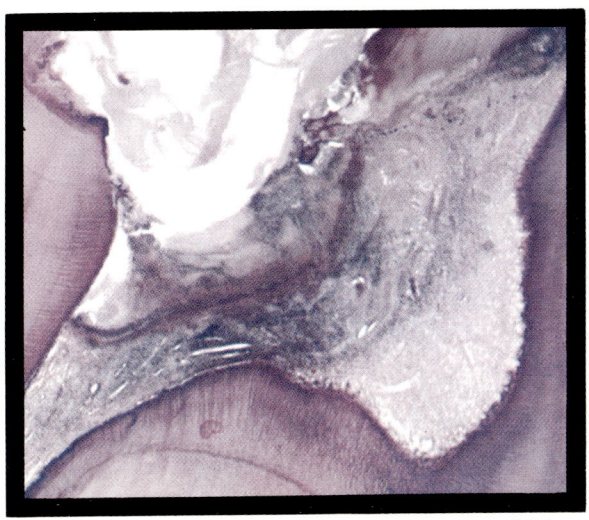

Chronic Ulcerative Pulpitis   X 23

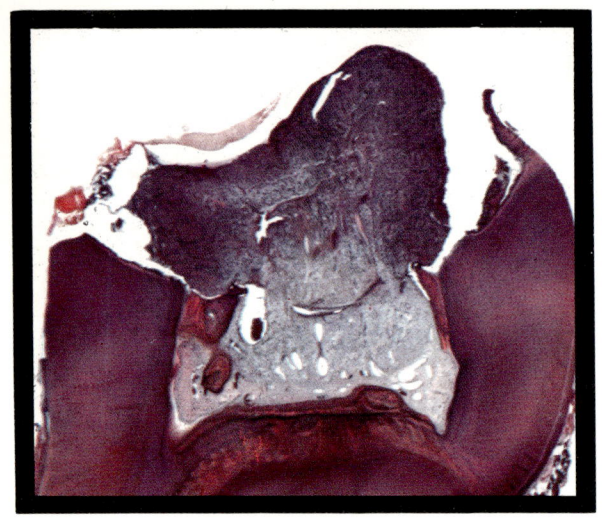

Chronic Hyperplastic Pulpitis (Pulp Polyp)   X 12

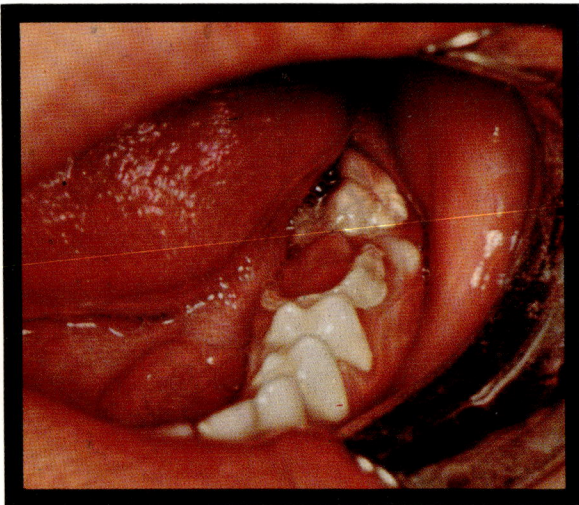

Pulp Polyp

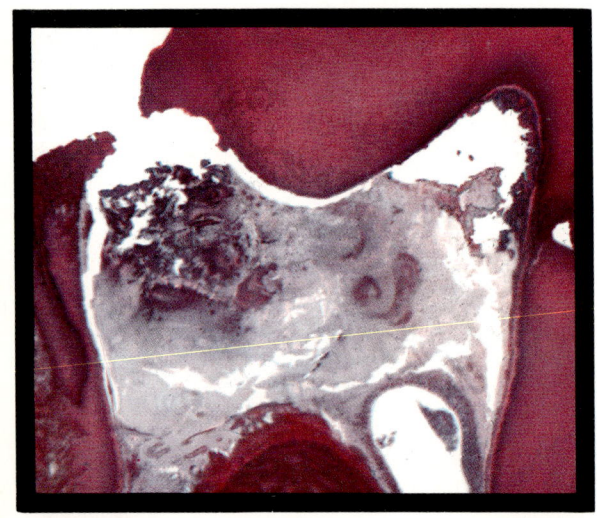

Necrotic Pulp   X 22

Pulpitis (Cont.)

(Top) Chronic hyperplastic pulpitis (pulp polyp) occurs only when the coronal pulp is widely exposed and an exceptionally good blood supply is available. Because of the latter requirement this lesion develops only in young individuals, especially in teeth that have large apical foramina. In the case shown there is a marked proliferation of granulation tissue extending outward to form a polypoid mass. The lower portion of the coronal pulp is relatively free of inflammatory cells. Frequently the surface of a pulp polyp becomes epithelized. This probably happens when epithelial cells are scraped off the tongue or cheek by the sharp edges of the carious tooth and transplanted onto the well-vascularized granulation tissue of the polyp. In hyperplastic pulpitis the potential recuperative ability of pulp tissue is well demonstrated. It is apparent that when the pulp has a good blood supply and room to expand because of wide exposure, it will remain vital and make a valiant attempt at healing even when subjected to extensive irritation.

(Center) A pulp polyp in the 1st molar of a 15-year-old patient. It extends upward almost to the line of occlusion. Because of the smooth, shiny surface it may be concluded that this polyp is covered by epithelium. Such a lesion should not be confused with hyperplastic gingival tissue which has grown into a large carious area. Pulp polyps are not particularly sensitive to touch, but they do bleed easily unless covered by epithelium.

(Bottom) Complete necrosis of the pulp in a deciduous molar tooth. Nuclear staining is absent, and the pulp chamber is filled with amorphous material and colonies of microorganisms. Total death of the pulp may result from the diffusion of chemical substances through the pulp, from thrombosis initiated by various types of total pulpitis, or from trauma severe enough to cause a loss of vascular continuity. The color of a tooth with a necrotic pulp may differ from that of adjacent normal teeth. This discoloration, which varies from yellow to gray or black, is due to staining of the dentinal tubules by pigments which are derived from the breakdown of red blood cells and the end products of protein degradation.

SEQUELAE OF PULPITIS

Pulpal inflammation that is not eliminated by resolution, endodontics or surgery usually results in periapical inflammation. This inflammatory reaction is most frequently caused by irritants emanating from the pulp although trauma also may cause periapical inflammation. The irritants from the pulp may be microorganisms, bacterially produced toxins, or products of protein degradation. Because of the injuries caused by agents other than microorganisms, periapical inflammation may or may not be an infection. The character of the tissue response depends upon the causative agent and the capacity for response of the individual's cells. Sequelae of pulpitis include dental granuloma, periodontal cyst, periapical abscess, gingival abscess, extra-oral fistula, cellulitis, osteomyelitis (p. 118) and actinomycosis (p. 117).

(Top) Chronic productive periodontitis (dental granuloma) at apex of a bicuspid tooth. A large area of bone is replaced by granulation tissue in which there are numerous inflammatory cells. In such a lesion repair is taking place, but exudation continues because cells are still being injured. If the irritating factor is eliminated, healing can occur.

(Center) If the chronic productive periodontitis involves a portion of the periodontal membrane that contains epithelial rests (see pp. 16, 34), this epithelium may be stimulated to proliferate. Such an area of epithelial proliferation is apparent at the top of this photomicrograph of a dental granuloma.

(Bottom) A periodontal cyst (closed epithelial-lined space containing fluid or semifluid) forms when a mass of epithelial cells in a dental granuloma proliferates to such a degree that the central cells outgrow their vascular supply, become necrotic and liquefy. (See pp. 34-36.) Once a cyst has formed, periapical curettage is necessary in addition to proper pulp canal therapy if the periapical tissues are to regenerate. Curettage is important only in removing the epithelial lining of the cyst. If a cyst is allowed to remain even after the original inflammatory irritant is eliminated, it may continue to enlarge by accumulation of fluid within the cyst and will destroy the surrounding tissue by pressure.

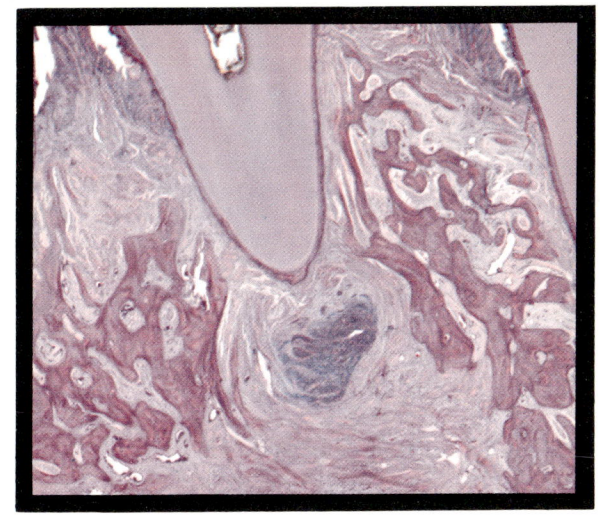

Dental Granuloma X 8

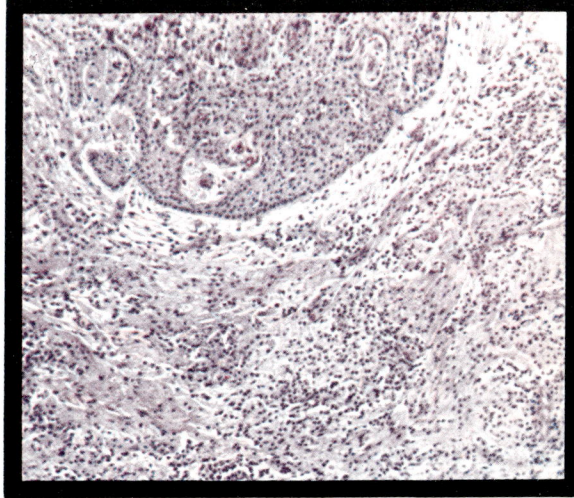

Proliferating Epithelium in Dental Granuloma X 90

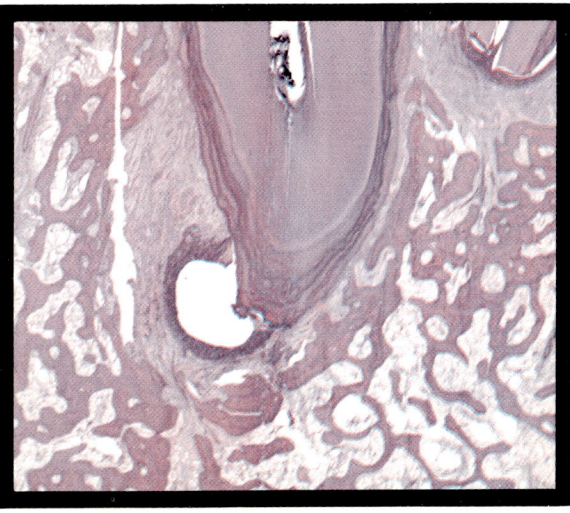

Periodontal Cyst X 8

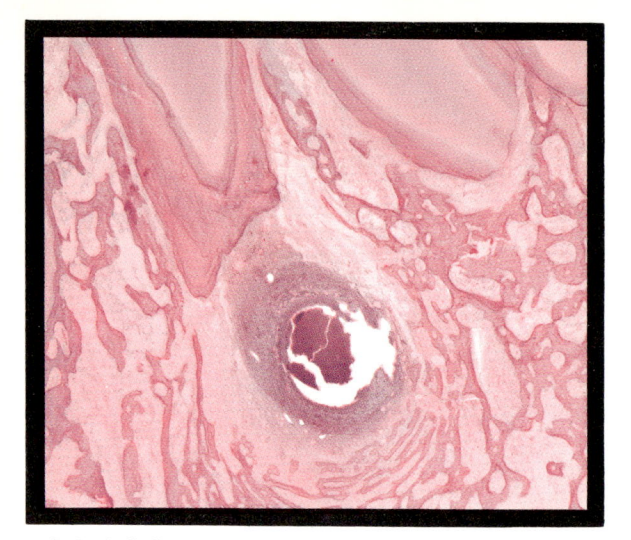

Periapical Abscess   X 8

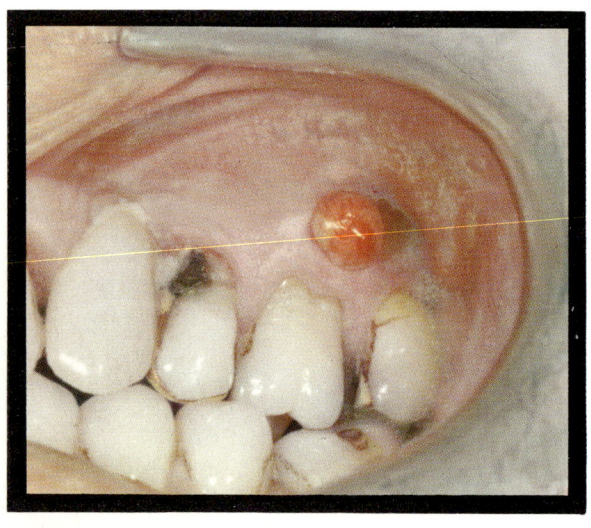

Gingival Abscess (Parulis)

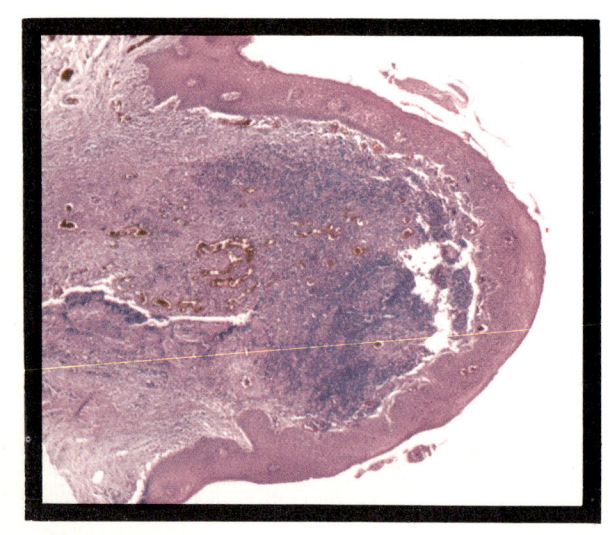

Gingival Abscess   X 28

Sequelae of Pulpitis (Cont.)

(Top) An abscess (localized collection of pus) in the periapical region of a bicuspid tooth. In the central portion of the inflammatory focus is a cavity partially filled with liquefied tissue debris and polymorphonuclear neutrophils. This type of lesion forms when an inflammatory exudate containing many polymorphonuclear neutrophils is able to confine an irritant of great intensity that has killed numerous cells. The great numbers of polymorphonuclear neutrophils liberate a large amount of a proteolytic enzyme which liquefies the necrotic tissue (both fixed tissue and dead leukocytes), forming a semiliquid material, pus. The wall of an acute abscess is composed only of inflammatory cells, whereas fibrous tissue is found in the outer wall of a chronic abscess.

(Center) The contents of the periapical abscess may be under great pressure due to an active inflammatory process forming additional pus. The pressure tends to force the pus into the surrounding tissue, and it naturally progresses along the lines of least resistance. It may burrow through the buccal cortical plate and emerge in the gingival mucosa. Accumulation of pus in this location, as shown in the illustration, is termed a parulis, or gingival abscess. If the pressure continues to increase, the parulis will rupture, pus will be evacuated, and the gingival swelling will regress. The evacuating tract thus formed may epithelize, resulting in a permanent, draining sinus, or its peripheral portion may heal and a gingival abscess again develop. A parulis may also result from extension of a periodontal abscess, which is formed when pus is trapped in the wall of a narrow periodontal pocket.

(Bottom) Photomicrograph of a gingival abscess similar to the one seen in the center picture. In the plane of this section the covering epithelium is intact, and just below it is a mass of inflammatory cells. In one region, near the apex of the specimen, is a partially clear area containing pus. The horizontal slit extending to the left border of the picture is part of the inflammatory tract which led to the periapical lesion.

Diseases of the Teeth and Supporting Structures

Sequelae of Pulpitis (Cont.)

(Top) This patient had a periapical abscess of the mandibular left 2nd molar. In this case the pus, influenced by gravity and following the line of least resistance, burrowed through the bone in a region that led to the masticator space. Finally it extended into the subcutaneous tissue, and an abscess was formed in the skin.

(Center) Marked swelling of the left side has resulted from extension of periapical inflammation. A diffuse nonsuppurative inflammatory process of this type is characterized by abundant serous exudation into the loose tissues. While it is commonly called "cellulitis," this is actually an edema which may resolve without suppuration, or which may progress to true cellulitis with diffuse suppuration, or in which an abscess may develop.

(Bottom) A phlegmon is an intense inflammatory process which spreads through tissue spaces over a wide area and is difficult to control. It is caused by microorganisms of high virulence and characterized by an exudate in which polymorphonuclear neutrophils predominate. Complications may arise when the spreading inflammation involves vessel walls. This causes roughening of the ordinarily smooth intima, and elements of the blood adhere to it, forming a thrombus (thrombophlebitis). Microorganisms frequently invade the vessel wall, enter the thrombus and continue to multiply (septic thrombosis). Once the clot is infected, it tends to soften, and fragments of it may break off and enter the general circulation, causing septicemia. By this same mechanism, septic thrombosis of the cavernous sinus may occasionally occur from a periapical infection when certain veins are involved. The prognosis of cavernous sinus thrombosis, as well as of phlegmonous inflammation, is better now than it was before the advent of antibiotics. The photomicrograph is a section from the floor of the mouth in a fatal case of phlegmonous inflammation. The two dark-staining ovoid areas are veins. Inflammatory cells have invaded the vessel walls. The lumina are partially occluded by septic thrombi.

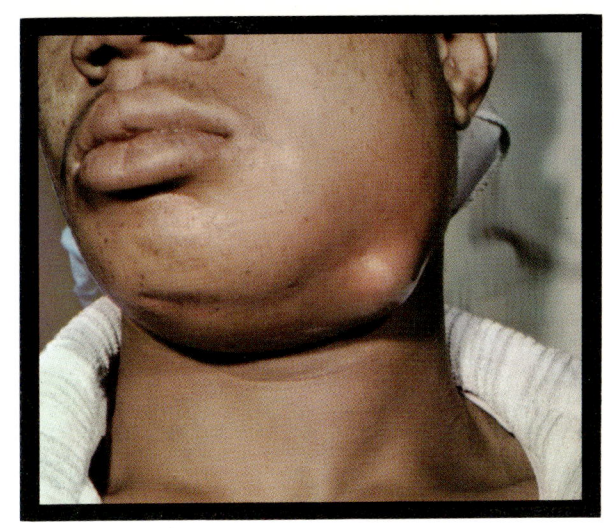

Cutaneous Abscess

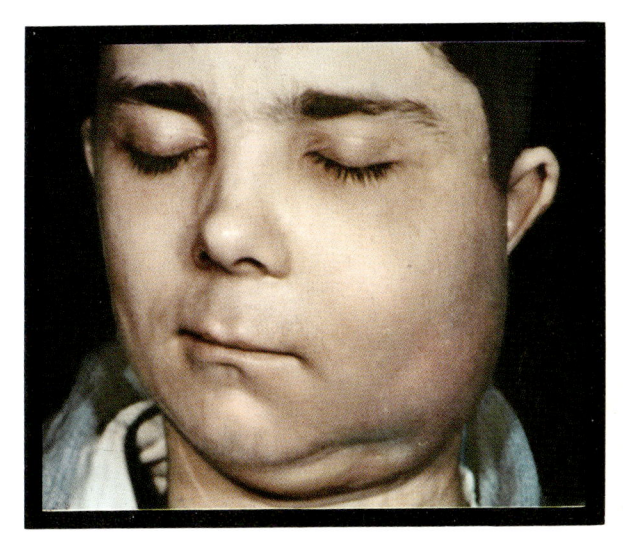

"Cellulitis"

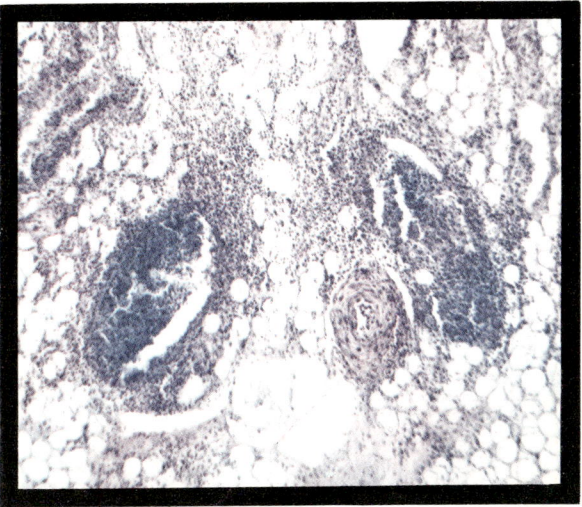

Thrombophlebitis X 80

76 Diseases of the Teeth and Supporting Structures

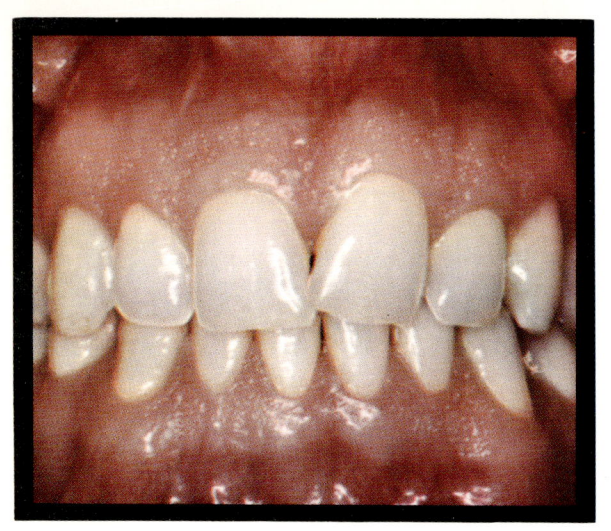

Normal Gingiva

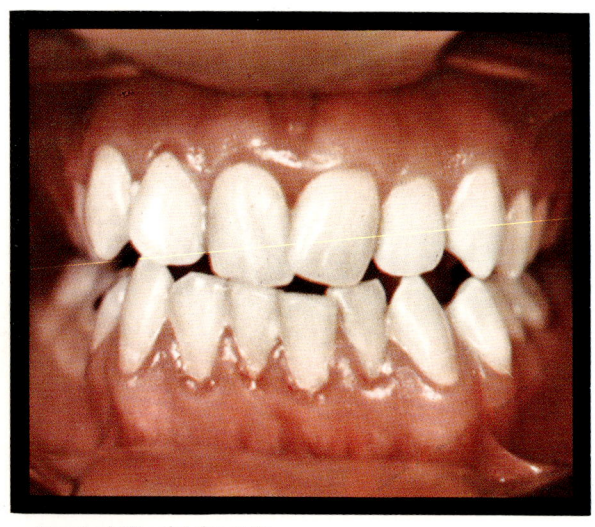

Marginal (Simple) Gingivitis

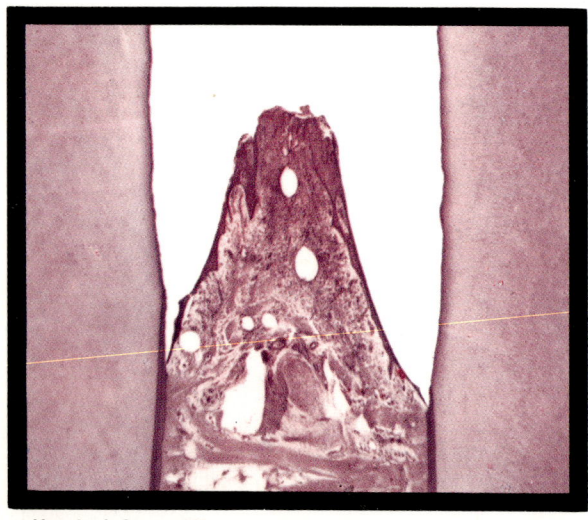

Marginal Gingivitis, Interdental Papilla   X 24

NORMAL GINGIVA

The gingiva is the soft tissue surrounding the teeth and covering the adjacent alveolar process. The portion coronal to the epithelial attachment is free gingiva, while the remainder is attached gingiva. The gingival crevice or sulcus, normally not more than 2 mm. in depth, is located between the tooth and the free gingiva (see p. 3). The part of the gingiva that occupies the interdental space is the interdental papilla.

(Top) Firm, healthy gingiva that is relatively normal (for age 40 years) showing characteristic sharp-edged free margins which approximate the contour of the cemento-enamel junction. The pale pink, stippled gingival tissue is readily differentiated from the adjacent red vascular vestibular mucosa. The contour of the attached gingiva reflects the contour of the surface of the alveolar process.

Any survey of gingival tissue should include observations of color, form, density and depth of the sulcus. Knowledge of the appearance of normal gingiva is prerequisite for recognition of the different types of periodontal disease.

MARGINAL (SIMPLE) GINGIVITIS

(Center) A mild inflammation of the free gingiva, exhibiting two of the cardinal signs of inflammation: redness (rubor) and swelling (tumor). These changes, which result from congestion and exudation, are most marked in the lower anterior region and about the necks of the maxillary right central and lateral incisors.

(Bottom) The clear areas on either side of this interdental papilla were occupied by the enamel which has been lost in preparing the specimen. The epithelium at the top of the papilla has been destroyed but still lines the sulci on either side. The large clear areas are dilated vessels and the dark-blue-staining material, most prominent near the tip, is chiefly inflammatory cells, identified under higher magnification as lymphocytes and plasma cells. The inflammation does not extend below the transseptal fibers extending between the teeth at the bottom of the picture.

Marginal Gingivitis (Cont.)

(Top) A rather severe case of marginal gingivitis resulting from the irritating effect of soft and hard accretions on the teeth. There is alteration of color, form and density of the gingiva. The inflammation is most marked about the maxillary left cuspid and lateral incisor, where an accumulation of materia alba is evident. Lack of home care and the diminished cleansing action of food, due to irregularity of the teeth, were important etiologic factors. In marginal gingivitis the gingival sulcus is often increased in depth. In uncomplicated gingivitis this is due to gingival enlargement rather than to deepening of the gingival sulcus by apical positioning of the gingival cuff (epithelial attachment).

(Center) The patient shown above after removal of soft and hard deposits and institution of proper home care. The treatment is incomplete, but marked improvement is evident. Most of the gingiva has a pale pink color and a dull, stippled surface, and the gingival margins are thinner. These changes occur rapidly after local irritants are removed, but if the disease is not treated, it may progress rapidly into periodontitis.

ACUTE HERPETIC GINGIVOSTOMATITIS

(Bottom) Characteristic gingival response to initial infection by the herpes simplex virus. The primary infection, which occurs most frequently in children, is also characterized by malaise, pyrexia, lymphadenitis and pharyngitis. Small vesicles which may form on the gingiva in this disease are often not seen because they rapidly macerate, producing painful ulcers. The entire gingiva is intensely red, but this may go unobserved because of the presence of desquamating epithelium, which forms a grayish membranous covering. This epithelial debris can be removed easily without hemorrhage resulting, and the red color is then strikingly apparent. In the case shown there is redness at the gingival margins of some teeth, and the membrane may be observed in other areas. A herpetic ulcer is apparent in the labial mucosa (lower left foreground). (See pp. 110-111 for recurrent herpes.)

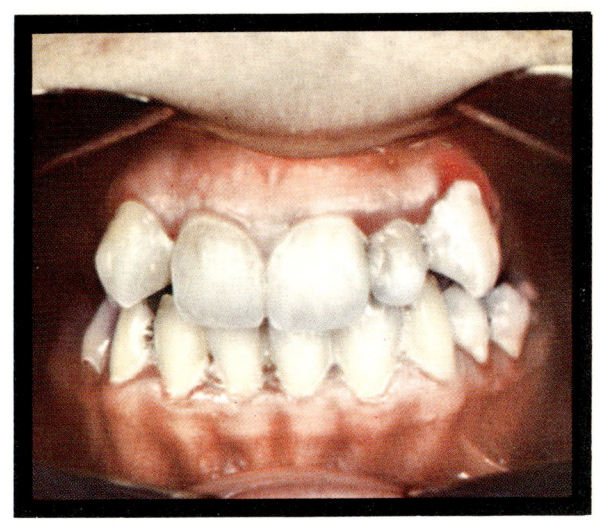

Severe Marginal Gingivitis, Before Treatment

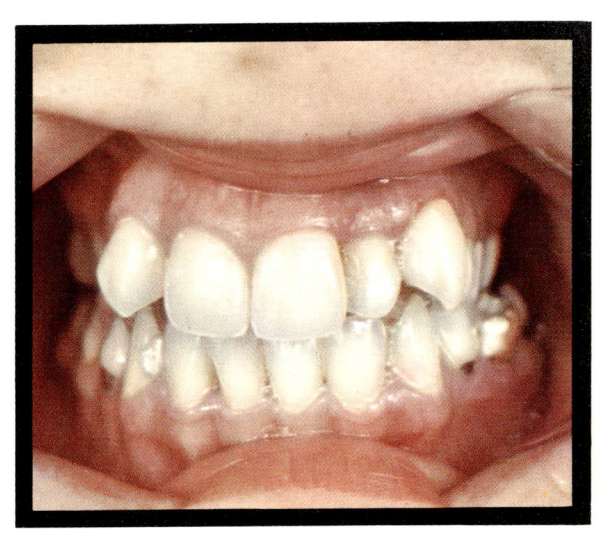

Same Case as Above, After Prophylaxis

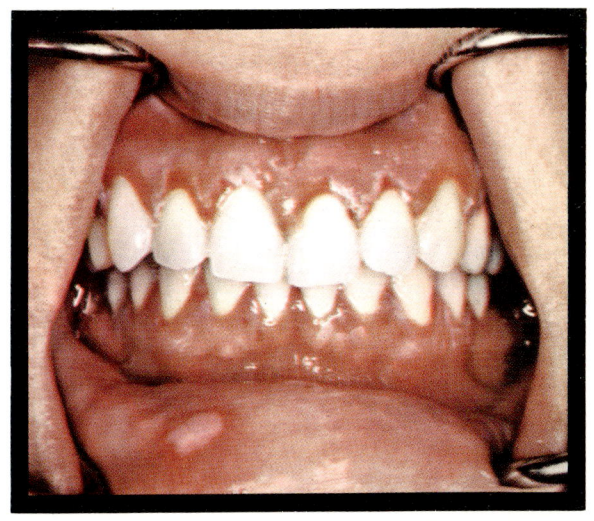

Acute Herpetic Gingivostomatitis

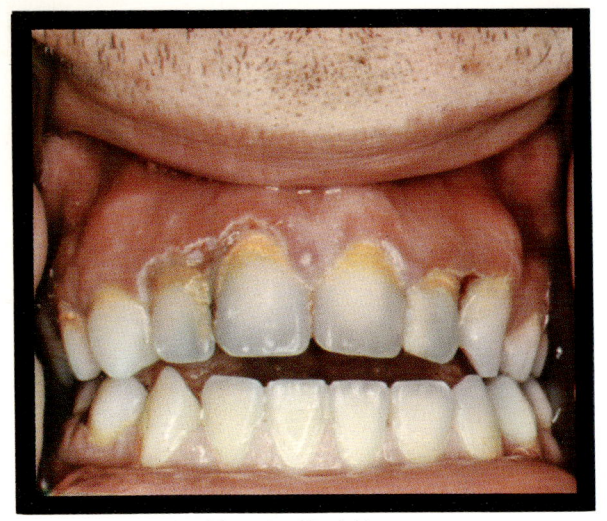

Acute Necrotizing Ulcerative Gingivitis

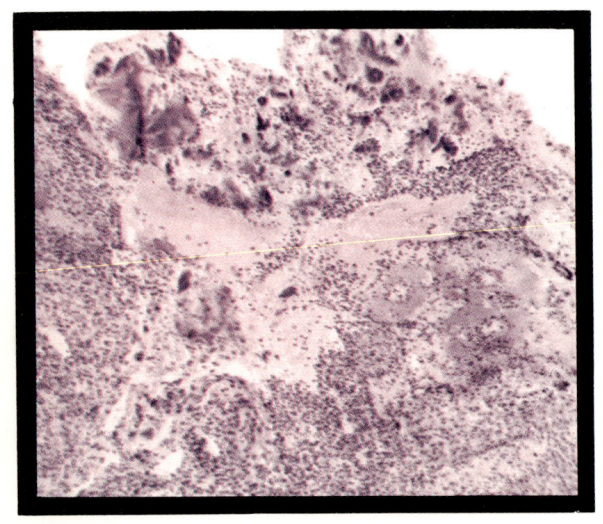

Gingival Papillae, Necrotizing Ulcerative Gingivitis   X 85

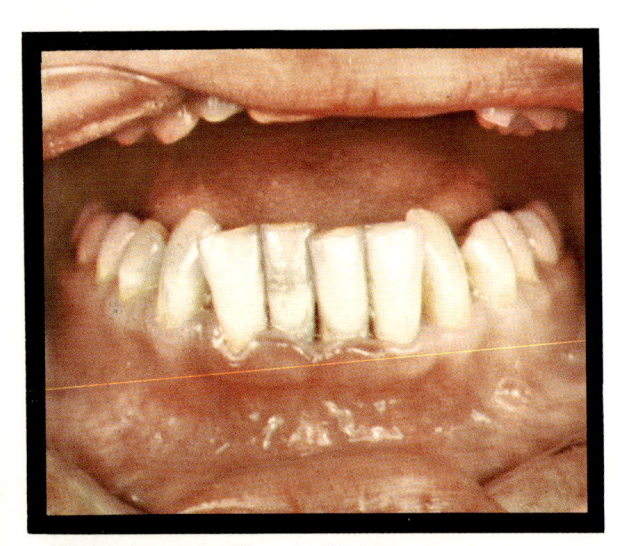

Chronic Necrotizing Ulcerative Gingivitis

NECROTIZING ULCERATIVE GINGIVITIS

(Vincent's Infection)

Necrotizing ulcerative gingivitis (ulceromembranous gingivitis, Vincent's infection, or trench mouth) is a noncommunicable inflammatory disease of the gingiva resulting from local irritation and the effects from fusiforms and spirochetes. The organisms, which are components of the normal oral flora, invade the gingival tissue when its resistance is lowered.

(Top) The acute phase of the disease is characterized by redness, swelling, ulceration, bleeding and pain. The grayish pseudomembrane that usually covers the ulcerated surface can easily be removed, leaving a raw, bleeding base. The ulceration is often limited to the interdental area but may extend onto the labial or lingual gingiva about the necks of the teeth. The disease is also seen frequently in the region of partially erupted 3rd molars. If therapy is inadequate, the acute stage may subside and the condition become subacute or chronic. In severe cases there is a fetid odor and a foul taste in the mouth. The treatment of choice is complete elimination of the local irritants by careful and thorough prophylactic procedures. Mild medicaments used locally, as well as antibiotic therapy, may serve as adjuncts to treatment but are of no value if used independently of scaling and polishing. Caustics are contraindicated.

(Center) Gingival specimen from an area of active necrotizing ulcerative gingivitis. It shows the characteristic intercellular coagulation necrosis with the formation of a false membrane containing numerous colonies of organisms. Intense inflammatory response is evident at the base of the ulcer.

(Bottom) Typical picture of chronic necrotizing ulcerative gingivitis which follows untreated or improperly treated acute cases. The gingival margin, rather than being scalloped, appears as nearly a straight line. This alteration is due to destruction of interproximal and labial marginal gingiva. An attempt at repair may produce pseudopapillae which extend above the interproximal craters, thus obscuring the tissue destruction in these areas.

Diseases of the Teeth and Supporting Structures 79

GINGIVAL ENLARGEMENT

All generalized nonneoplastic increase in gingival bulk is classified as gingival enlargement, while focal enlargements are specifically designated. Enlargements due to inflammation may be manifest as hyperemia, hyperplasia, fibrosis, etc. Included among the causes of gingival enlargements are hormonal imbalances of puberty and pregnancy, heredity, Dilantin and leukemia. Inflammation may be associated with any of these enlargements.

(Top) Pubertal enlargement is associated with disturbed hormonal balance at puberty. It usually is preceded by some degree of marginal gingivitis. The papillae increase in size, and the gingival margins are thickened as a result of hyperemia and edema. The tissues are soft and bleed readily. Removal of local irritants may produce some improvement, but reestablishment of hormonal balance is essential for complete resolution. This gingival disease is more common in girls than in boys.

(Center) Enlargement of the gingiva associated with pregnancy is similar, clinically and histologically, to pubertal enlargement. It is associated with hormonal activity of pregnancy but, as in pubertal enlargement, usually has local irritating factors contributing to its initiation. Hormonal therapy is not indicated. The disease occurs in about 5 per cent of pregnant women. The enlargement usually subsides after parturition, but local therapy is desirable, along with good oral hygiene, to aid in controlling the associated gingivitis. A few patients with gingival enlargement of pregnancy develop so-called pregnancy tumors (see p. 90).

(Bottom) The most characteristic histologic feature of hormonal gingival enlargement of puberty or pregnancy is the marked vascularity of the tissues, as shown here. The lesion resembles a granuloma pyogenicum. The excessive vascularity accounts for the bright red color, and the hyperemia and edema for the enlargement. Obviously, since the enlargement may resolve when the hormones are in normal relationship, gingivectomy is not indicated during pregnancy or puberty for this type of enlargement.

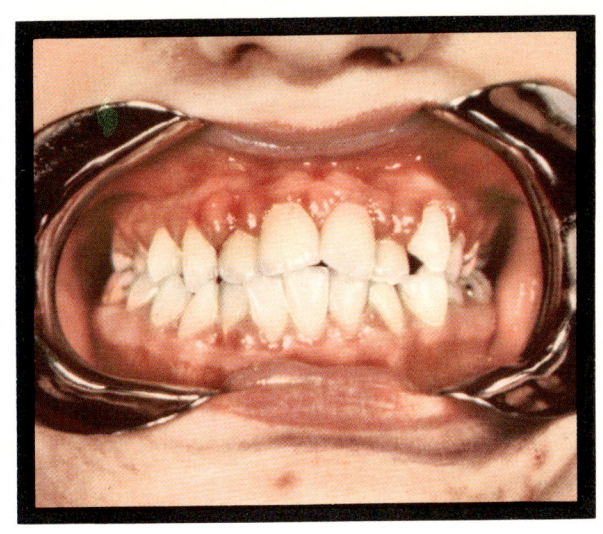

Pubertal Enlargement

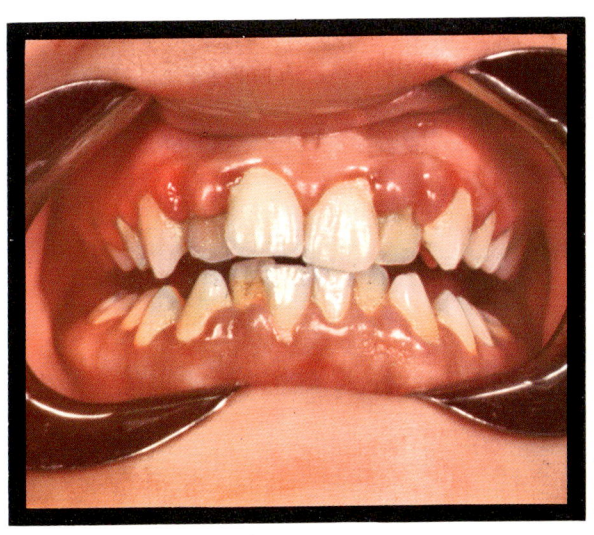

Gingival Enlargement of Pregnancy

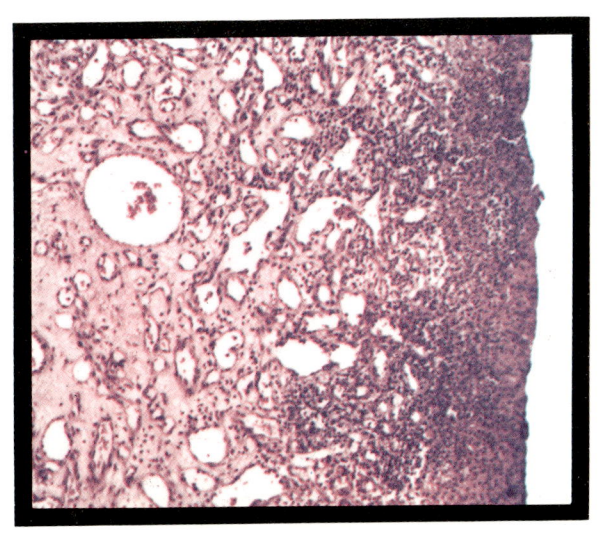

Hormonal Enlargement, Gingival Papilla   X 90

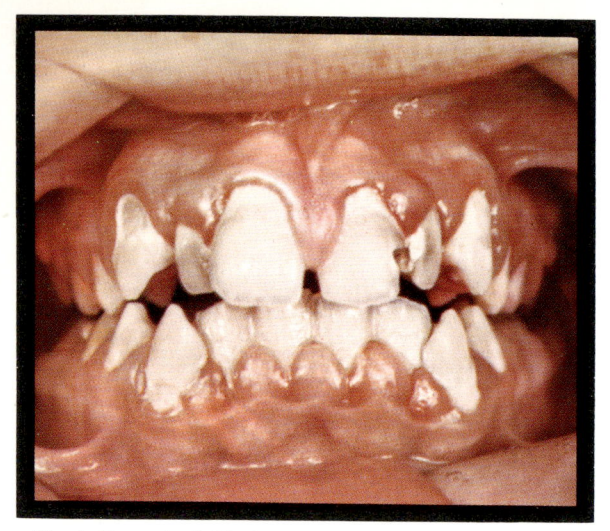

Simple Hyperplastic Gingivitis

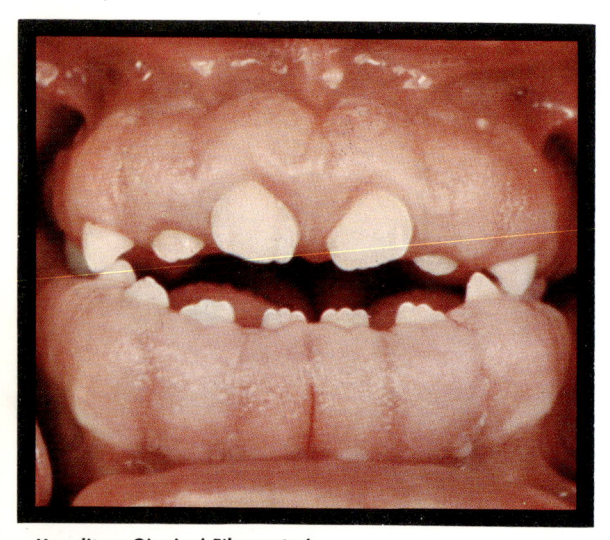

Hereditary Gingival Fibromatosis

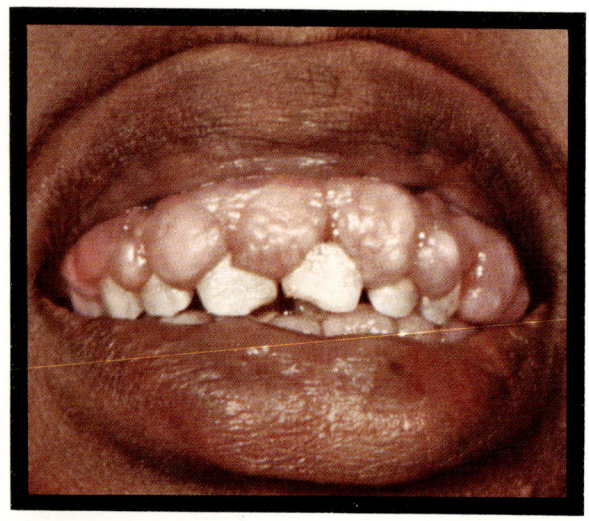

Dilantin Enlargement

Gingival Enlargement (Cont.)

(Top) Simple hyperplastic gingivitis results from long-continued local irritation. It may be considered a chronic form of simple marginal gingivitis in which the body's response to the continuous irritation is a productive type of inflammation. In simple marginal gingivitis the affected tissue is soft and spongy, the swelling being due to the inflammatory exudate; whereas in simple hyperplastic gingivitis the extensive enlargement of the tissue is firm, being the result of subepithelial fibrosis. In the case illustrated the papillae are markedly increased in size, gingival margins are blunt, and crevices increased in depth. Treatment consists of removal of local irritants, use of periodontal packs, massage and gingivoplasty.

(Center) In hereditary gingival fibromatosis, usually initiated at the time of eruption of the teeth, the individual has a great genetic propensity for the proliferation of connective tissue in response to minor irritation. Once started, the increase in size of the gingiva is conducive to further local irritation, so that the process becomes progressively more severe. Removal of local irritants may bring improvement, but gingivoplasty is necessary to produce physiologic contour. Once the excess tissue has been removed, it will be possible to maintain exceptional oral hygiene, which will retard regrowth of tissue.

(Bottom) Dilantin enlargement, which closely resembles hereditary gingival fibromatosis both clinically and histologically, occurs in some individuals who are using Dilantin Sodium for the control of epilepsy. In this type of gingival disease Dilantin markedly stimulates connective tissue proliferation, resulting in a progressive gingival enlargement that may eventually cover the teeth completely. It is believed that in most instances local irritation is an initiating factor, though this point is in dispute. This disease is quite rare in edentulous areas. Gingivoplasty in the presence of continued Dilantin therapy is indicated when there is soft tissue impingement during mastication, but it does not result in a cure.

Diseases of the Teeth and Supporting Structures

Gingival Enlargement (Cont.)

(Top) In this gingival specimen, from a patient with Dilantin enlargement, inflammatory cells are seen near the floor of the gingival sulcus (lower left), but the predominant feature is the excessive subepithelial fibrosis. The connective tissue proliferation has caused the gingival tissue to be bulbous and the free margin to be blunt. This photomicrograph could not be distinguished from one of hereditary gingival fibromatosis or possibly from one of simple hyperplastic gingivitis, although in the latter there is often more epithelial hyperplasia, more inflammatory exudate and less extensive fibrosis.

(Center) Leukemic enlargement is due to infiltration of the tissues by leukemic cells and usually is associated with severe gingivitis. The gingival color frequently is deep red to purple, and the enlarged tissue may stand away from the teeth, resulting in deep, wide sulci. Edema and hyperemia associated with the gingivitis add to the size of the gingiva. Because of the purpuric tendency (p. 163) there is often severe, spontaneous gingival hemorrhage. Necrosis of the gingiva and adjacent tissues is not uncommon. Early necrosis may be misdiagnosed as necrotizing ulcerative gingivitis. Leukemic enlargement may be seen in any type of leukemia but most commonly in monocytic and, then, myelogenous types. There is no diagnostic characteristic difference in the gingival changes associated with different types of leukemia. Local therapy consists of careful removal of hard and soft deposits and establishing a good oral hygiene. Surgical procedures are contraindicated.

(Bottom) Low-power view of gingival specimen *(left)* shows the very heavy infiltration of leukemic cells. The crevicular lining is ulcerated. Under higher magnification *(right)* the atypical leukocytes are seen. The type of cellular infiltration will vary with the type of leukemia (myelogenous, lymphocytic, monocytic), but it is difficult to determine the type of leukemia by examination of gingival biopsy alone. Gingival biopsy is not suggested as a routine diagnostic procedure when leukemia is suspected.

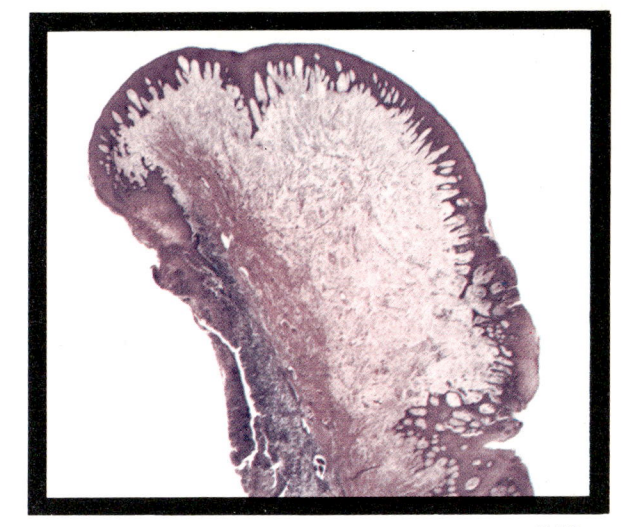

Dilantin Enlargement — X 12

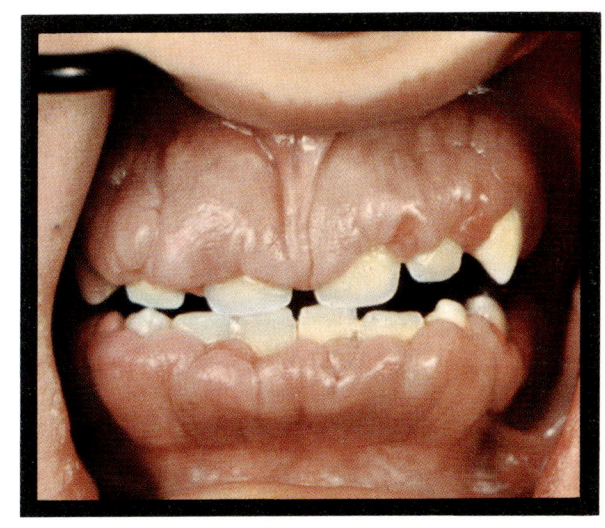

Leukemic Enlargement, Gingiva

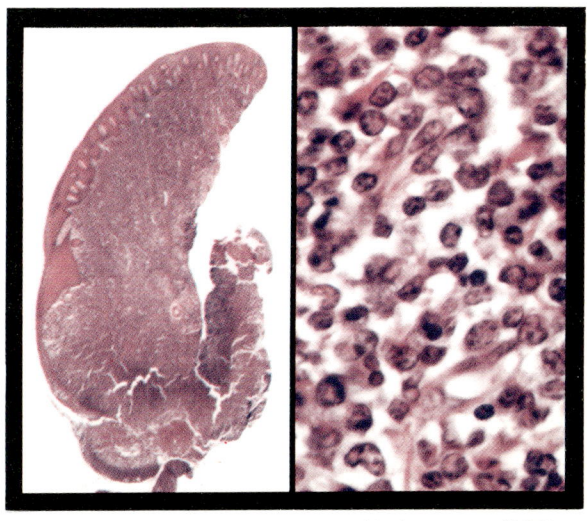

X 11 — Leukemic Enlargement, Gingiva — X 560

82 *Diseases of the Teeth and Supporting Structures*

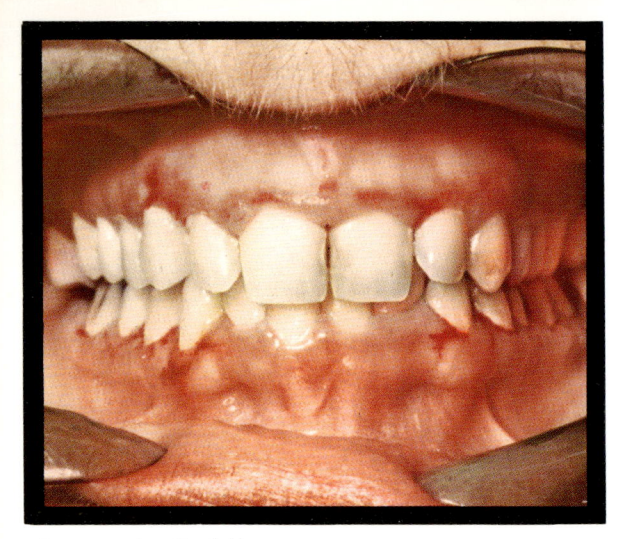

Desquamative Gingivitis

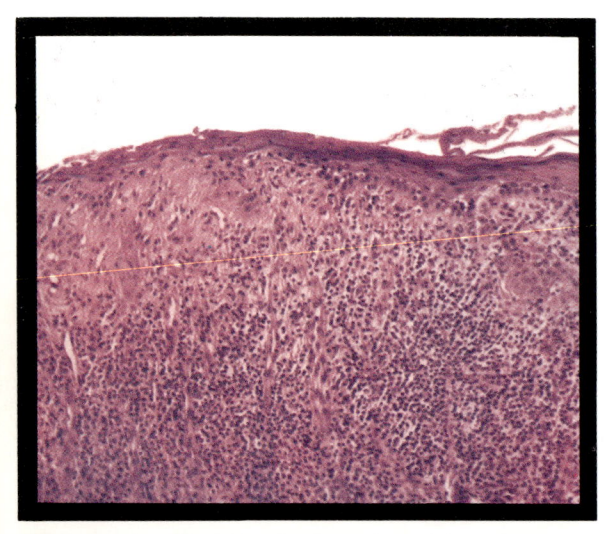

Desquamative Gingivitis, Specimen from Edge of Red Area X 100

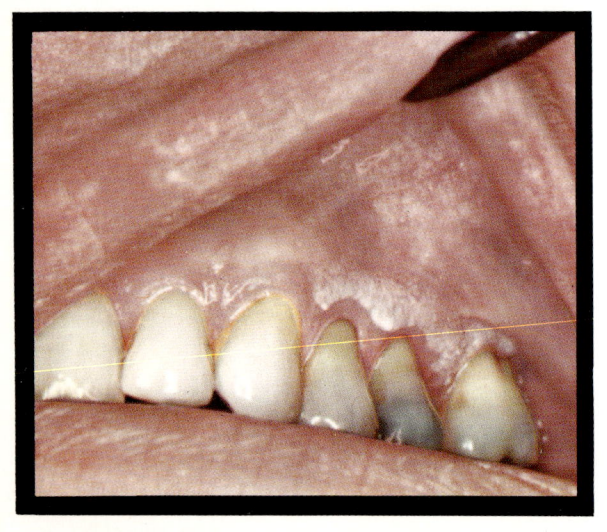

Atrophic Senile Gingivitis

DESQUAMATIVE GINGIVITIS

("Gingivosis")

(Top) Desquamative gingivitis is characterized by a bullous or vesicular process that causes the epithelium to "desquamate" readily. When the surface is rubbed carefully, a thin vesicle forms and may be ruptured by the very act of rubbing. More vigorous rubbing pulls off the epithelium, leaving a red, shiny, sensitive surface. An airblast introduced into the gingival sulcus usually produces an air-filled bleb. The disease, which occurs most frequently in middle-aged women, may be due to hormonal imbalance, emotional factors, allergy or other stresses. Areas of regeneration and desquamation may give a mottled appearance to the gingiva. Cyclic changes are typical and make evaluation of therapy difficult. In the illustration, several small red denuded areas are apparent. In some cases, at a certain stage of the disease, the entire gingiva may be red and raw from the desquamation. This type of gingival disease should be differentiated from erosive lichen planus of the gingiva.

(Center) An intense inflammatory infiltrate extends to the surface epithelium, making it difficult to distinguish between epithelium and corium. At the left there is almost no epithelial covering. Homogenization of the collagen is seen. A thin layer of epithelium is evident more centrally, and at the right actual desquamation is apparent. Clinically, the area at the left would be red, blending into a gray region at the right.

ATROPHIC SENILE GINGIVITIS

(Bottom) Chronic atrophic senile gingivitis is a condition seen in postmenopausal women. It is characterized by atrophy of gingival mucosa, with focal areas of hyperkeratosis. There is usually some gingival recession. In the case pictured the mucosa is thin, shiny, and pale in color. Above the molar and premolar teeth there is a grayish-white rough area of hyperkeratosis. The changes, both clinical and microscopic, are similar to those seen in chronic atrophic senile vaginitis, which is sometimes a concomitant finding. Hormonal therapy, though frequently suggested, is usually of questionable benefit.

Diseases of the Teeth and Supporting Structures

PERIODONTITIS

Periodontitis, an inflammatory disease involving all the tooth-supporting structures, is the sequel of untreated or improperly treated gingivitis. Destruction of the periodontal fibers and resorption of the alveolar crests are the characteristic findings. Local irritation due to poor oral hygiene is the primary cause, although poorly made dental restorations with lack of proper contour, contacts and margins are equally irritating. Occlusal trauma, endocrine disturbances, allergy and some deficiencies may be contributing factors, altering the course and progress of the disease.

(Top) Clinically, periodontitis appears as a severe gingivitis with the additional feature of deepened gingival sulci due to apical movement of the epithelial cuff without equal change in the level of the gingival margin. The presence of such a deep gingival sulcus (the true pocket) resulting from loss of supporting tissues, is pathognomonic of periodontitis.

(Center) These radiographs show two types of destruction of the periodontium seen in periodontitis. On the left the destruction is of a horizontal nature, with the bone loss uniform on an entire segment of the teeth (advanced, above; early phase, below). On the right are vertical pockets, the one below extending to the apex of the mesial root. A pocket is described as infrabony when it extends below the level of the alveolar crest.

(Bottom) The drifting of a tooth or teeth (as the maxillary anteriors, here) is often considered as the first clinical evidence of periodontosis. Widening of the periodontal membrane and lack of pocket formation are also signs of the disease. Periodontosis is described as a degeneration of the periodontum related to systemic factors and evidenced by noninflammatory degeneration of the periodontal membrane and resorption of the alveolar bone. Occlusal trauma may be a factor in migration of the teeth, and eventually, as in this patient, periodontitis is superimposed with pocket formation. The existence of periodontosis as an entity is in dispute.

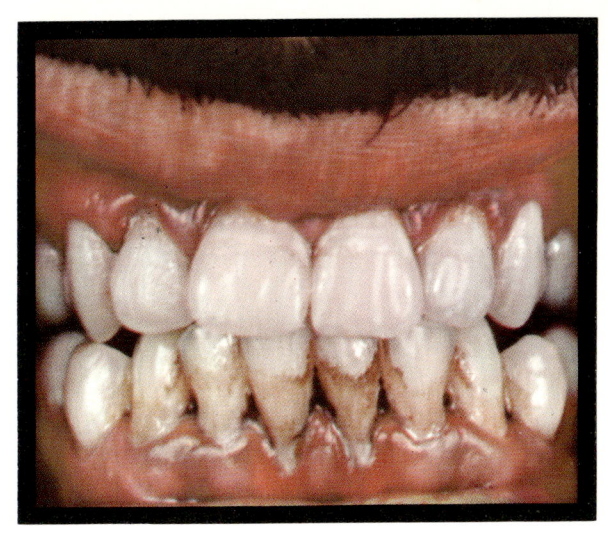

Periodontitis

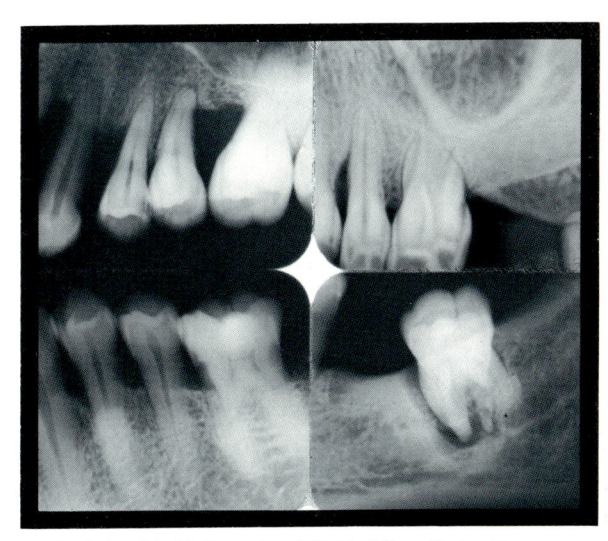

Periodontitis, Horizontal and Vertical Bone Destruction

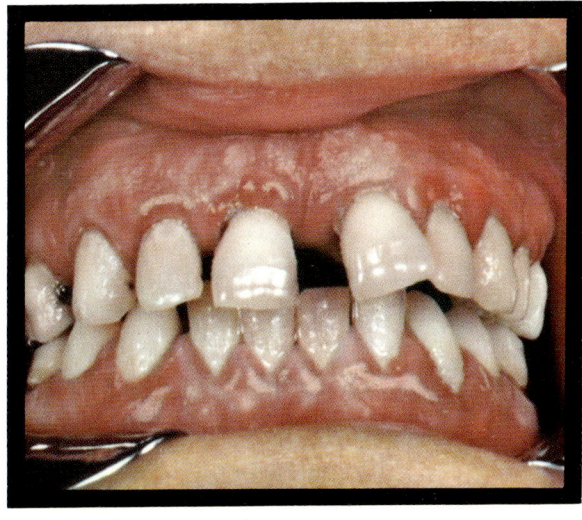

Tooth Migration (Periodontosis)

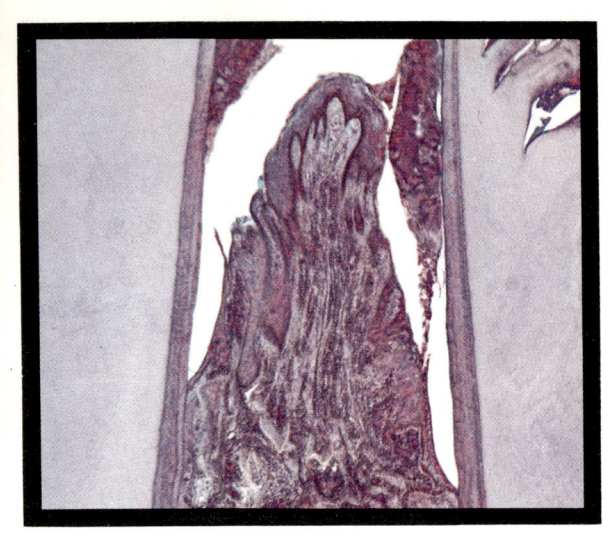

Periodontitis, Shallow Pockets   X 33

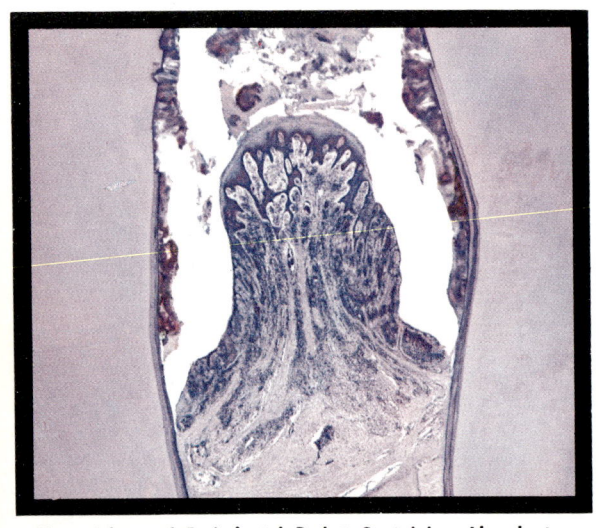

More Advanced Periodontal Pocket Containing Abundant Calculus   X 20

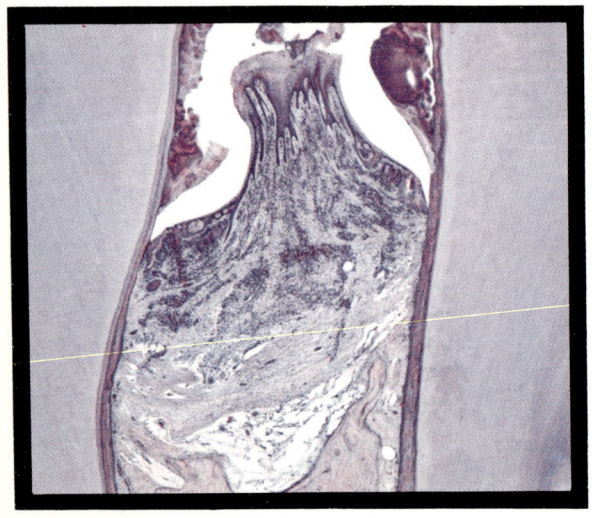

Advanced Periodontitis, Shallow Pockets   X 20

PERIODONTAL POCKETS

Periodontitis is a progressive disease beginning as a gingivitis and spreading into the underlying tissues, where it causes destruction of the periodontal membrane and the supporting bone. If left untreated, it leads to looseness of the teeth and ultimately to exfoliation. The inflammation may extend directly into the periodontal membrane, destroying the fibers and causing bone resorption because of lack of stimulation by the fibers; or the disease may first attack the alveolar bone crest with secondary involvement of the periodontal membrane. Pressure from gingival edema may initiate alveolar crest resorption. When the periodontal fibers are lost, the epithelial attachment (stimulated by the inflammatory process) proliferates apically, and a periodontal pocket is formed. At first the inflammation may be aseptic, but calculus, which is ever-present in pockets, will soon cause minute ulcerations of the crevicular epithelium, and microorganisms and toxins will invade the underlying tissue. This intensifies the inflammatory process with increased tissue destruction.

(Top) Calculus extends to the bottom of 2 comparatively shallow pockets on either side of a gingival papilla. The papillae in this and the 2 pictures below have shrunken in processing the specimens, and the epithelial attachments are now separated from the cementum. The calculus is in the pockets alongside the crevicular epithelium, with the epithelial attachments below. The inflammatory process extends below the epithelial attachments.

(Center) Calculus is seen on the cementum at either side of an inflamed papilla. The epithelial attachments were extremely narrow. The crevicular epithelium lining the pockets is ulcerated, and the intense inflammatory reaction extends to the transseptal fibers, which appear to be deterring its progress into the deeper portions of the periodontal membrane.

(Bottom) Although the epithelial attachments have progressed far apically, the pockets are shallow because the gingival crest has moved in the same direction. There is much loss of alveolar bone, and the inflammatory cells are infiltrating the reconstituted transseptal fibers. Note the irritating calculus.

Periodontal Pockets (Cont.)

(Top) The epithelial attachment is far down on the cementum, and the surface of the root is covered with calculus. The epithelium lining the pocket is irregular in pattern, and proliferating projections of this epithelium surround masses of granulation tissue in which there are numerous inflammatory cells. There is a complete loss of arrangement of the periodontal fibers, and much of the alveolar process has been resorbed.

(Center) An infrabony pocket is seen on the left extending below the level of the alveolar crest. The papilla is blunt and folded, and relatively few inflammatory cells are present. The width of the periodontal membrane (on the left) is increased, and there is disorganization of the principal fibers. In the same area the vessels are more numerous and dilated. The interdental septum is markedly resorbed, and fibrosis of some of the marrow spaces is apparent. In this case both vertical and horizontal loss of supporting structures has occurred.

(Bottom) Two teeth with periodontitis in different stages are shown in this photomicrograph. There is marked vertical bone loss next to the tooth at the left with a deep pocket extending far below the alveolar bone crest. The intense inflammation beneath the pocket epithelium makes it difficult to distinguish the epithelial boundary. Connective tissue fiber bundles extend from the alveolar bone crest down along the bone's surface to insert into the cementum below the base of the pocket. Such a pocket is a good candidate for treatment by subgingival curettage. After removal of the pocket epithelium, the residual periodontal membrane participates in organization of the blood clot and regeneration of alveolar bone and fibers. Debris trapped in such narrow, deep pockets may initiate a periodontal abscess. On the left side of the tooth to the right, well oriented periodontal fibers are present on the apical half of the root. Above the alveolar crest there is marked inflammation, but the epithelial attachment has not moved far apically. At the far right a deep pocket is seen, and there is more bone loss. Pocket depth may vary at different places on the same tooth.

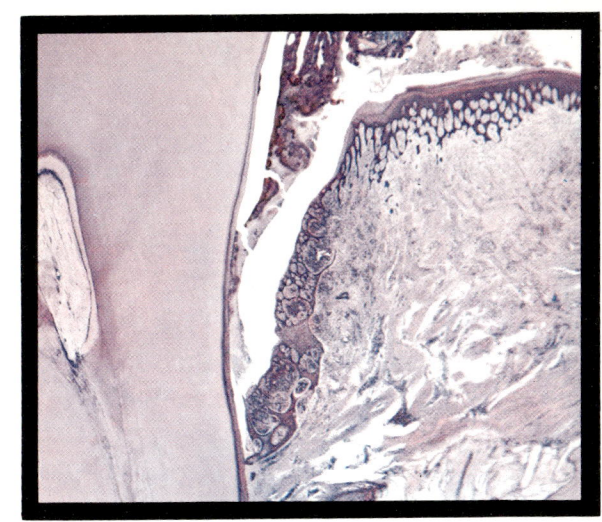

Advanced Periodontitis, Deep Pocket   X 16

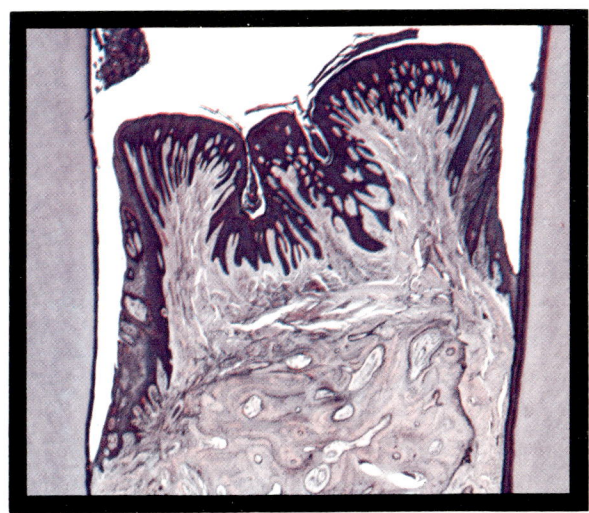

Infrabony Pocket   X 17

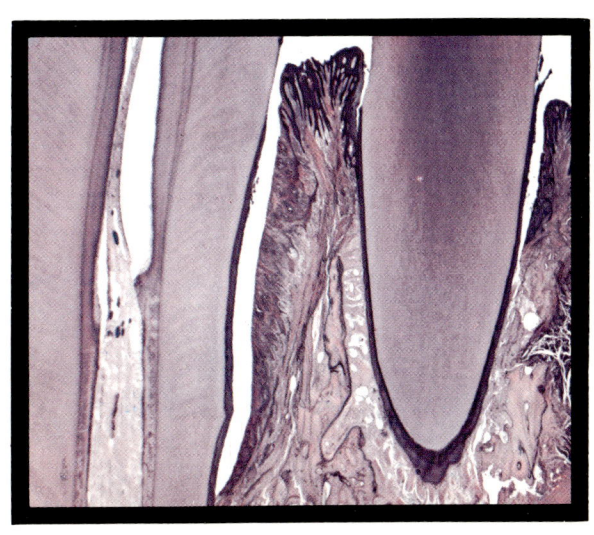

Advanced Infrabony Pocket   X 10

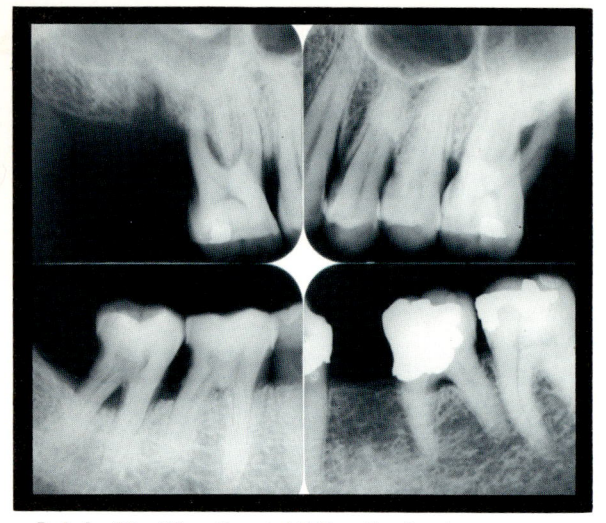

Periodontitis, Bifurcation and Trifurcation Involvement

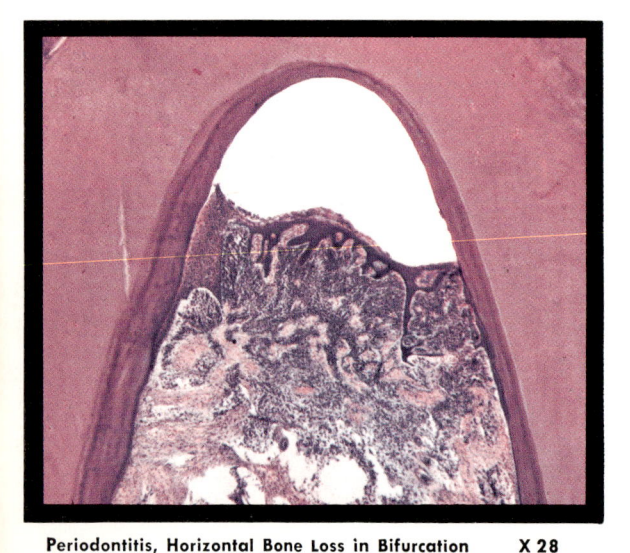

Periodontitis, Horizontal Bone Loss in Bifurcation   X 28

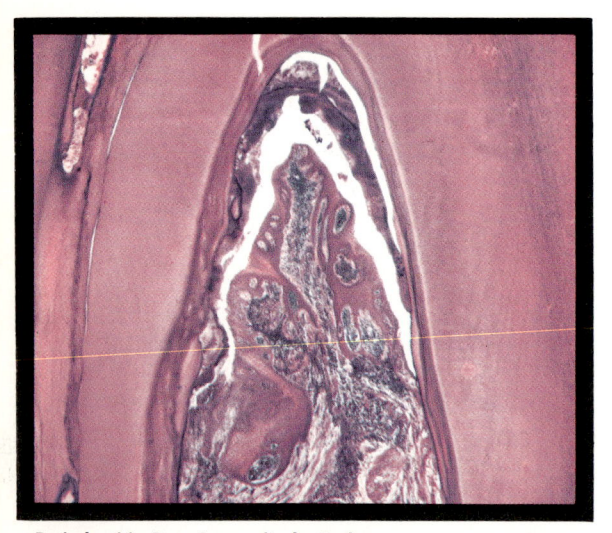

Periodontitis, Deep Interradicular Pockets   X 22

PERIODONTAL DISEASE INVOLVING INTERRADICULAR AREAS

When periodontitis has advanced to the degree of involving the interradicular area, it is usually advisable not to attempt treatment of that particular tooth. It is important, therefore, to be cognizant of all such areas when analyzing a case and deciding on a plan of treatment. Bifurcation or trifurcation involvement, however, is frequently overlooked, both clinically and radiographically. Inflammatory hyperplasia of gingival tissue may mask the interradicular destruction. In radiographs these areas of decreased density may not be discerned because of improper angulation or the superimposition of radiopaque tissues.

(Top) The upper left film demonstrates that the deep pocket about the distal buccal root extends into the trifurcation. In the lower left radiograph a horizontal type of bone loss is evident, and there is interradicular involvement of both molars—slight in the 1st and advanced in the 2nd. The upper right film illustrates interradicular involvement of the 1st molar and extensive bone loss about the distal buccal root. At the lower right, the molar with the large restoration has a radiolucent area between the roots. This destruction resulted from extension of buccal and lingual pockets.

(Center) Photomicrograph demonstrates advanced horizontal destruction with complete exposure of the bifurcation. The epithelial attachment is comparatively broad on both of the root surfaces. Beneath the irregular covering epithelium is granulation tissue in which there are numerous inflammatory cells. This granulation tissue fills the space formerly occupied by the periodontal membrane and the interradicular bony septum.

(Bottom) This photomicrograph illustrates the histologic appearance of a tooth in which a deep labial or lingual pocket extends into the bifurcation. Calculus and soft tissue nearly fill the interradicular area, so that clinically the gingival level might appear normal. If a probe were passed into the crevice, however, the marked destruction would be readily evident. In bifurcation involvement of this configuration, pus is frequently trapped.

Diseases of the Teeth and Supporting Structures

TRAUMATISM

Trauma from occlusion exists when abnormal masticatory force has caused injury to the dental pulp, the temporomandibular joint or the periodontium. It may be a contributing factor and occasionally an initiating factor in periodontal disease. The signs, symptoms and pathologic changes related to occlusal trauma are due mainly to disturbances in circulation. In the periodontal tissues there may be edema, congestion, hemorrhage, thrombosis, necrosis, atrophy, degeneration, resorption of bone and cementum, and repair.

(Top) Clinical appearance of the gingiva in one stage of traumatism. There is excessive incisal wear and moderate but generalized gingival recession. The gingival margins are thick, and some of the interdental papillae are slightly bulbous, although they do not fill the embrasures. Stillman's clefts are apparent in the region of the lower central incisors, the one below the left central being more advanced. These fine vertical clefts are produced by atrophy of the labial gingiva, together with extension of adjacent hyperplastic tissue into the area of recession.

(Center) McCall's festoons (most apparent in this case about the lower anterior teeth) are seen frequently in traumatism but are not pathognomonic of it. These semilunar enlargements of the free gingival margin are the result of compensatory hyperplasia and degeneration of free gingival fibers. Other signs and symptoms of occlusal traumatism are increased mobility of teeth, loss of interproximal contacts, sensitivity of teeth, gingival cyanosis, and disturbances of the temporomandibular joint.

(Bottom) Abnormal force, applied in this case in a distal lingual direction, has caused drifting and spacing of the bicuspids, irregular vertical bone loss, wedge-shaped thickening of the periodontal spaces, and uneven thickness of the lamina dura. If excessive horizontal force is applied in a plane that can be visualized in a radiograph, the typical findings are a cervicolateral wedge-shaped widening of periodontal space on one side and an apicolateral widening on the opposite side.

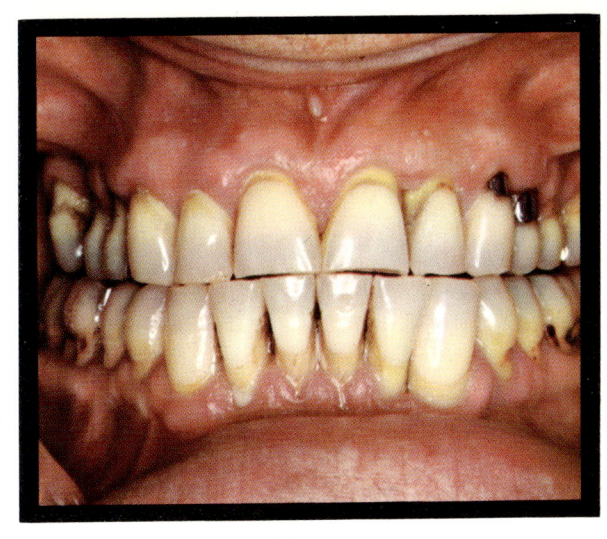

Traumatism, Stillman's Clefts

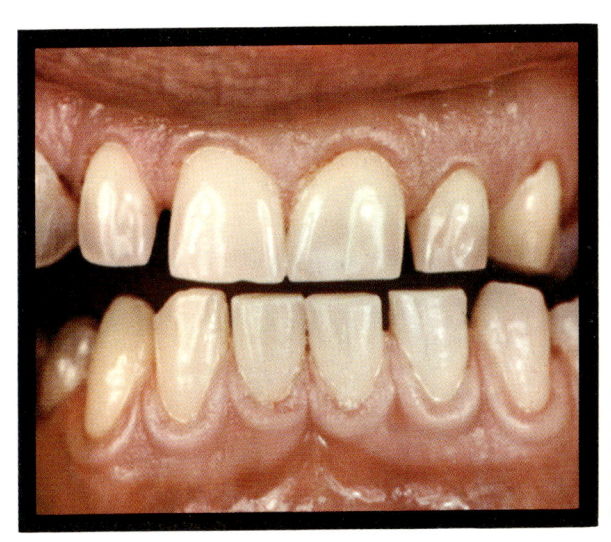

Traumatism, McCall's Festoons

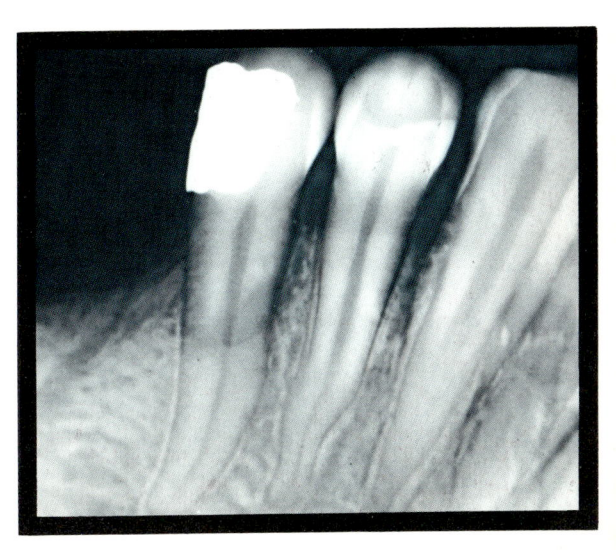

Traumatism

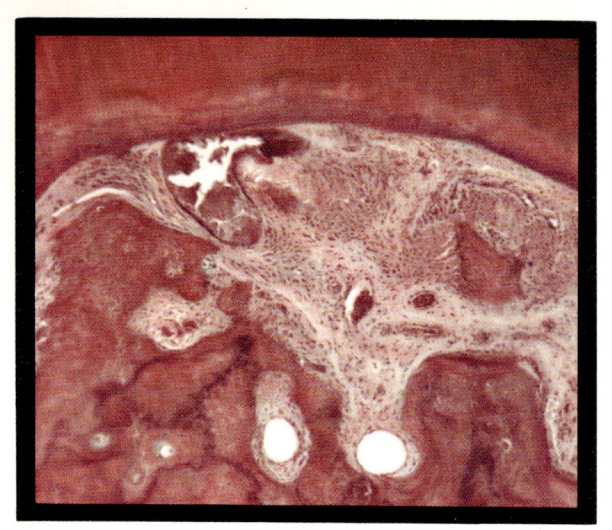

Traumatism, Early Changes X 40

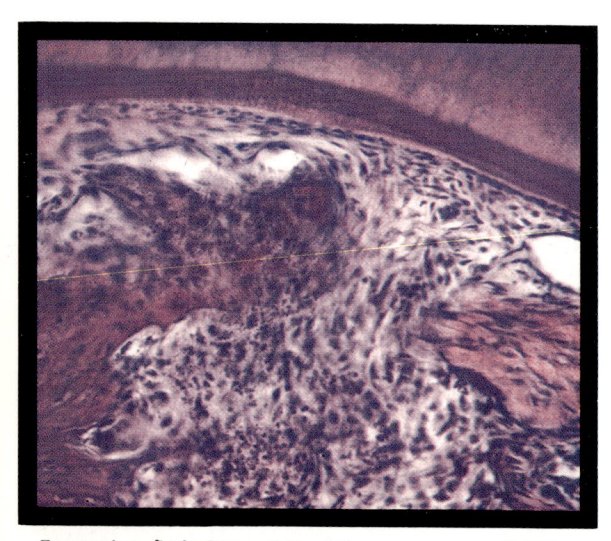

Traumatism, Early Stage of Resolution X 120

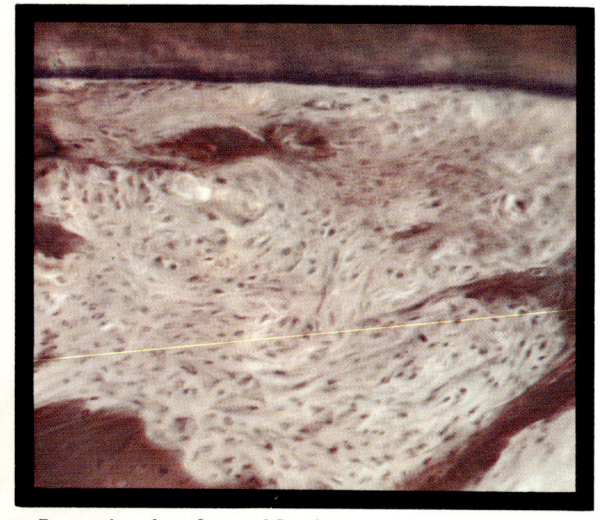

Traumatism, Late Stage of Resolution X 190

Traumatism (Cont.)

A tooth may change position in the jaw without deleterious effect in well-regulated orthodontic treatment, in physiologic mesial drift and in response to mild alteration of masticatory forces. In these instances there is a slow resorption of the alveolar bone on one side of the tooth and a compensating deposition in response to tension on the opposite side. If a tooth is subjected to severe abnormal stress, however, the periodontal membrane may be compressed markedly, causing impairment of the circulation, which in turn results in degeneration or necrosis. Bone is resorbed extensively in the pressure area and replaced temporarily by granulation tissue. This combination of changes is favorable for the extension of gingival inflammation and may result in sudden deep pocket formation unless the traumatic force and local irritants are eliminated and the tooth stabilized.

(Top) Bifurcation area of a molar tooth showing early changes of traumatism. At extreme left there is hyalin degeneration of the compressed periodontal membrane. Near this area is a large thrombosed vessel (hemorrhage associated with this vessel in other sections). In most of the photomicrograph the periodontal space is widened due to resorption of the crest of the interradicular septum. In this region young connective tissue and some residual periodontal fibers are present.

(Center) In this case the periodontal membrane and a portion of the bone are replaced by granulation tissue in which there are numerous inflammatory cells. Osteoclastic resorption of the remaining bone is evident. If epithelial rests were present in such an area, they might be stimulated to proliferate.

(Bottom) Healing stage of traumatism from region along the lateral root surface (picture rotated 90°). Nearly all of the lamina dura and some of the alveolar process have been resorbed. The fibrous connective tissue replacing the periodontal membrane and extending into the marrow spaces is free of inflammatory cells and shows some degree of maturity. It is loose and, as yet, shows no functional orientation. (Compare normal periodontum, p. 6).

FIBROUS (FIBROID) EPULIS

Epulis is a term applied to discrete gingival enlargements, including benign neoplasms. In fibrous (fibroid) epulis fibroblastic proliferation predominates. The lesion is due to a low-grade irritation of long duration which results in an exuberant overgrowth of granulation tissue with fibrous organization. It is similar to the fibrotic nodules produced by cheek chewing (p. 138). It is not a true neoplasm but is an exaggeration of the repair process. Surgical removal usually is indicated.

(Top) A slightly lobulated fibrous epulis located between the maxillary right cuspid and the lateral incisor. It is firm, pedunculated and light pink in color. The surface of these lesions may be ulcerated because of trauma. They may slowly increase in size if the irritating factor (usually in the gingival sulcus) is still present.

(Center) This photomicrograph is a low-power view of the epulis seen in the top picture. At the upper left is a portion of the alveolar mucosa, and at the other end of the cut surface is part of the interdental papilla. The oval nodule arising from the gingiva is composed of dense fibrous connective tissue. This particular lesion is of long duration and static. In other instances histologic examination might reveal more epithelial hyperplasia and young proliferating connective tissue heavily infiltrated with inflammatory cells. A fibrous epulis is sometimes referred to as a gingival fibroma, but in no sense is it a true neoplasm. It is not necessary to sacrifice teeth in the removal of this lesion, for it has a superficial origin. It may recur, however, if the base is not completely excised and the source of irritation eliminated.

(Bottom) In the central portion of this gingival enlargement an extensive amount of trabecular bone is evident. Ossification occurred because young connective tissue cells differentiated into osteoblasts. In addition to ectopic bone formation, mucoid degeneration and dystrophic calcification are relatively frequent findings in fibrous epulides.

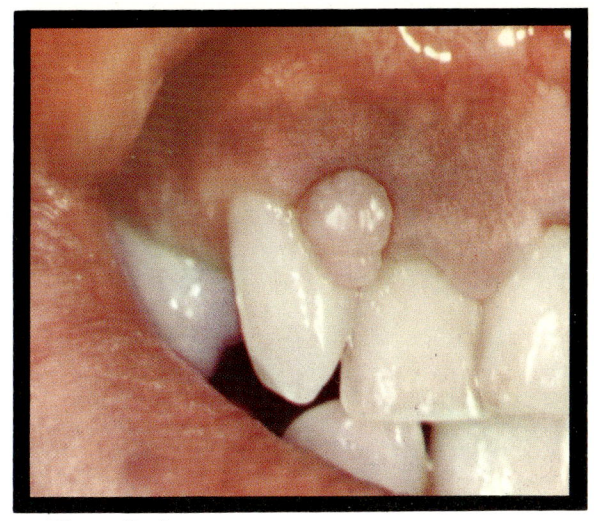

Fibrous Epulis

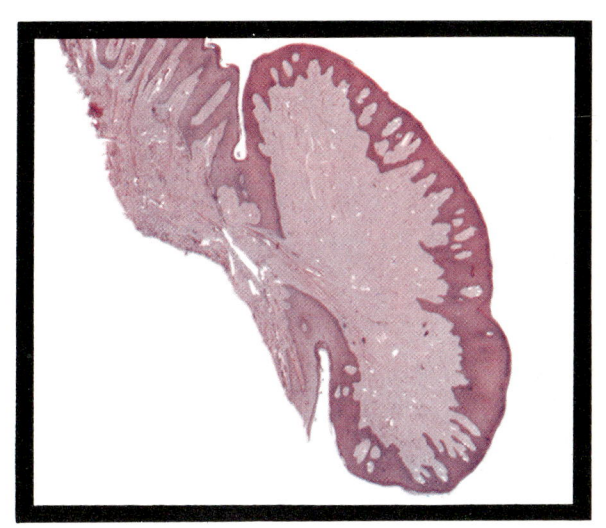

Fibrous Epulis   X 17

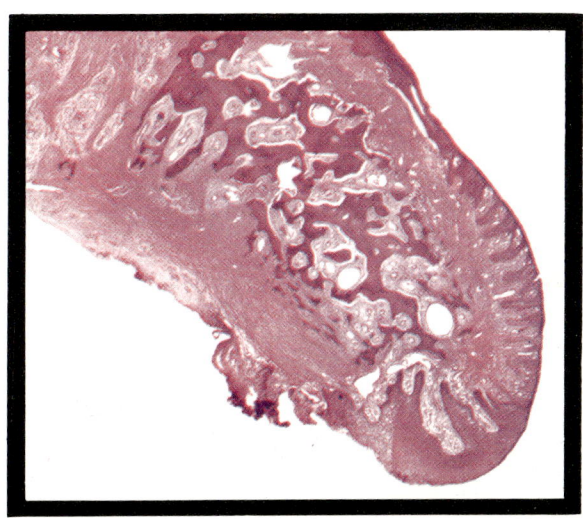

Fibrous Epulis with Ossification   X 20

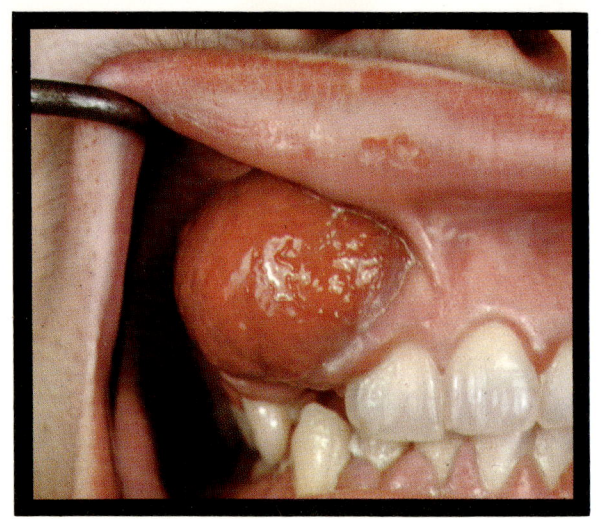

Giant Cell Epulis

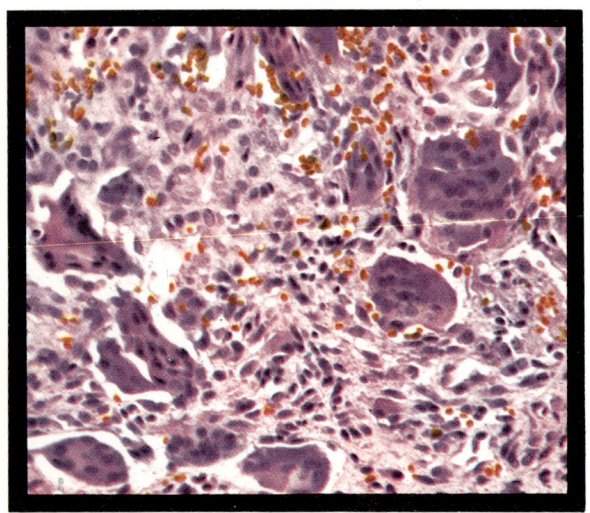

Giant Cell Epulis   X 230

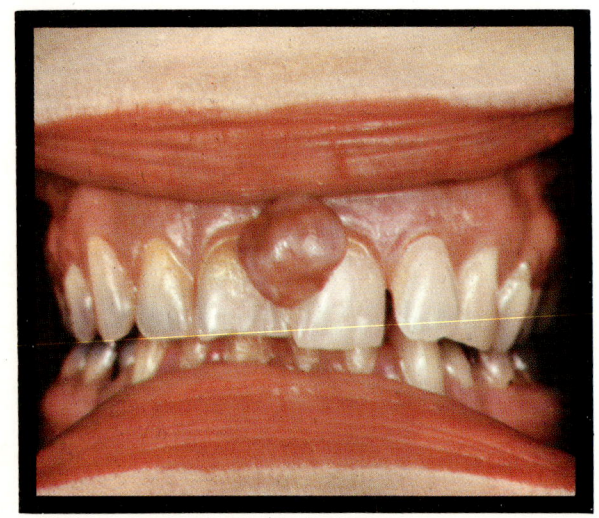

Pregnancy "Tumor," 2 Months Postpartum

GIANT CELL EPULIS

(Giant Cell Reparative Granuloma)

(Top) Giant cell epulis (peripheral giant cell reparative granuloma), once erroneously termed a giant cell sarcoma, is a nonneoplastic enlargement characterized by proliferating fibroblasts forming a stroma containing numerous multinucleated giant cells. Clinically, the lesion usually is soft, sessile or slightly pedunculated and purple to deep red in color. It is often fairly large and has a relatively high incidence in children. It may become ulcerated and bleed readily. This entity may involve the periodontal membrane but also occurs in edentulous areas. Occasionally it may cause superficial bone destruction. It recurs rapidly if not completely removed. Sometimes the lesions stop growing, fibrose and become indistinguishable from fibrous epulides.

(Center) This photomicrograph demonstrates the spindle cell stroma and the multinucleated giant cells which are typical of this lesion. Other characteristic features of this entity are hemosiderin-filled macrophages and numerous red blood cells located in sinusoidal spaces and extravascularly. Whether the giant cells are osteoclasts or of the foreign body type is in dispute. A histologically similar lesion in the jaws, designated as a central giant cell tumor or giant cell reparative granuloma, is indistinguishable from a "brown tumor" occurring in hyperparathyroidism (p. 129).

GRANULOMA GRAVIDARUM

(Pregnancy "Tumor")

(Bottom) Granuloma gravidarum is a discrete red, soft, lobulated blastomatoid enlargement of the gingiva which occurs in 1 to 2 per cent of patients having pregnancy gingivitis. This lesion, which bleeds easily because of its marked vascularity, cannot be distinguished histologically from pregnancy gingivitis (p. 79) or granuloma pyogenicum (p. 119). Excision should be delayed, if possible, until the tumor partially involutes (after parturition); removal during pregnancy may result in quick recurrence. In the case illustrated the preexisting gingivitis has subsided, and the lesion has decreased markedly in size.

4
Diseases of the Oral Mucosa and the Jaws

INTRODUCTION

Diseases of the oral mucosa may be divided into those of local origin and those that reflect systemic disease, although general factors may influence the course and even the initiation of diseases of local origin, and local factors may determine whether a given general disease will show local manifestations and how the lesions will progress.

Systemic infections which may show oral lesions include syphilis, tuberculosis, measles and primary herpes. Such generalized metabolic disturbances as anemia, avitaminosis, hyperparathyroidism and acromegaly may produce oral lesions. Diseases of obscure origin such as scleroderma, pemphigus, lupus erythematosis and lichen planus may have oral signs or symptoms.

Many disturbances of local origin are due to physical or chemical irritants. Among these are cheek-chewing lesions, hyperplasias from denture irritations, amputation neuromas and drug burns. Radiation, coal-tar products of tobacco, and electrogalvanism are other local irritants that may be of etiologic importance. Localized infections include osteomyelitis, actinomycosis, thrush and, in some instances, sialadenitis. Benign migratory glossitis (geographic tongue) and periadenitis mucosa necrotica recurrens are examples of noninfectious inflammations of local origin.

Not all of the diseases of the oral mucosa and jaws are included in this chapter. Neoplasms, disturbances in development and those relating to the supporting structures of the teeth are discussed elsewhere, and, obviously, many are omitted in a book of limited size.

Diagnosis must be established before definite treatment may be instituted. The diagnosis may be quite obvious, or it may be necessary to carry out definite steps before the disease can be recognized. A detailed history is taken and recorded. The lesion should be examined carefully, both visually and manually, and its characteristics recorded. X-ray examination is essential when calcified tissues are involved. With the history and the clinical and x-ray examination completed, several possible diagnoses may come to mind, and then it may be necessary to ask additional specific questions or to seek assistance through the use of the biopsy technic or from specific laboratory tests. Even though the diagnosis of a given lesion may appear simple, the capable clinician will seek complete information and think carefully before he makes his decision.

It is important to be able to recognize the cause of a given oral disease and to distinguish lesions of local origin from those with generalized causes. To do this it is necessary to have a thorough knowledge of those systemic diseases which produce oral lesions and of the appearance of the locally produced disturbances. The treatment for diseases of local origin, obviously, is quite different than that for diseases of systemic origin, although many lesions of systemic origin require local, as well as systemic, therapy. Failure to recognize the systemic origin of oral ulcers resulting from agranulocytosis may lead to delay in initiating proper therapy and thus jeopardize the patient's life. Oral lesions of pernicious anemia left undiagnosed or misdiagnosed may delay therapy until irreversible neurologic changes have occurred. The dentist, as the member of the health services team responsible for the oral cavity, must accept his obligation to diagnose and treat diseases of the oral mucosa and jaw bones.

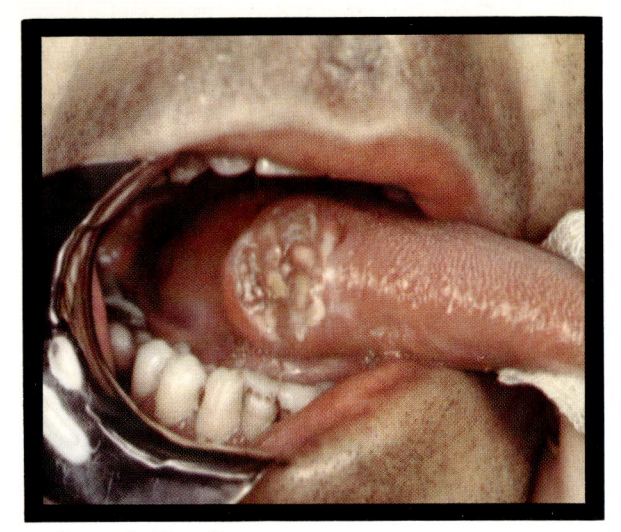

Traumatic Ulcer, Tongue

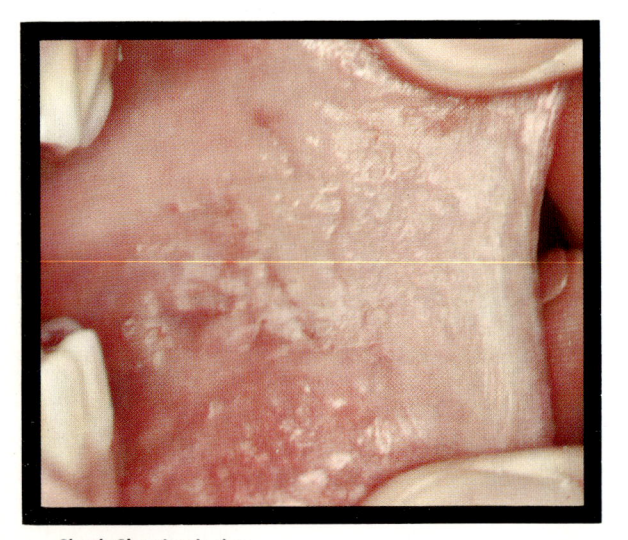

Cheek Chewing Lesion

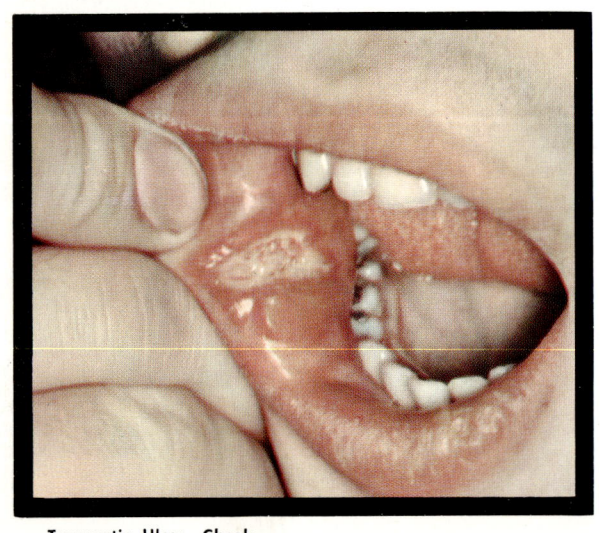

Traumatic Ulcer, Cheek

CHEEK AND TONGUE CHEWING

(Top) Three weeks before this picture was taken the patient severely lacerated his tongue while chewing. The area of injury became secondarily infected, and this large ulcerated lesion with a raised, rolled border developed. The surrounding tissue was firm to palpation. Such a lesion cannot be differentiated clinically from carcinoma (see p. 156) and should be considered malignant until proved otherwise by histologic examination. This lesion healed following penicillin therapy, but that treatment was not instituted until it had been established that the lesion was inflammatory and not neoplastic. In cases such as this in which there is a strong clinical impression of malignancy, it is good practice to have 2 negative biopsy reports, the 2nd biopsy being done because of the possibility that the 1st was not from a representative area.

(Center) Some individuals have a nervous habit of nibbling on the cheek mucosa unconsciously. As demonstrated in the illustration, this may produce a thin, rough keratotic film in the area irritated. Fragments of epithelium, attached at one end, are often seen in these cases due to continual nibbling on the same area. Grasping these shreds of tissue with the teeth and stripping them off leaves red, raw, eroded areas. Patients usually deny the nibbling habit, but the lesions resulting from it are generally very characteristic.

(Bottom) A large ulcerated lesion which resulted from a single act of trauma. It is not uncommon for most people at some time or other to bite the cheek inadvertently while chewing. Lesions produced by these injuries are usually not severe, and they heal rapidly. In the case illustrated, however, the teeth probably penetrated deep into the tissue, causing vascular damage. The thrombosis that followed deprived the area of its nutrient supply, and necrosis resulted. This type of lesion tends to be expansile for a few days after the injury. Due to secondary infection and the extensiveness of these lesions, they usually heal slowly, with the production of abundant granulation tissue. Because of their persistence and their indurated borders, they may simulate carcinoma clinically.

Diseases of the Oral Mucosa and Jaws

Cheek and Tongue Chewing (Cont.)

(Top) The soft, linear streak of parakeratin seen in the buccal mucosa at the occlusal line is frequently termed linea alba. These lesions usually occur in individuals with thick cheeks that are closely adapted to the buccal surfaces of the teeth. The line may be initiated by irritation from rough buccal cusps. This condition may be intensified by the habit of sucking and chewing on the cheeks.

TRAUMATIC (AMPUTATION) NEUROMA

This entity is not a neoplasm, as the name might imply, but an exaggerated response to nerve injury. Peripheral nerves have a great propensity for regeneration. When such a nerve is severed, both parts degenerate—the peripheral end completely, and the proximal portion back to the first node of Ranvier. After degeneration is completed, the stump of the nerve begins to grow along its old course and, if not impeded, will completely reinnervate the part. If the regenerating nerve tissue meets some obstruction such as dense scar tissue, it may continue to proliferate locally, and a nodule of nerve and scar tissue may be formed. The mass thus produced is a traumatic neuroma. If sensory nerves are involved, pain is felt upon pressure. Traumatic neuromas frequently occur in amputation stumps. The most common oral site is over the mental foramen in edentulous mouths, but they may occur wherever a tooth has been removed.

(Center) A tangled mass of nerve and scar tissue forming an ovoid enlargement at the end of a nerve. This appeared as a slowly enlarging, painful nodule in the neck following by 2 years the dissection of cervical lymph nodes in the treatment of carcinoma, metastatic from the tongue.

(Bottom) Photomicrograph of a portion of the above neuroma demonstrating the intermingling nerve elements and scar tissue. The reddish-purple areas are dense fibrous connective tissue; the light-lavender-staining components are nerve fascicles. With the stain used, the axon cylinders are not apparent at this magnification. The small, dark-staining, wavy, spindle-shaped structures are Schwann cell nuclei.

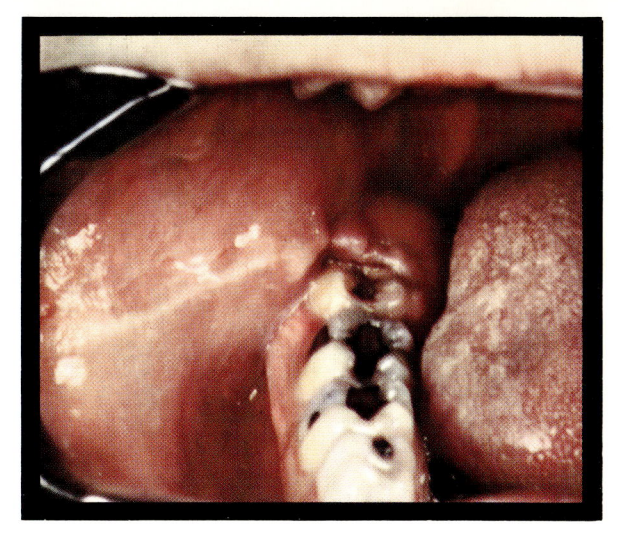

Linea Alba

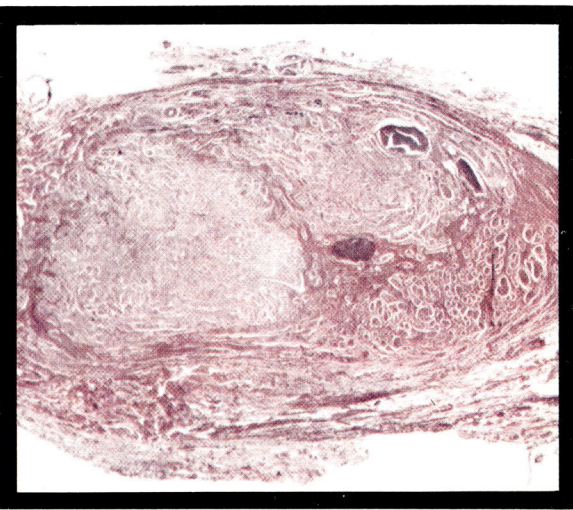

Traumatic Neuroma   X 12

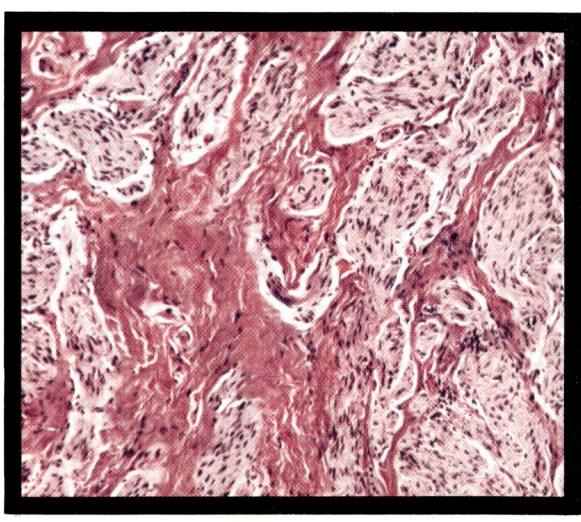

Traumatic Neuroma, Higher Magnification of Same Specimen   X 100

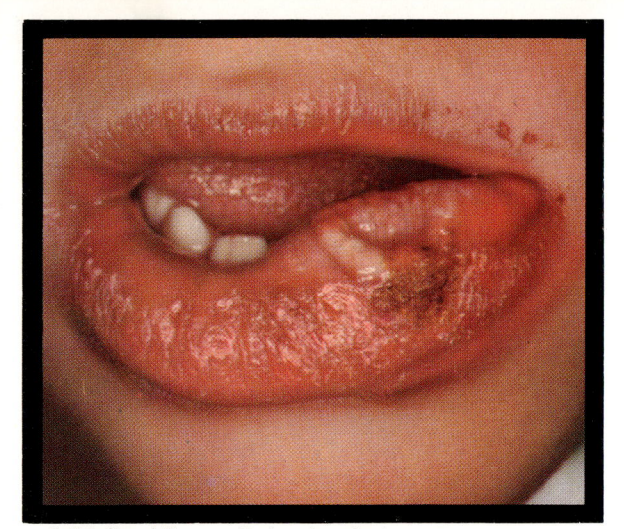

Self-Inflicted Trauma During Anesthesia

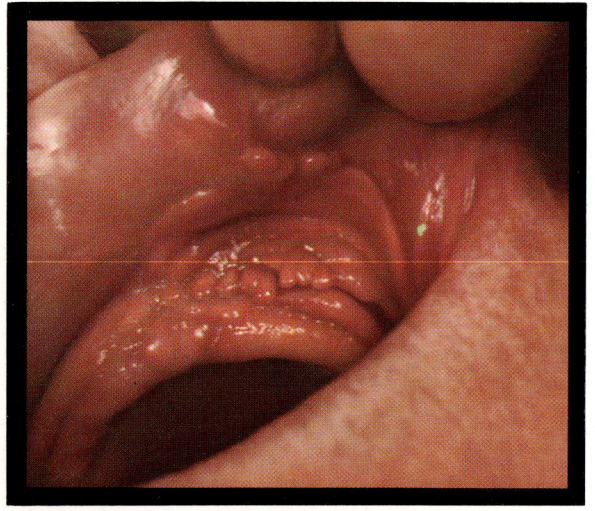

Inflammatory Hyperplasia, Alveolar Mucosa

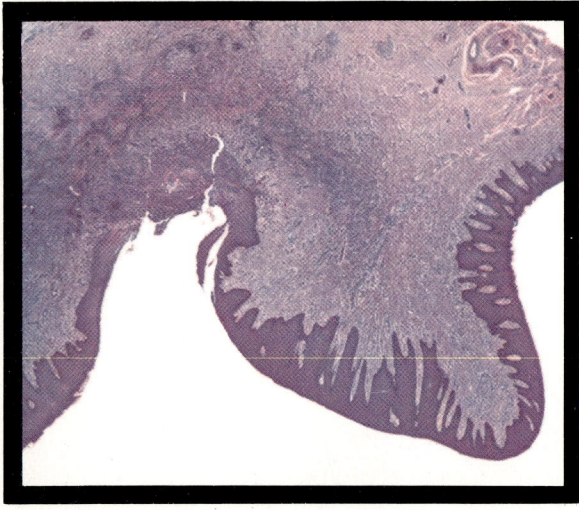

Inflammatory Hyperplasia, Alveolar Mucosa   X 13

SELF-INFLICTED TRAUMA DURING ANESTHESIA

(Top) This lesion resulted from biting the lip while it was anesthetized. Such a penetrating wound with superficial secondary infection is occasionally found in children following their first experience with mandibular block anesthesia. The child may bite the anesthetized lip inadvertently while eating or, fascinated with the tingling sensation, may playfully chew on it much harder than he realizes because no pain is felt. In most instances neither the patient nor the parents may be aware that the wound was self-inflicted and may believe that some accident occurred during dental treatment. Emphatically forewarning both the child and the parents of the injury that can be produced by biting the lip will often prevent its occurrence.

HYPERPLASIA FROM DENTURE IRRITATION

(Center) The numerous curtainlike folds of excess tissue are the result of wearing an ill-fitting maxillary denture. Originally there may be a small ulcer (denture cut), but as the soft tissue continues to be irritated by the denture flange, a productive inflammation results. This type of hyperplasia is frequently seen about the anterior part of a full maxillary denture when the patient has natural anterior mandibular teeth but no posterior replacements. Inflammatory hyperplasia of this sort, while basically similar to that occurring elsewhere in response to chronic irritation, is commonly termed epulis fissuratum because of the cleft or clefts found in the enlargement.

(Bottom) A fissure which accommodated the edge of a denture is apparent along the lower border of this cross-sectioned biopsy specimen. At the bottom of this deep crevice there is ulceration. The whole specimen is heavily infiltrated with inflammatory cells. The bulbous enlargement at the right would be seen clinically as a fold of tissue hanging over the periphery of the denture. The covering epithelium is slightly hyperplastic, but this soft tissue enlargement is mainly the result of fibrous tissue proliferation and inflammation.

Hyperplasia from Denture Irritation (Cont.)

(Top) Inflammatory papillary hyperplasia of the palatal mucosa is frequently observed under ill-fitting dentures, especially those having a relief chamber. The hyperplasia is produced in response to irritation from movement of the denture and from accumulating debris. The polypoid masses are usually intensely red, soft and freely movable. If the denture is not worn for several days, the inflammation will subside, and the size of the papillomatous nodules may be reduced. They seldom disappear completely and should be removed surgically.

(Center) This is a photomicrograph of a section of tissue removed from the palate in the above case. The surface epithelium along the lower border of the specimen is hyperplastic, and long, slender rete pegs extend into the corium, which is quite vascular and very heavily infiltrated with inflammatory cells. It is apparent that there has been a proliferation of connective tissue which has contributed to the formation of the papillomatous masses. Some of these may show dyskeratosis in the epithelium and, rarely, frank carcinoma.

TRAUMATIC BONE LESION

(Bottom) Traumatic bone lesions (hemorrhagic or extravasation cysts) are localized areas of bone necrosis that are purported to result from intramedullary hematomas which do not become organized. The intra-osseous hemorrhage is believed to be related to a traumatic incident in an area of the bone which has hemopoietic marrow. In specific cases, however, a history of trauma may be impossible to obtain. These bone lesions, which occur in young individuals, are asymptomatic and are usually discovered during a routine radiographic examination. They are frequently found near the apex of teeth but are not related to periapical inflammation. The teeth in the vicinity test vital, and thus these lesions may be differentiated from periodontal cysts. Exposure of a traumatic lesion reveals a dry bony cavity containing no cystic lining. The cortical bone over the lesion may be thin but usually is not expanded.

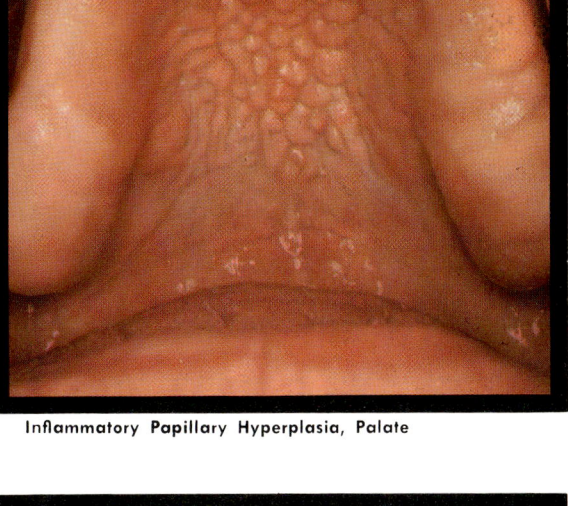

Inflammatory Papillary Hyperplasia, Palate

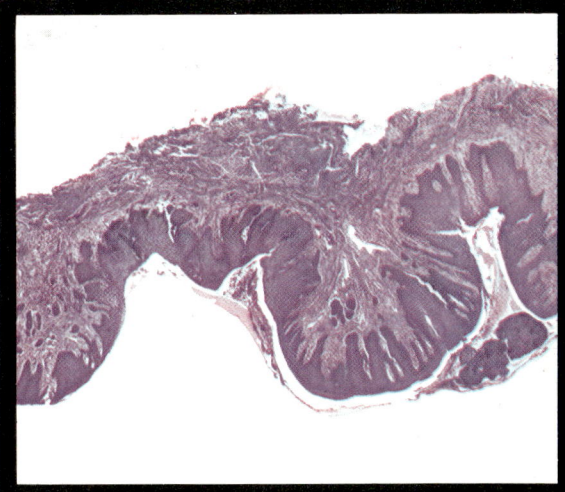

Inflammatory Papillary Hyperplasia   X 17

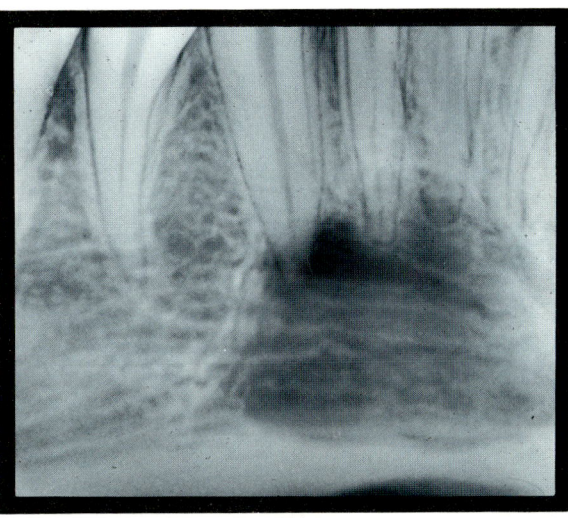

Traumatic Bone Lesion, Mandible

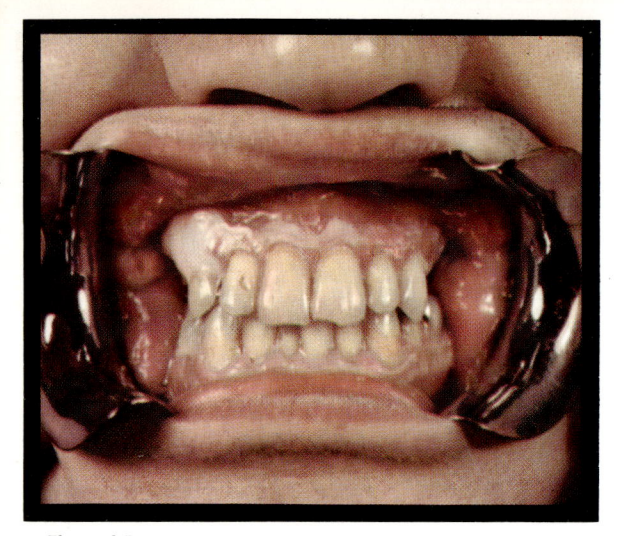

Thermal Burn, Impression Material

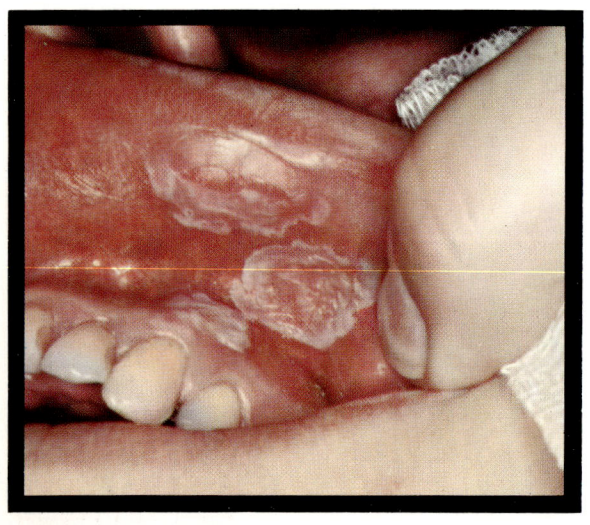

Chemical Burn, Aspirin

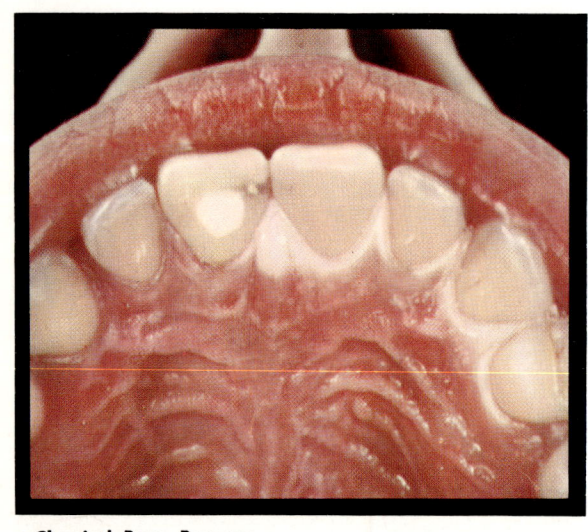

Chemical Burn, Pyrozone

THERMAL BURNS

(Top) Extensive thermal burns do not often occur in the oral cavity, principally because of its inaccessibility to most of the severe thermal hazards. Minor burns, as from very hot beverages or foods, occasionally occur on the palatal or labial mucosa even though this tissue is somewhat protected from thermal injury by its moist surface. Severe sloughing of the oral mucosa from flash burns is occasionally seen in combat personnel. Burns of varying degrees of severity may result from careless application of the cautery, using dental instruments which are too hot, dropping hot wax on the tissues, or using impression material which is at too high a temperature. In the patient shown, the coagulation of the gingival mucosa resulted from taking an impression with hydrocolloid material which was at a temperature sufficiently high to injure the tissue. Within 24 hours all of the coagulated material sloughed, exposing the underlying bone.

CHEMICAL BURNS

(Center) The placing of an aspirin tablet in the mucobuccal fold for alleviation of dental pain is a common but unwarranted practice. It usually results in the coagulation of cytoplasm, producing a discrete white area corresponding roughly to the size and shape of the tablet. The lesions are generally superficial unless the aspirin tablets are used repeatedly in this improper manner. If powdered aspirin is applied, a larger area of the mucosa will be involved. Chemical burns may also be produced by numerous other substances; the most frequently encountered are caused by sodium perborate, phenol, toothache drops and zinc chloride. The lesions are not specific for each drug, and it is necessary to question the patient to determine the causative agent.

(Bottom) This chemical burn was produced by Pyrozone which was being used for bleaching the pulpless maxillary right central incisor. The coagulated tissue is apparent along the gingival margins of all the upper left anterior teeth. The pattern of the affected area corresponds to the typical distribution of a liquid escaping through an improperly adapted rubber dam.

Diseases of the Oral Mucosa and Jaws

GALVANISM

(Top) A galvanic current may be generated in the oral cavity between two dissimilar adjacent metals, with saliva acting as an electrolyte. Occasionally this current may temporarily be of sufficient magnitude to cause injury, as in the case illustrated. This patient experienced intense pain and developed an ulcer on the gingiva following insertion of an amalgam in the mandibular 2nd molar which approximated the gold restoration in the 1st molar.

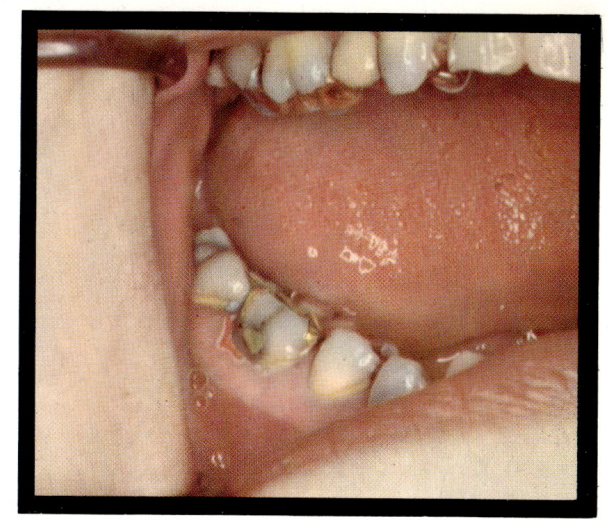

NICOTINIC STOMATITIS

(Center) In this moderately advanced case of nicotinic stomatitis, numerous red dots—the inflamed and dilated orifices of salivary gland ducts—are apparent throughout the whitened palatal mucosa. Earlier the mucosa is intensely red; later it becomes pale, due to a slight increase in cornification. In advanced cases the palatal tissue is more heavily cornified, and nodules appear. A few of these nodules (which are related to hyperplasia of the underlying glands, to retention of saliva and to fibrosis) are seen in this case in the anterior palatal region. Nicotinic stomatitis is observed most frequently in pipe smokers but does occur in individuals who use cigars or cigarettes. The mucosal changes are caused by heat and the irritating effect of the combustion products of tobacco. The intensity of these changes is dependent on the manner of smoking, the quantity of tobacco used, and the sensitivity of the individual.

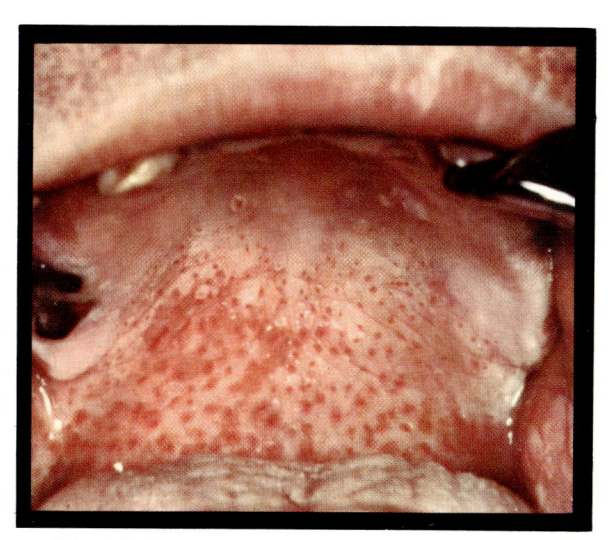

(Bottom) Numerous umbilicated nodules, typical of an advanced case, are evident in the posterior gland-bearing areas. The entire palatal mucosa, except under the partial denture, has a white, cooked appearance. Individuals who wish to continue smoking can prevent further irritating effects of tobacco by wearing an appliance that will cover the palate. Nicotinic stomatitis is a definite clinical entity. The histologic findings, though not pathognomonic, include hyperplasia of surface epithelium with deep, broad, fused rete pegs; hyperkeratosis; dilatation of gland ducts; squamous metaplasia of the ductal epithelium; and sialadenitis of minor glands.

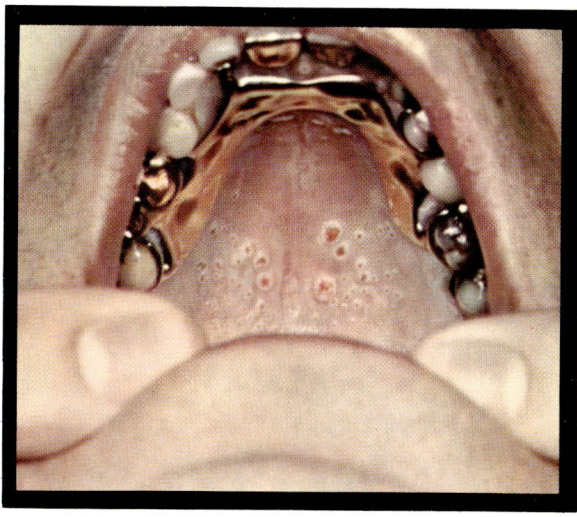

Galvanism

Nicotinic Stomatitis

Nicotinic Stomatitis, Advanced Stage

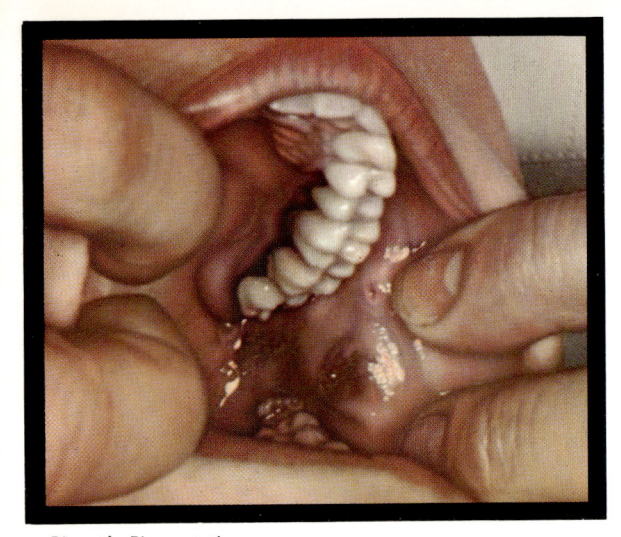

Bismuth Pigmentation

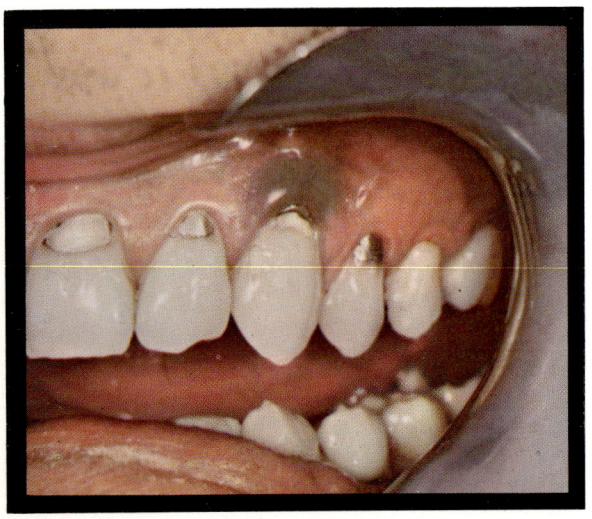

Localized Argyrosis (Amalgam Tattoo)

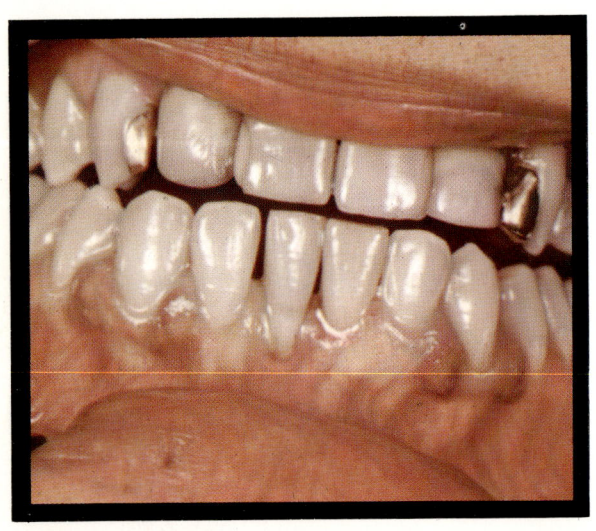

Atabrine Pigmentation

PIGMENTATION

(Top) Oral pigmentations resulting from the generalized absorption of metals are usually caused by bismuth, silver or lead. Lead may be accidentally inhaled or ingested, while the other two are usually introduced into the body intentionally for therapeutic purposes. The patient shown had been receiving bismuth for treatment of syphilis. A dark-blue pigmentation can be seen in the lingual gingiva, the buccal mucosa and the retromolar area. The degree of coloration in these cases is associated with the state of oral hygiene. Decomposing debris about the teeth furnishes hydrogen sulfide, which, when coming in contact with the soluble bismuth salt in the body fluids, leads to the formation of blackish insoluble bismuth sulfide, which is deposited in the tissues. The tongue and buccal mucosa may also become pigmented when these tissues are irritated by accretions or rough areas on the teeth.

(Center) The nonelevated grayish-blue area in the gingiva near the maxillary left cuspid is due to the incorporation in the tissues of silver amalgam filling material. The pigmentation is caused by the formation of an insoluble silver salt which is deposited in the collagen fibers of the lamina propria. Histologically, the pigment is seen as minute brownish-black granules. There is little, if any, tissue reaction to this foreign material, and it is not necessary to remove these pigmented areas except for cosmetic reasons. Localized argyrosis is frequently seen in edentulous areas, probably resulting from the accidental incorporation of amalgam into the tissues during extraction. Occasionally amalgam dust may be implanted in soft tissue by the disking of a tooth containing an amalgam restoration. Generalized argyrosis may result from prolonged ingestion and absorption of silver salts. In such cases the skin of the entire body has a metallic gray color.

(Bottom) The yellowish-brown gingival pigmentation in the cuspid regions is the result of taking the antimalarial drug Atabrine. A yellowish color to the oral mucous membrane as part of a generalized pigmentation may also occur in jaundice, carotenemia, hemochromatosis and Addison's disease.

Diseases of the Oral Mucosa and Jaws

Pigmentation (Cont.)

(Top) Melanin pigmentation of the oral mucosa not associated with pathologic changes is usually termed "physiologic pigmentation." It may occur in individuals of any racial or national origin, being seen occasionally in light-skinned people, commonly in those having darker complexions, and most frequently in Negroes. Physiologic pigmentation is most often observed on the labial and buccal aspects of the gingiva (melanosis gingivae). Other areas involved, in order of frequency, are the buccal mucosa, hard palate, tongue, lips and soft palate.

(Center) This section of tissue was taken from a pigmented area in the oral mucosa. Careful examination of the basal epithelial cells will reveal that they contain a brownish-staining material, melanin, which is not ordinarily apparent in routine histologic sections of oral mucous membrane. In very heavily pigmented areas the melanin, which is formed in special cells in the basal layer (melanocytes), would be seen not only in basal epithelial cells but also in the prickle cells and in phagocytes in the corium. Pigmentary changes sometimes occur in mucous membrane as well as skin following inflammatory reactions. This photomicrograph is of such a case, but the histologic findings in Addison's disease, physiologic pigmentation or Peutz-Jeghers syndrome would be similar.

(Bottom) Excessive melanin pigmentation in and about the oral cavity may be associated with a generalized intestinal polyposis. This relatively rare combination of findings, Peutz-Jeghers syndrome, has been observed most frequently in dark-skinned individuals and appears to be inherited. The melanin spots in this syndrome are most evident on the lips and buccal mucosa but may be present in other portions of the oral cavity, on the face (especially about the mouth) and on the digits. The patient shown, a 21-year-old Mexican, had had 2 operations for removal of intestinal polyps. Circumoral pigmentation was first noted at the age of 2. The spots became more numerous as the patient grew older.

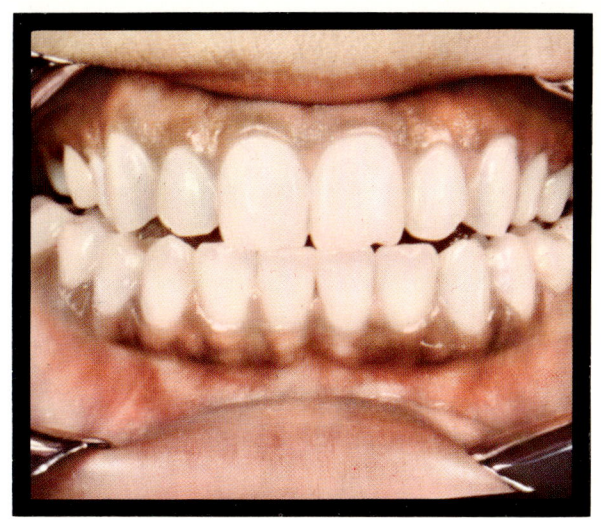

Physiologic Pigmentation (Melanosis Gingivae)

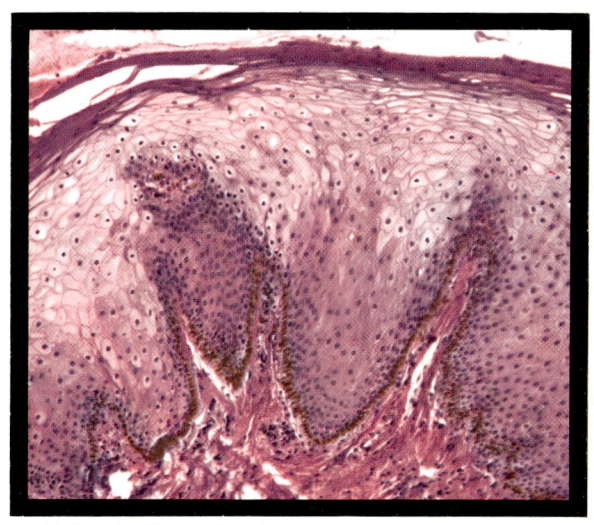

Melanosis, Mucous Membrane   X 100

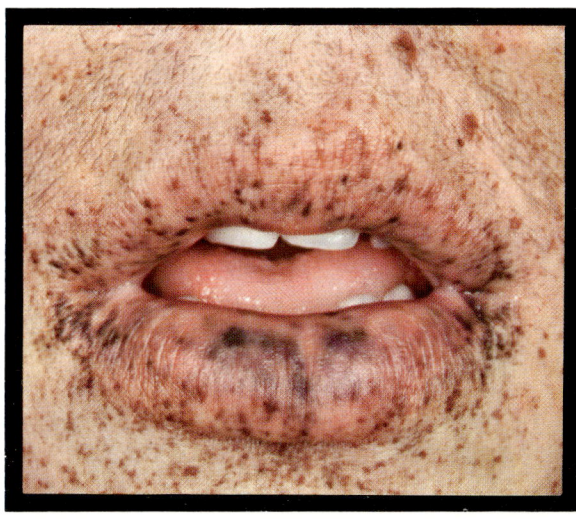

Melanin Pigmentation Associated with Intestinal Polyposis

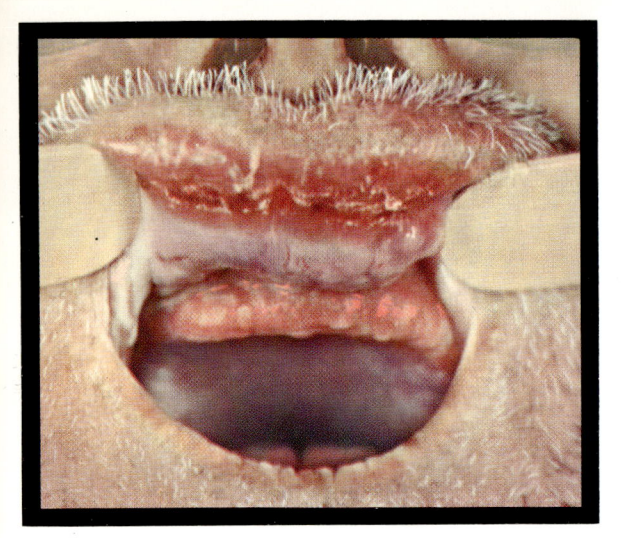

Acute Radiation Reaction, Mucous Membrane

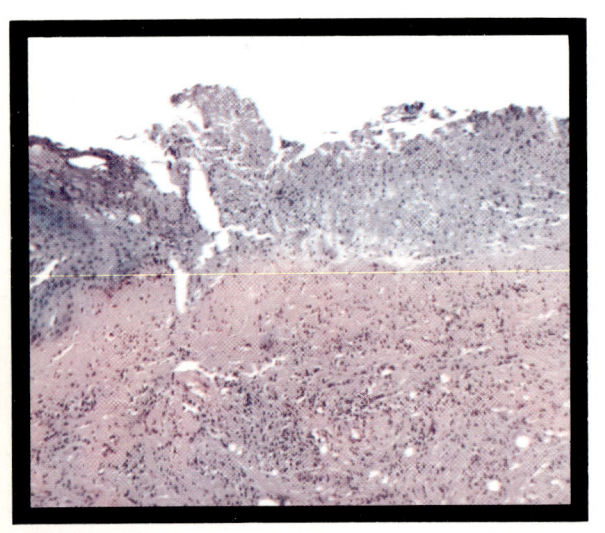

Radiation Effect, Mucous Membrane X 90

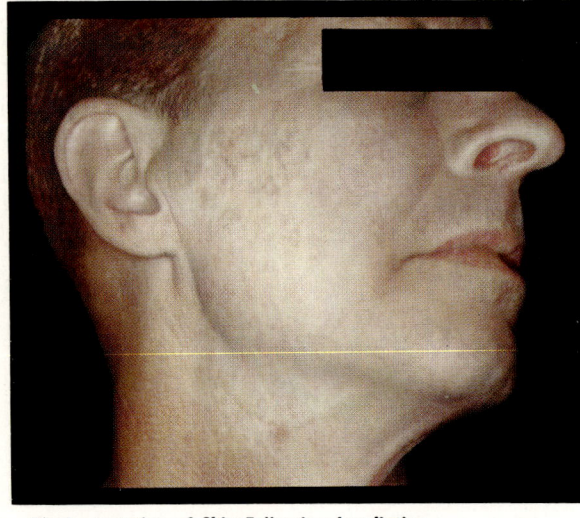

Depigmentation of Skin Following Irradiation

RADIATION EFFECT, SOFT TISSUE AND BONE

Ionizing radiation is of value in treating neoplasms because it injures tissue. In the killing of malignant cells, unless the tumor is exceptionally radiosensitive, some degree of injury to normal tissue occurs. The undesirable effects accompanying radiation therapy are related to the type of radiation, the dosage, the division of the dosage, the amount of shielding, and the susceptibility of the individual. Cells may be killed or their functions may be impaired, intercellular substance may degenerate, blood vessels may sclerose or become telangiectatic. There is no immediate indication of damage to skin or mucous membranes. It is only after a period of approximately 2 weeks that evidence of injury is apparent. The acute reaction following this latent period consists of redness and edema of the area involved. If the dosage is not too great, this reaction will subside, and the tissues eventually become relatively normal. When tissue is exposed to excessive radiation, progressive degenerative changes occur over a period of years, and carcinoma may develop.

(Top) A reddish-purple, edematous area is apparent in the vestibular mucosa. This acute radiation reaction occurred 21 days after the institution of intra-oral x-ray irradiation for treatment of carcinoma on the mandibular alveolar ridge.

(Center) This is a section of mucous membrane that had been injured by ionizing radiation. The covering epithelium on the upper border of the photomicrograph is necrotic. There is homogenization of the collagen in the upper corium, and mucoid degeneration is apparent near the lower border of the picture.

(Bottom) Six years before this picture was taken the patient was treated through the right cheek for intra-oral carcinoma by x-ray irradiation. The residual effects of the radiation are demonstrated by the zone of depigmentation in the lateral aspect of the face and upper neck. In the depigmented area there is also atrophy of the skin and a loss of secondary skin structures. Typical spiderlike, telangiectatic vessels are apparent just anterior to the ear. (See also p. 63, top.)

Diseases of the Oral Mucosa and Jaws

Radiation Effect, Soft Tissue and Bone (Cont.)

(Top) When bone is heavily irradiated, its blood vessels may become sclerosed with a resultant impairment of the blood supply and reduced vitality. Such bone may be asymptomatic for years if the overlying mucosa is intact or if it is not injured. The partially devitalized bone has markedly reduced resistance to infection and poor healing power. Thus trauma or surgical procedures followed by infection may result in extensive, progressive osteomyelitis which will not respond to the usual therapeutic procedures. This particular form of postirradiation osteomyelitis often is called osteoradionecrosis. Some authorities prefer to reserve that term for aseptic necrosis of bone following irradiation, using the designation "radiation osteitis" when infection intervenes. The patient at the right has had heavy irradiation of the maxilla followed by osteoradionecrosis. (See p. 63 for the effect of radiation on teeth.)

(Center) This patient had received intensive x-ray radiation for an intra-oral carcinoma. He remained asymptomatic for years until after extraction of an anterior mandibular tooth. Healing did not occur, and progressive, painful necrosis of the mandible developed. Because periodontal and periapical infections produce bone changes and initiate osteoradionecrosis, the teeth are critical when radiation therapy is to be used in the head and neck region (see p. 63). When intensive irradiation is contemplated and the jawbones and salivary glands cannot be adequately shielded, the teeth should be extracted prior to irradiation. Extraction of teeth from heavily irradiated bone should be avoided, but if extraction is essential, pre- and post-operative antibiotic therapy may reduce the hazard of osteoradionecrosis.

(Bottom) Fingers of a 50-year-old dentist who, early in his practice, had exposed them to an excessive amount of radiation by holding periapical films in patients' mouths. Several years after he discontinued this habit the skin of the fingers gradually became tense, dry and atrophic. Hyperkeratotic and ulcerative lesions appeared. Skin from the right index finger was removed, and the area was grafted. The lesion was a squamous cell carcinoma.

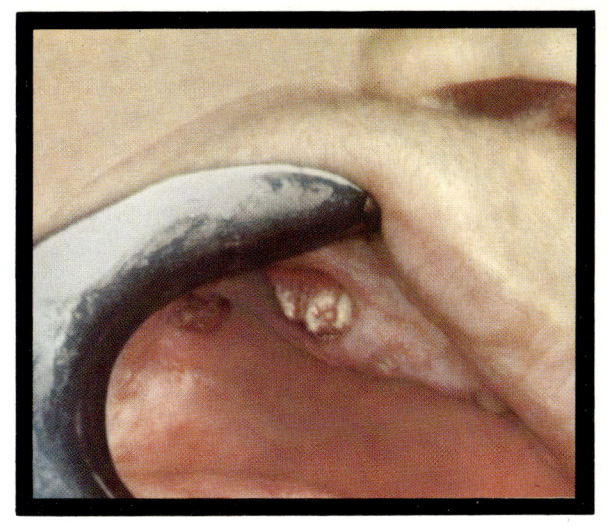

Osteoradionecrosis, maxilla

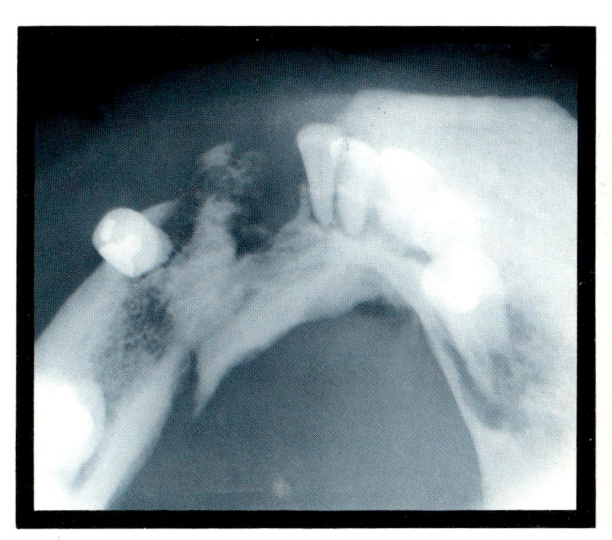

Osteoradionecrosis, mandible

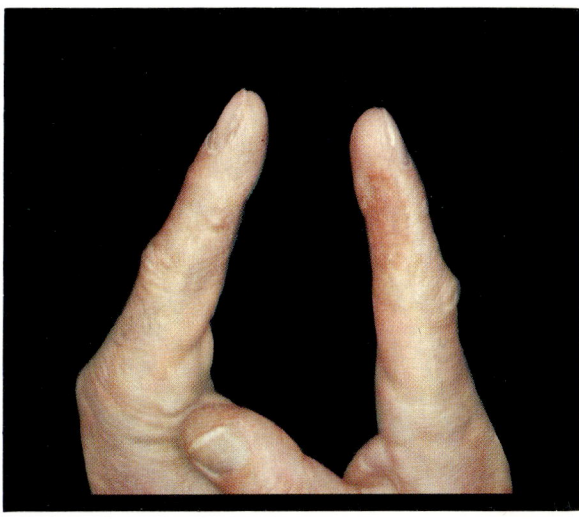

Radiodermatitis, Fingers

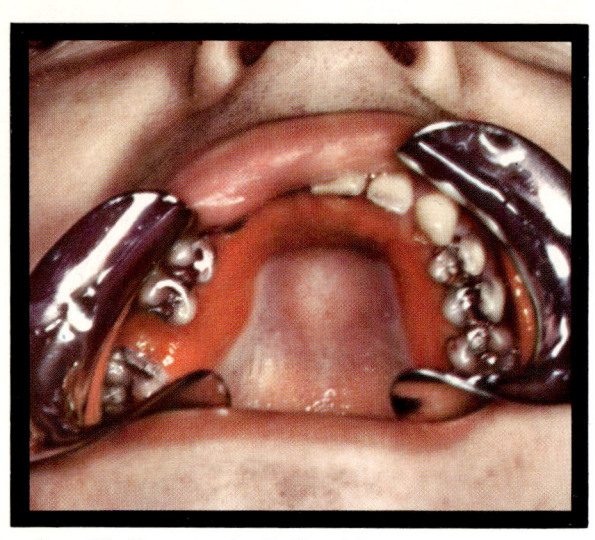

Stomatitis Venenata, Acrylic Material

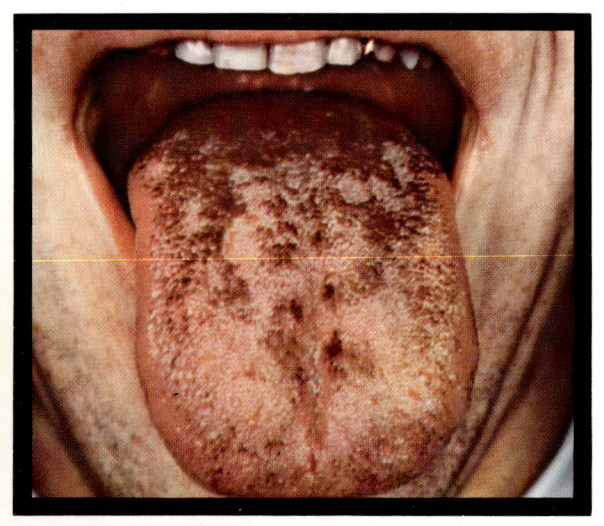

Hairy Tongue Associated with Antibiotic Therapy

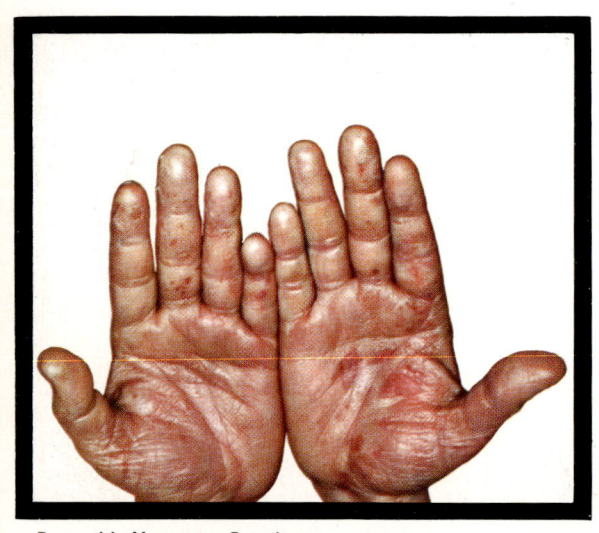

Dermatitis Venenata, Procaine

DRUG IDIOSYNCRASY

Certain individuals react to drugs differently than do the majority of people. Such reactions in the oral cavity are termed "stomatitis venenata" if due to contact with a drug, or "stomatitis medicamentosa" if the offending agent has been used systemically.

(Top) Marked redness of the oral mucosa is sharply limited to the area in contact with an acrylic partial denture. The denture was strapped to the patient's arm below the axilla, and erythema was present in the contact area within 24 hours. Such contact sensitivity is rare, and the diagnosis should not be made unless a patch test on the skin or mucosa is positive. Scrapings from the suspected denture are adequate for the test. Inflammation beneath dentures usually results from poor oral hygiene or mechanical irritation rather than from such sensitivity.

(Center) The most common oral change related to antibiotic therapy is an extensive black or yellow coating of the tongue. This coating does not usually develop unless the drug has been used for at least a week. It generally persists for several days and then frequently desquamates, leaving the tongue red and sore. The excessive tongue coating is not caused by hypersensitivity but is related to the predominance of fungi in the oral flora. When the flora again becomes balanced, the tongue returns to normal. The patient shown received chloromycetin for 3 weeks, at the end of which time the coat was uniform over the entire dorsal surface. The picture was taken a week later, after some desquamation had occurred.

(Bottom) In years past, when procaine was the most widely used local anesthetic, an appreciable number of dentists were susceptible to contact with it. This picture was taken 36 hours after spilling procaine on the hands. The reaction is not specific for procaine but may occur from contact of any anesthetic or other substance to which an individual is hypersensitive. The first manifestations are usually redness and swelling. Later there may be vesiculation, erosion and ulceration. Skin sensitivity may be determined by patch testing.

Diseases of the Oral Mucosa and Jaws

Drug Idiosyncrasy (Cont.)

(Top) Marked enlargement of the upper lip caused by a localized vascular change which allowed the sudden escape of an excessive amount of fluid into the tissue. The patient experiences this reaction each time that he receives a local anesthetic. Angioneurotic edema may also occur in individuals who are sensitive to other drugs or to various cosmetics or foods. This type of reaction is most common in the cheeks, lips and eyelids. The swelling does not usually last longer than 1 or 2 days. It may be reduced by the administration of adrenalin or antihistamines, but ordinarily this is not necessary. With severe laryngeal edema tracheotomy may be necessary.

(Center) A few drops of penicillin solution accidentally splashed on this dentist's face while he was giving an injection to a patient. This individual normally has a slender face, but here the cheeks are swollen, the nose and upper lip are enlarged, and the upper eyelids are puffy and red. The presence of papular lesions is also apparent on the cheeks. The picture was taken 36 hours after his contact with the drug. This dentist also experiences a severe reaction to the parenteral administration of penicillin.

(Bottom) Stomatitis medicamentosa which followed by 48 hours the administration of Pyridium for an infection of the urinary tract. Swelling, superficial necrosis, and ulceration of the gingiva are seen. The buccal mucosa and pharynx were similarly affected, and the patient complained of intense pain. The stomatitis subsided spontaneously within a few days after discontinuing the use of the drug.

Any drug may cause abnormal reactions in susceptible individuals. Certain groups of drugs, however, such as the antibiotics, sulfonamides, barbiturates, halogens and salicylates, are responsible for the majority of unusual reactions. Drug idiosyncrasy should always be considered in the differential diagnosis of oral lesions. In some instances the substances responsible for the undesirable effects are readily ascertained, but usually considerable questioning, testing, and elimination of suspicious substances are necessary to determine the offending agent.

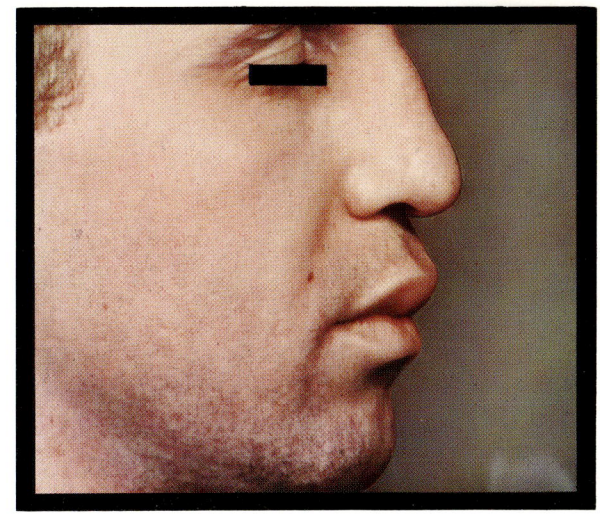

Angioneurotic Edema, Lip

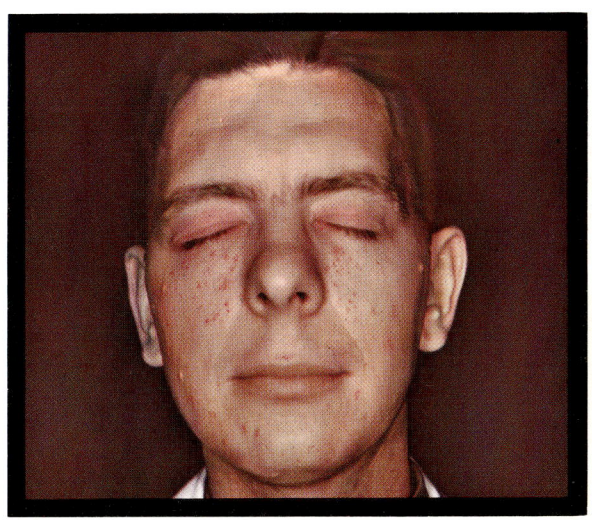

Dermatitis Venenata, Penicillin

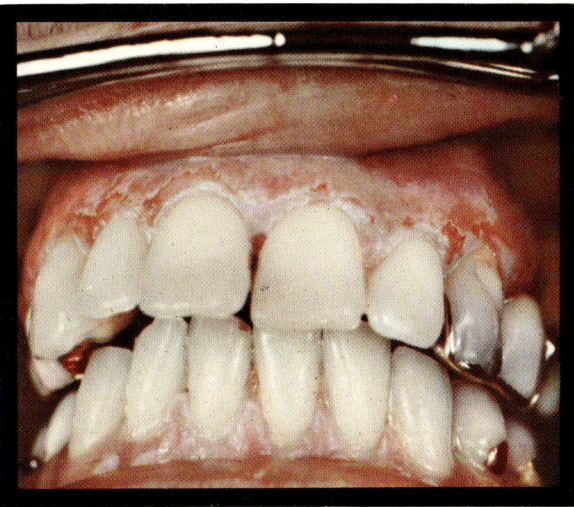

Stomatitis Medicamentosa, Pyridium

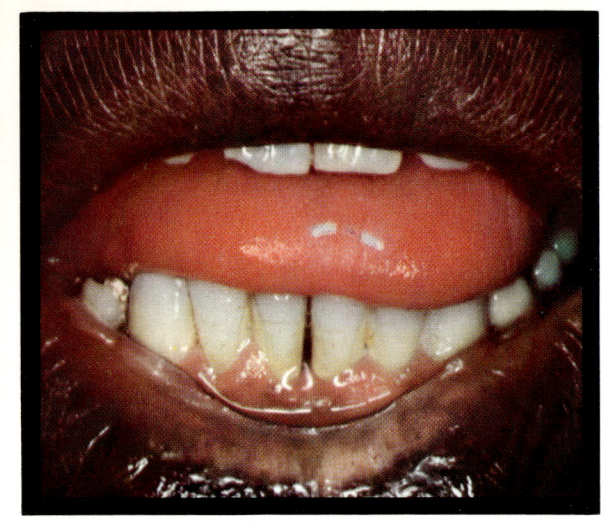

Keratotic Areas, Tip of Tongue

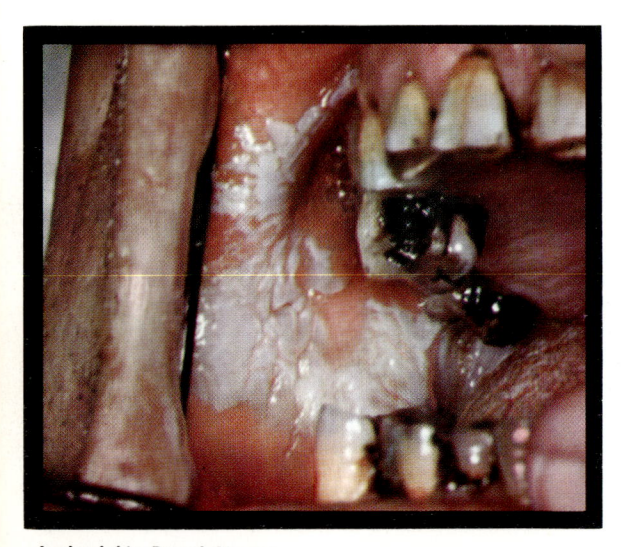

Leukoplakia Buccal Mucosa

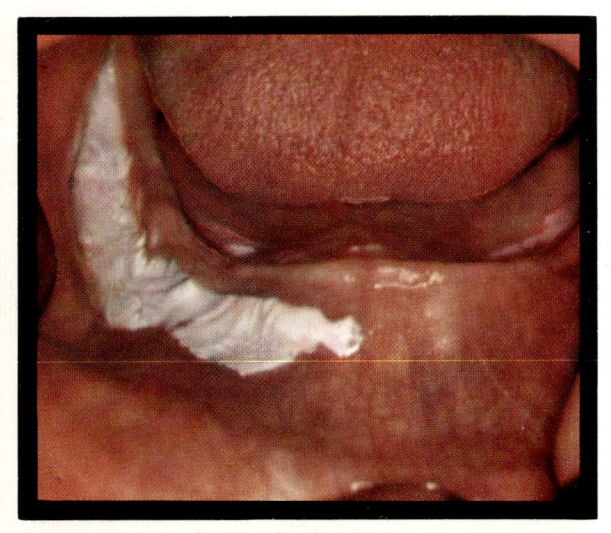

Leukoplakia of the Alveolar Mucosa

KERATOSIS AND LEUKOPLAKIA

There is much confusion concerning the use of the term leukoplakia. Some use it as a clinical term to designate a white plaque in accordance with the primary meaning of the word; others use it to mean a lesion with certain histologic features such as hyperkeratosis or dysplasia (dyskeratosis). While these differences in viewpoint cannot be settled arbitrarily, it is highly important that the therapist and the diagnostician thoroughly understand each other's use of the term in any specific case. Since hyperkeratosis, parakeratosis, dyskeratosis and acanthosis are identified histologically rather than clinically, these terms will be reserved in this Atlas for histologically recognized entities and the term leukoplakia will be applied arbitrarily to a white, opaque, leathery-appearing plaque not identifiable clinically as some other white lesion (such as lichen planus, drug burn, solar cheilosis, white spongy nevus, carcinoma, etc.). If the lesion shows hyperkeratosis, dyskeratosis or other changes histologically, they will be so designated in the laboratory diagnosis. The irritations which produce leukoplakia may also be factors initiating carcinoma, and in this sense all leukoplakia possibly may be considered as "premalignant." The degree of actual cellular change toward malignancy will be indicated by the appearance of the tissue and will serve as a more definitive guide to the therapist.

(Top) Two small white lesions resulted from the tongue rubbing against calculus on the lower anterior teeth. Upon removal of the calculus, the lesions disappeared. The use of the term keratosis for these is presumptuous but probably justified.

(Center) A diffuse area of leukoplakia in the buccal mucosa of a tobacco chewer. The pouch created by the wad of tobacco is apparent opposite the maxillary molar region. The involved area is soft and pliable, and a biopsy revealed only increased surface keratinization.

(Bottom) A very thick, extensive area of leukoplakia in the mandibular alveolar mucosa. The clinical appearance may suggest carcinoma, but histologic examination showed it to be a benign hyperkeratosis.

Keratosis and Leukoplakia (Cont.)

(Top) In the photomicrograph at the left, which is a section of a white patch, it is apparent that the epithelium, except for a heavy parakeratin layer, varies little from normal. (See p. 2.) The epithelial cells stain uniformly and do not vary in size and shape. There is little, if any, interference with their orderly maturation. Because of the degree of surface keratinization it is evident that this lesion would have appeared clinically as a very thick white patch and might have been considered precancerous. The photomicrograph on the right, a portion of another white patch, reveals a flattening of the rete pegs and a heavy parakeratin layer, but no epithelial changes which would suggest that the lesion might become malignant.

(Center) The white lesion in this case is thick, extensive, leathery and fissured. Histologic examination revealed epithelial alterations which might be construed as indicating the possibility of future carcinomatous change. The question of what white patches should be biopsied is often asked. Histologic examination should be made of all such lesions which persist after removal of local irritants unless there is absolutely no doubt of the diagnosis. Occasionally the most innocent-looking white area is found to have malignant potentialities when examined microscopically. Even individuals with extensive clinical experience frequently do not rely on clinical evaluation alone.

(Bottom) Epithelial changes suggestive of premalignancy are hyperchromatism, loss of polarity, increase in number of mitotic figures, and irregularity of size and shape of nuclei. These changes are implied in the term malignant dyskeratosis, although literally dyskeratosis signifies only disordered keratin formation. Probably dysplasia is the better term. In the specimen illustrated there are a few hyperchromatic cells in the lower malpighian layer and some loss of polarity. To the left, atypical budding is seen at the tip of one rete peg. While these changes are minimal, they are sufficient to indicate that changes which may progress to malignancy have occurred.

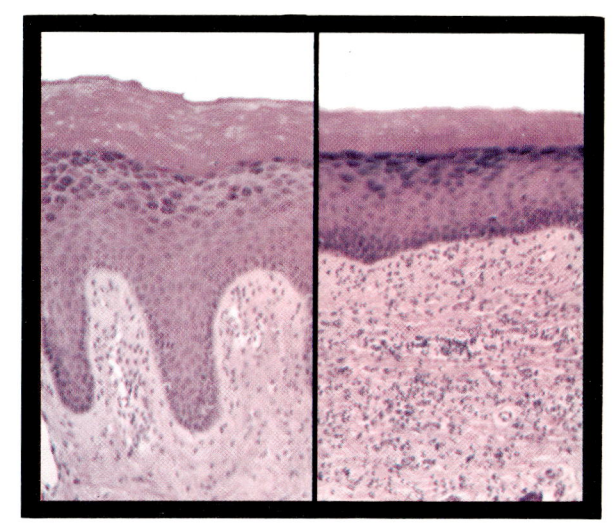

Focal Keratosis   X 90

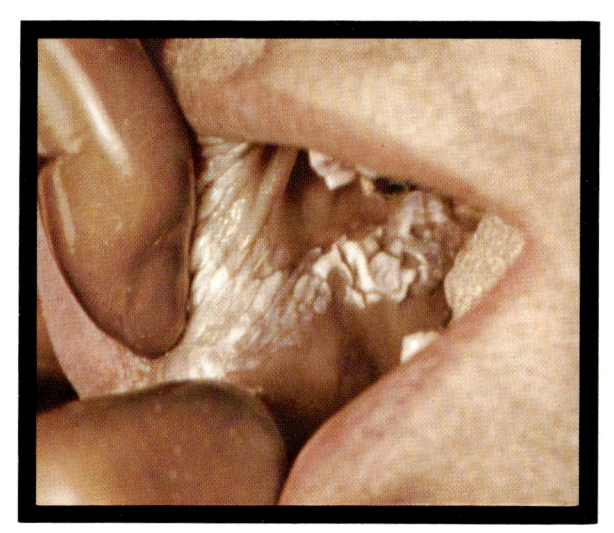

Leukoplakia, Buccal Mucosa

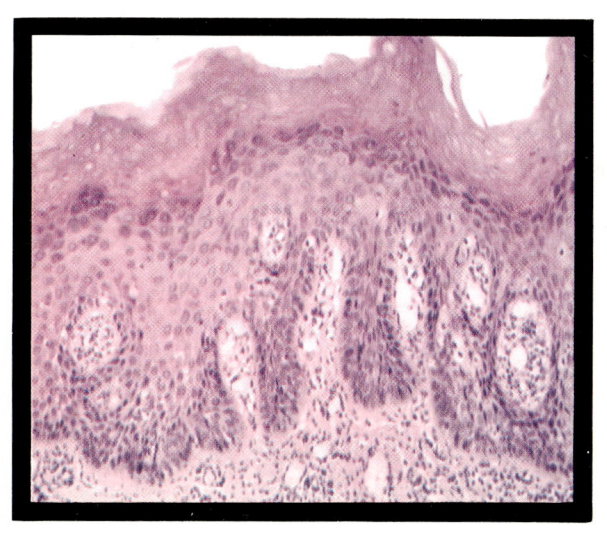

Mild Dysplasia   X 180

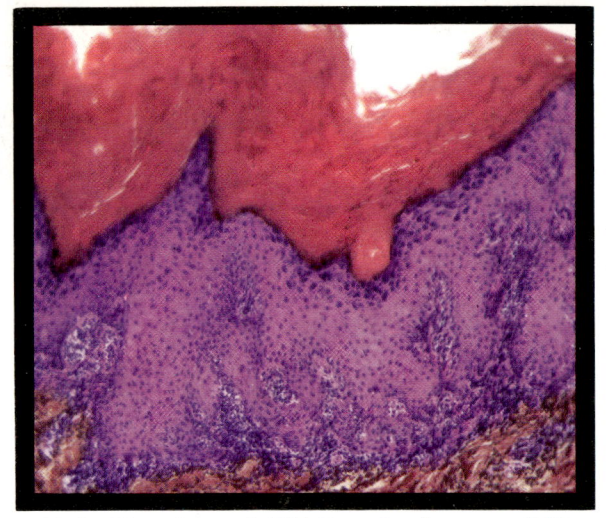

Marked Hyperkeratosis With Some Atypia X 80

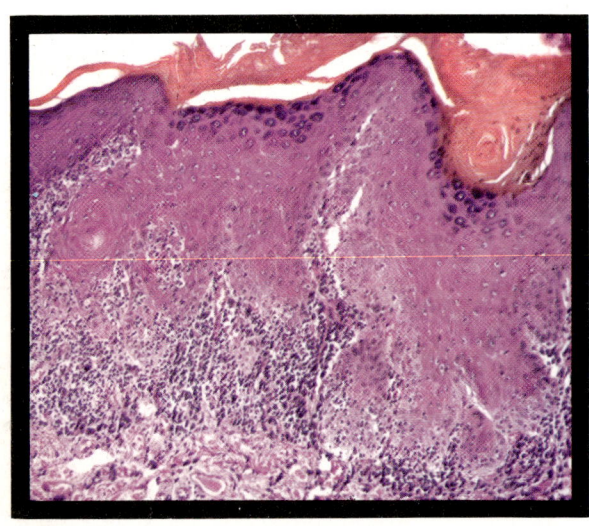

Keratosis and Severe Dysplastic Change X 85

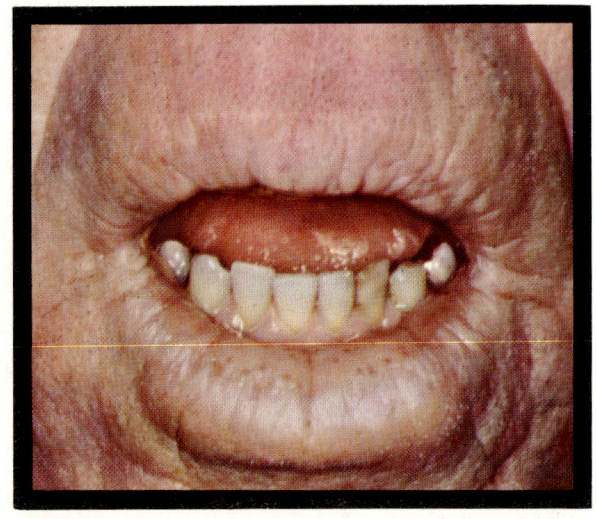

Solar Cheilosis

Keratosis and Leukoplakia (Cont.)

(Top) Histologic examination in this case reveals an extreme degree of keratinization, a prominent granular layer, a disorderly arrangement of cells in the lower malpighian layer, and an irregular downward proliferation of the rete pegs. The basal layer is somewhat difficult to identify because of its invasion by inflammatory cells. Irregularly shaped cells with hyperchromatic nuclei (better seen at higher magnification) are present in the lower layers of the epithelium.

(Center) In this specimen the parakeratin layer is increased, and there is a very atypical downgrowth of epithelium. The cells in this downgrowth are large and show altered staining characteristics. No basal layer is apparent, and the line of separation between epithelium and corium is indistinct. Undoubtedly there would be much disagreement as to whether this is early squamous cell carcinoma or premalignancy. In borderline cases all the material submitted should be thoroughly sectioned and examined. When this is done, indisputable evidence of carcinoma is frequently discovered. Because the changes that are exhibited in the photomicrograph are the most severe that could be found in this case, the diagnosis of severe dysplasia was made. In lesions of the lip, the differentiation between severe dysplasia and early carcinoma is of academic significance only, because the treatment is similar for both.

SOLAR CHEILOSIS

(Bottom) The degenerative changes in the vermilion portion of the lips of this patient are associated with exposure to the elements, mainly the actinic rays of the sun. The lips, which are covered by a thin, white, keratotic film, have an atrophic appearance. Numerous red, pinpoint erosive areas are present in the exposed portion of the lower lip. Solar cheilosis occurs most frequently in fair-skinned individuals, especially redheads. In advanced cases vermilionectomy is advisable, for this condition predisposes to carcinoma. Treatment in cases of mild involvement consists of applying anti-actinic creams to prevent further degenerative changes.

Diseases of the Oral Mucosa and Jaws

Solar Cheilosis (Cont.)

(Top) Photomicrograph of two different areas from a lipshave (vermilionectomy) specimen removed from a patient with typical clinical characteristics of solar cheilosis. In the left picture the epithelium is markedly atrophic, being only a few cells thick. A thin layer of keratin is seen on the surface. In the right photomicrograph there is a very heavy parakeratin layer, and the epithelium is proliferating into the corium in an atypical manner. In areas such as this, carcinoma may develop. In both photomicrographs there are light-blue-staining homogeneous masses in the underlying connective tissue. These masses are composed of degenerated collagen and elastic tissue.

WHITE SPONGE NEVUS

(Center) This familial disease, which is also referred to as congenital keratosis and as familial white folded gingivostomatosis, is characterized by extensive thick, keratinized lesions in the oral mucosa. The keratinized areas have a shiny, opalescent surface, which may be pebbly or filamentous in character. The lesions are soft and spongy and are often traversed by numerous deep grooves. Occasionally small vesicles are seen. The entire oral mucosa, as well as other mucous membranes, may be involved. This harmless disease should be distinguished from other keratotic oral lesions of more serious character. The diagnosis should be based on the history, clinical appearance and histologic findings.

(Bottom) The histologic findings are distinctive and diagnostic. The epithelium is quite hyperplastic, and the rete pegs are broad and fused. Parakeratin is present in varying amounts on the surface and, in some regions, extends deeply into the malpighian layer. A marked edema, both intracellular and extracellular, is evident in the prickle cell layer. Small vesicles are occasionally formed. Several of the prickle cells are devoid of nuclei and cytoplasm; others have small amounts of red cytoplasm around nuclei; and in others the nuclei are of normal size and dense red cytoplasm fills the cells. The detailed cellular changes cannot be seen at this magnification.

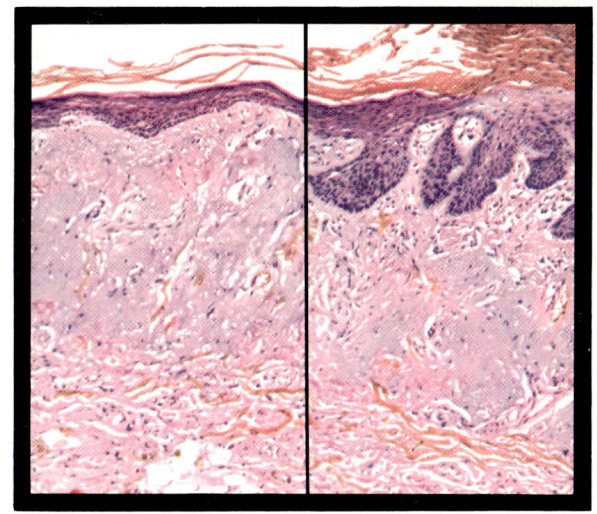

Solar Cheilosis   X 80

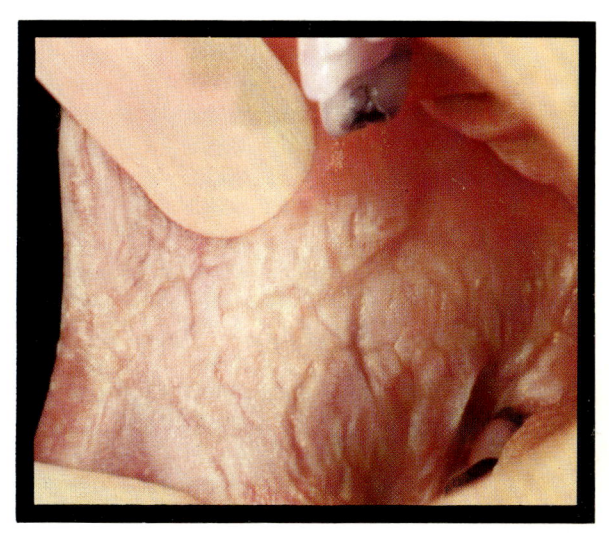

White Sponge Nevus, Buccal Mucosa

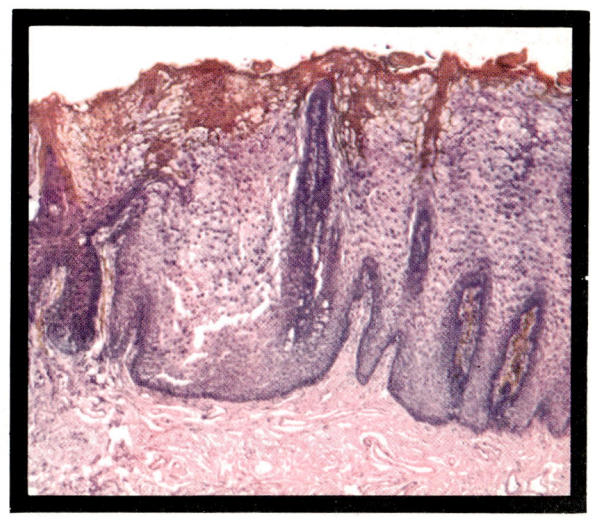

White Sponge Nevus, Biopsy Specimen from Above Case   X 40

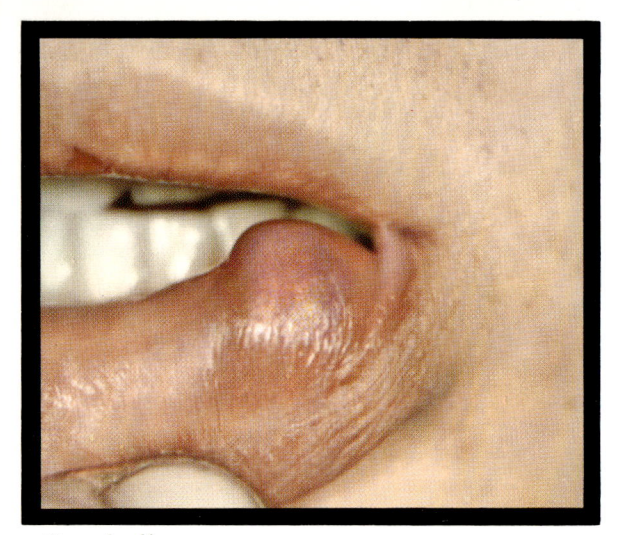

Mucocele, Lip

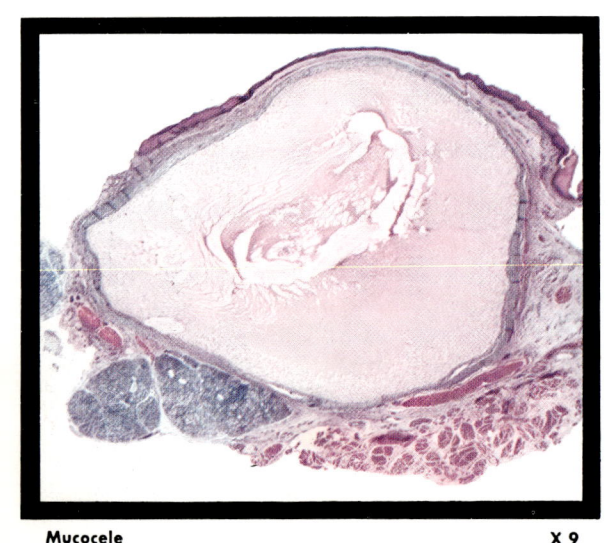

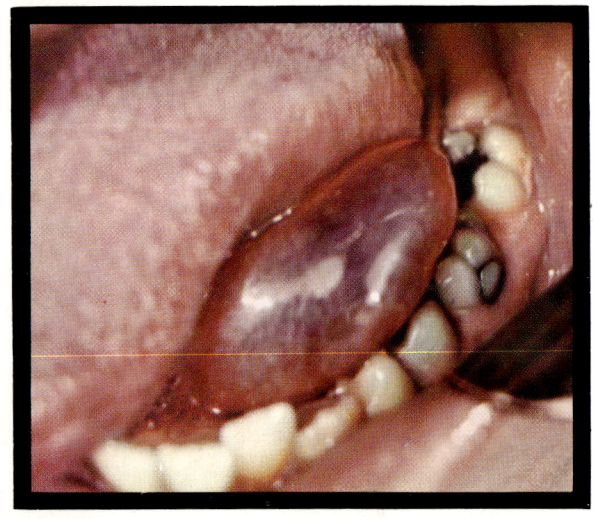

Mucocele   X 9

Ranula

MUCOUS RETENTION CYST

(Mucocele)

(Top) Spherical swelling of the lower lip due to an abnormal collection of mucin in the underlying tissues. This enlargement might be confused clinically with a mixed tumor of salivary gland origin (p. 150) or with a lipoma (p. 139). A mixed tumor, however, is quite firm to palpation. A lipoma is soft and may be yellow, whereas a mucocele is fluctuant and often has a slight bluish tinge. Oral mucoceles occur most frequently in the lower lip but may be found wherever there is salivary gland tissue. Trauma is the most likely cause of mucoceles. Mucin escapes into the tissues surrounding the gland, coagulates, causes an inflammatory reaction and is walled off by granulation tissue. Obstructing the duct in laboratory animals failed to produce similar lesions, and the results of experimentally severing salivary gland ducts in laboratory animals have been variable.

(Center) Topographic view of a superficially located mucocele. The surface epithelium (purple-staining border near top of picture) is very thin over the summit of the enlargement. The greater part of the specimen consists of a mass of light-bluish-pink-staining homogeneous material (mucin) confined by a capsule of fibrous connective tissue. Inferior to the mucocele are striated muscle fibers (red) and salivary gland tissue (blue). An epithelial lining may be present in small mucoceles but is seldom seen in large ones. Clinically, the lesion shown here would probably appear blue because it is located near the surface, but one more deeply situated would not exhibit that feature. Mucoceles of long duration sometimes become organized and then are represented by a fibrotic nodule.

(Bottom) A large mucous retention cyst located in the floor of the mouth is generally termed a ranula because of its supposed resemblance to the ventral surface of a frog. Ranulas are usually associated with the sublingual glands and may be unilateral, like the one pictured, or they may involve the whole floor of the mouth. When superficial they appear as blue or purplish-red enlargements. Occasionally they are congenital.

SIALOLITHIASIS

Stones may form in any of the major or minor salivary glands or their excretory ducts. The submandibular gland and Wharton's duct are by far the most frequently involved. The most common manifestation of ductal calculi, which do not generally cause a complete obstruction, is the enlargement of the gland during eating. The glandular swelling diminishes between meals as the entrapped saliva is gradually excreted. When such swelling occurs, there may be severe pain. Histologic examination of a decalcified stone reveals that calcified material has been deposited in circular layers. It is believed that the stones develop as a result of deposition of calcium salts into a nidus of organic material.

(Top) A relatively large salivary stone is apparent in Wharton's duct. The overlying tissue is distended, and capillaries are quite evident. Removal can be readily accomplished by stabilizing the stone and incising down to it. The wound should not be sutured, for obstruction of the duct is apt to result. Small stones in this location may sometimes be milked out of the duct.

(Center) Occlusal radiograph revealing ovoid, opaque areas which are salivary calculi in the submaxillary duct. When salivary stones are suspected, care should be taken in the angulation of the x-ray tube so that the mandible is not superimposed over the area in question.

SJÖGREN'S SYNDROME

(Bottom) This patient had changes and symptoms typical of the syndrome: dry eyes, and dryness of the upper respiratory tract including the mouth, nares and pharynx; and involvement of salivary glands (including palatal) and lacrimal glands. She also had rheumatoid arthritis. Biopsy of a greatly enlarged parotid gland revealed heavy infiltration with lymphocytes (obliterating almost all other structures) and a few scattered islands of squamous and ductal epithelium (benign lymphoepithelial lesion). These changes also may be seen in a single gland unassociated with the syndrome.

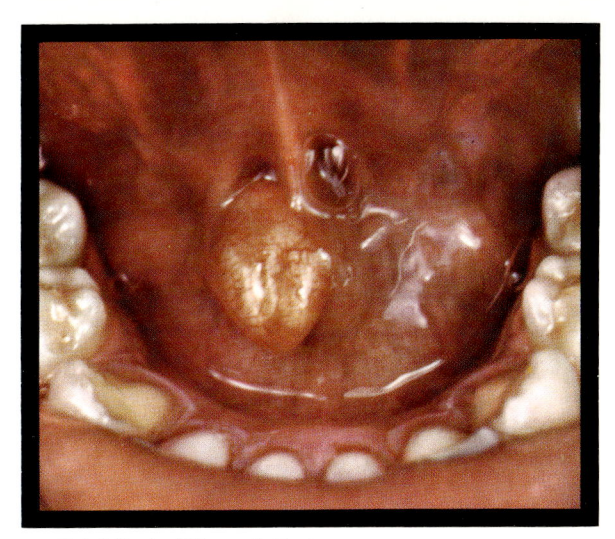

Sialolithiasis, Wharton's Duct

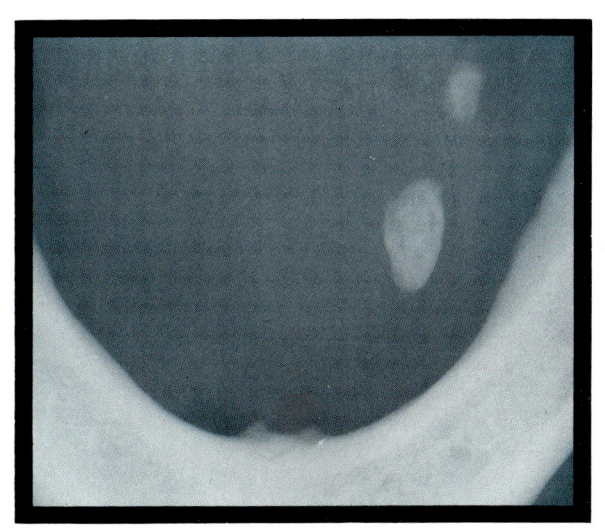

Salivary Calculi

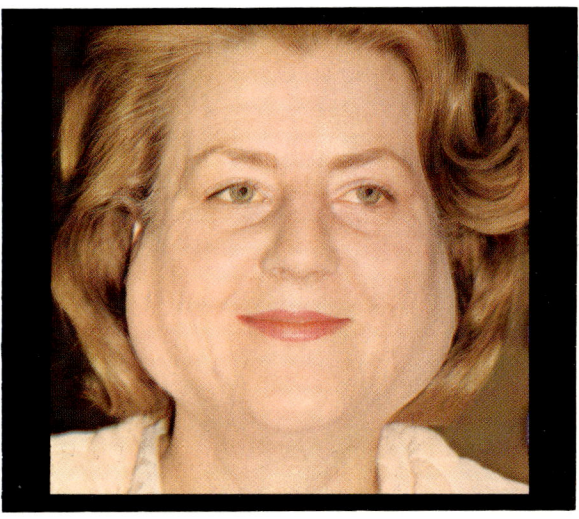

Sjögren's Syndrome

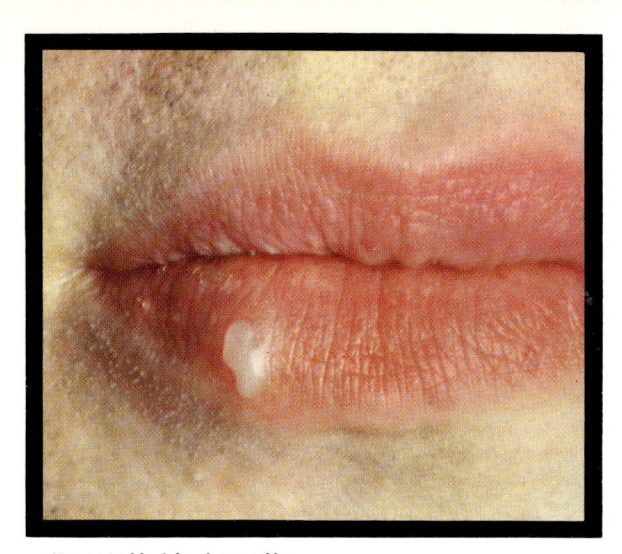

Herpetic Vesicle, Lower Lip

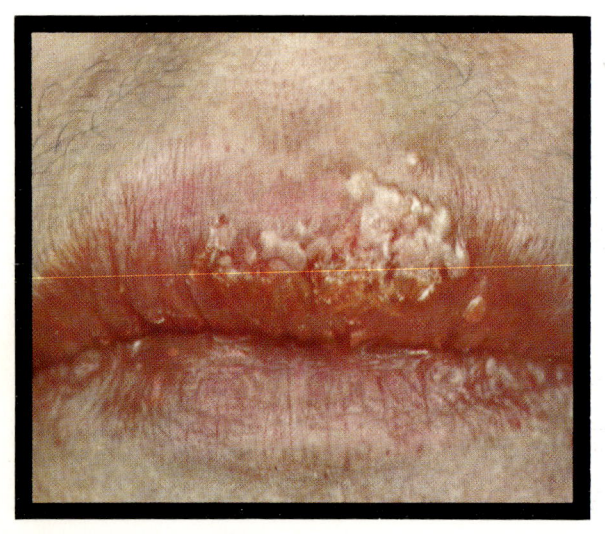

Herpes Labialis, Crusting

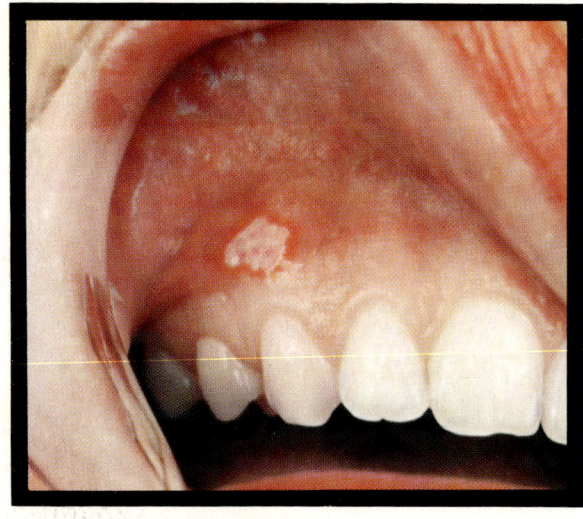

Solitary Herpetic Ulcer, Gingiva

RECURRENT HERPETIFORM LESIONS

These recurrent oral and labial lesions probably result from the reactivation of herpes simplex virus residual in the tissue from primary infection (p. 77). The intra-oral lesions are also known as recurrent aphthae, aphthous stomatitis, recurrent herpes, etc. There is some controversy as to whether or not all of these are, in fact, herpetic lesions so that the descriptive term "herpetiform" is used. Reactivation of the virus and appearance of the lesions may be associated with upper respiratory infection, tissue manipulation or trauma, fever, exposure to sunlight, gastrointestinal upsets and menstruation. The recurrent lesions usually are limited in extent, beginning with a slight swelling and a mild burning sensation, followed in a few hours by vesicle formation. In moist areas the thin-walled blisters rupture almost immediately, and on the lips they persist for only a few hours. Unless they become severely infected secondarily, the resultant ulcers remain superficial, healing in 10 to 14 days without scarring. Constitutional symptoms typical of primary herpetic gingivostomatitis are absent in the recurrent disease. Heavy doses of vitamin B complex, broad-spectrum antibiotics, repeated smallpox vaccination, and gamma globulin are suggested for control or elimination of recurrences.

(Top) Large vesicle of lip resulting from coalescence of smaller ones. In the vesicular stage the lesions of herpes may be dehydrated with absolute alcohol and ether, preventing rupturing and secondary infection. Healing time may be shortened thereby.

(Center) A typical conglomerate lesion of herpes labialis which was initiated by sunlight. Some of the vesicles have already ruptured, fibrin has been deposited, and a crust has been formed.

(Bottom) This gingival ulcer is characteristic of the herpetic lesion which occurs in moist areas. It is superficial and has a yellowish, fibrinous base. At the periphery remnants of the vesicle are still evident. The typical red, inflamed border is quite irregular. Lesions of this sort are characterized by intense pain which persists for several days.

Diseases of the Oral Mucosa and Jaws 111

EXANTHEMS

(Top) In chickenpox (varicella) the cutaneous eruption frequently is associated with coalescing vesicular oral lesions, as seen here in the palate. In measles (rubeola) small bluish white spots on bright red bases (Koplik's spots) may be seen, usually adjacent to Stensen's duct, during the late prodromal and early eruptive stage in most patients. Small petechial spots at the junction of the hard and soft palate may be seen in German measles (rubella) and sometimes in infectious mononucleosis.

PERIADENITIS MUCOSA NECROTICA RECURRENS

This rare condition is frequently confused with recurrent herpetic stomatitis. It may be differentiated from the latter disease, however, by the history and clinical findings. The patient usually complains that for a period of years he has had at least one lesion in the mouth at all times. These lesions start as small white plaques which increase in size. They then slough, leaving a craterous ulcer which is intensely painful. Because of the size and depth of the ulcer, healing is prolonged and may take 4 to 6 weeks. Scarring is usually evident in areas where there have been repeated lesions. Patients with periadenitis mucosa necrotica recurrens may be poorly nourished because the intense pain associated with the ulcers makes it difficult to take food. The disorder occurs in gland-bearing areas of the mucosa. Histologically, it is characterized by necrosis and inflammation in the region of the ducts of the accessory salivary glands. The cause is unknown.

(Center) On the lower lip near the corner of the mouth is a large, well-developed, depressed ulcer that is characteristic of this disease. It has begun to heal, and some fibrosis has occurred, as evidenced by the elevated tissue at the periphery of the lesion.

(Bottom) This patient was afflicted with the disorder periadenitis mucosa necrotica recurrens for 20 years. In the vestibular mucosa near the commissure are numerous firm, irregular elevations. These are fibrotic areas associated with the healing of ulcers that have formed repeatedly in this location.

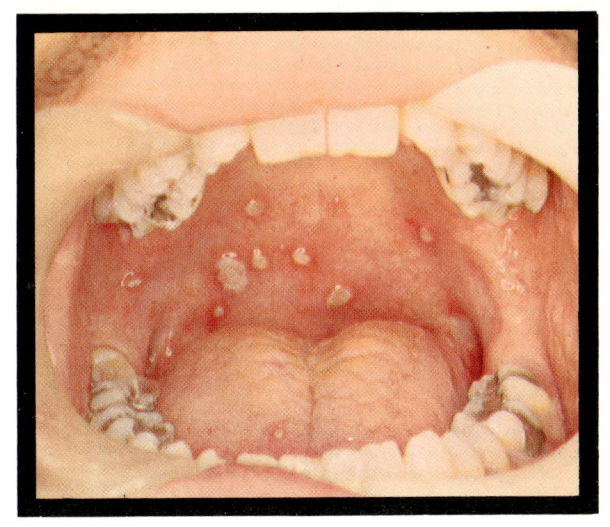

Chickenpox (Varicella), Palate

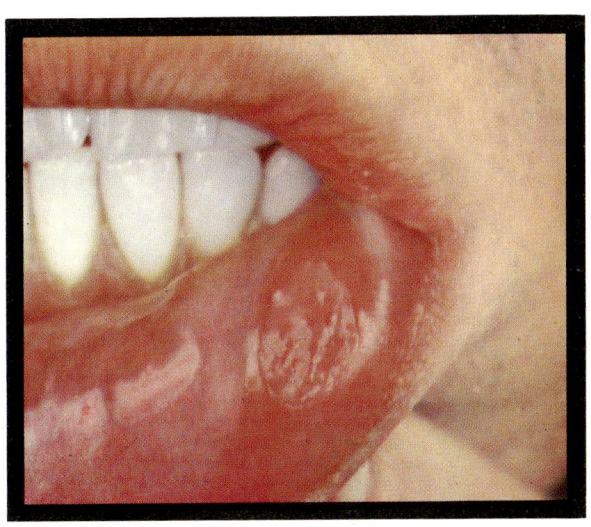

Periadenitis Mucosa Necrotica Recurrens

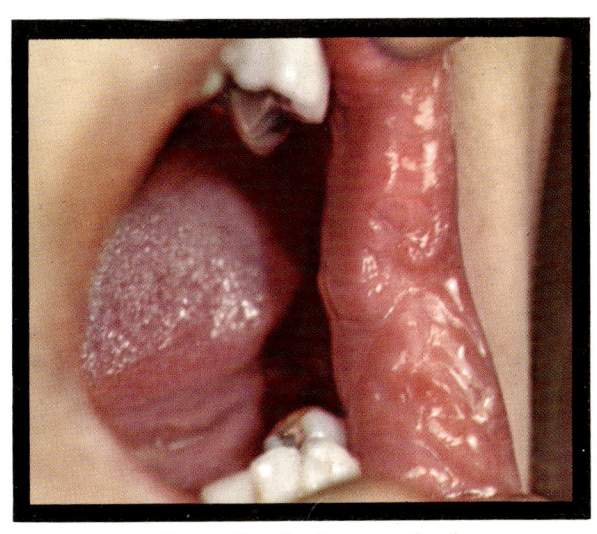

Periadenitis Mucosa Necrotica Recurrens, Scarring

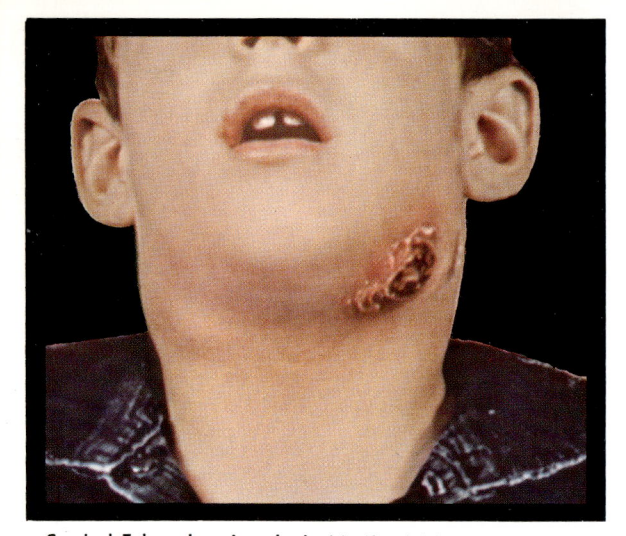

Cervical Tuberculous Lymphadenitis (Scrofula)

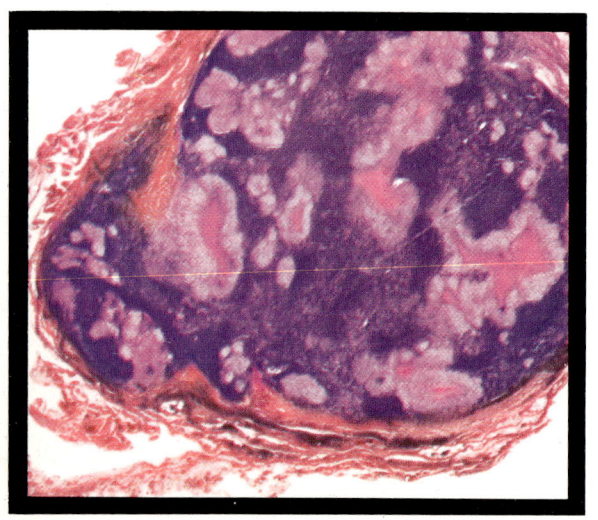

Tuberculous Lymphadenitis Caseation Necrosis   X 14

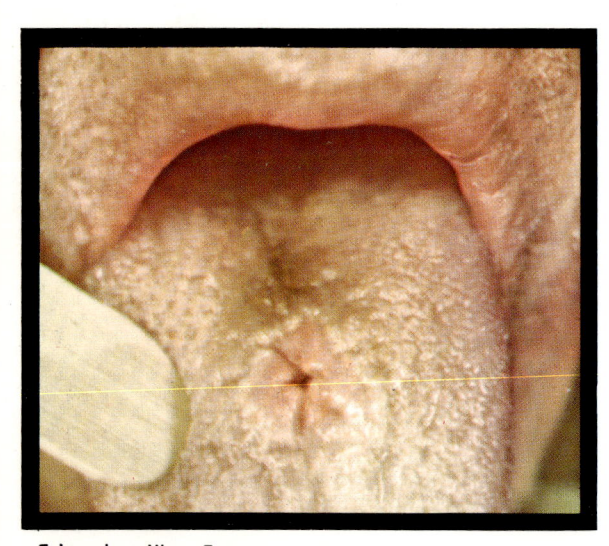

Tuberculous Ulcer, Tongue

TUBERCULOSIS

(Top) Bilateral cervical tuberculous lymphadenitis in a young boy. This form of the disease is due to infection with the bovine strain of tubercle bacilli, usually as a result of drinking milk from tuberculous cows. The microorganisms enter the body through the tonsillar tissue constituting Waldeyer's ring, and some of them reach the regional lymph nodes and produce secondary lesions. The involved nodes gradually enlarge; they are hard and discrete at first but later fuse, become soft (due to caseation necrosis) and finally rupture to the surface.

(Center) Extensive caseation necrosis, a typical finding in tuberculosis, is seen here in a lymph node. Grossly, this particular type of necrosis looks like cream cheese. Microscopically, it appears as a pinkish-red homogeneous mass with no evidence of cell outlines.

(Bottom) Tuberculous ulcer with a typical ragged, undermined border. This type of ulcer usually has a gelatinous base and is painful. Occasionally an oral tuberculous lesion is papular in structure. Oral lesions in this disease are usually associated with pulmonary tuberculosis and result from hematogenous spread of the infection or from inoculation of small abrasions by infected sputum. Lesions may occur anywhere in the oral cavity; they are rare, but if present, they frequently involve the tongue. They may occur as periapical lesions.

Tubercle bacilli (human or bovine strains) may enter the body by way of the respiratory tract, the alimentary tract or the skin. Infection of the lung by the human type of bacillus is by far the most frequent form of this disease in man. Many individuals have a tuberculous infection of the lung in early childhood. The primary focus is usually located in the midportion of the lung just beneath the pleura. Regional lymph nodes also become involved. The tuberculous nodes and the lung focus constitute the primary or juvenile complex. With recovery the individual usually has some degree of immunity to the tubercle bacillus, though in some cases a hypersensitivity is developed. Reinfection may occur in adult life.

Diseases of the Oral Mucosa and Jaws

Tuberculosis (Cont.)

The body's response to the tubercle bacillus results in the formation of a distinctive granulomatous lesion characterized by limited vascularity, epithelioid cells arranged in tubercles, lymphocytes, Langhans' giant cells and caseation necrosis. When the causative organisms enter the tissues, cells are killed. As a result, polymorphonuclear neutrophils are attracted to the area of injury. They ingest the bacilli but are killed or damaged by them. The polymorphonuclear neutrophils usually disappear in about 24 hours, and macrophages (scavenger cells) then infiltrate the area. They ingest and slowly digest the dead leukocytes and the tubercle bacilli. In the process, probably due to liberation of lipid material from the capsules of the bacilli, these macrophages change character and are then termed epithelioid cells. Epithelioid cells have abundant light-bluish-staining cytoplasm and centrally placed nuclei; they form a circular mass called a tubercle. A Langhans' giant cell often forms within the tubercle by the fusion of several epithelioid cells. In the granulation tissue at the edge and within the tubercle are numerous lymphocytes. At a certain stage caseation necrosis of the granulation tissue (not the original parenchyma) occurs in the central portion of the tubercle. If the macrophages are able to destroy the bacilli more rapidly than they can multiply, fibrous encapsulation of the area can occur.

(Top) Mucous membrane epithelium (upper right corner) and an ulcerated area *(left)*. In the dense, relatively avascular fibrous connective tissue are two lighter-staining areas which consist of coalesced tubercles.

(Center) Specific granulomatous reaction to tubercle bacilli. The upper circular area is formed by the fusion of 4 small tubercles. Langhans' giant cells are seen within the tubercles. Caseation necrosis is not evident.

(Bottom) Higher magnification of the lower tubercle seen in the center picture, showing epithelioid cells, lymphocytes and a typical Langhans' giant cell. In the inset, tubercle bacilli (red) are demonstrated in tissue stained by the Ziehl-Neelsen method.

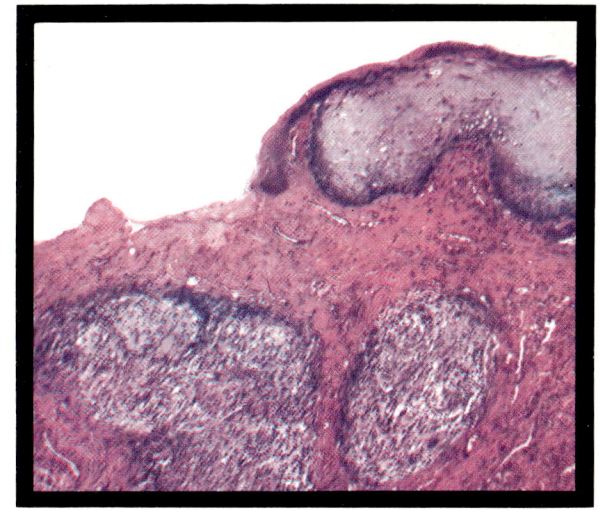

Tuberculous Ulcer   X 80

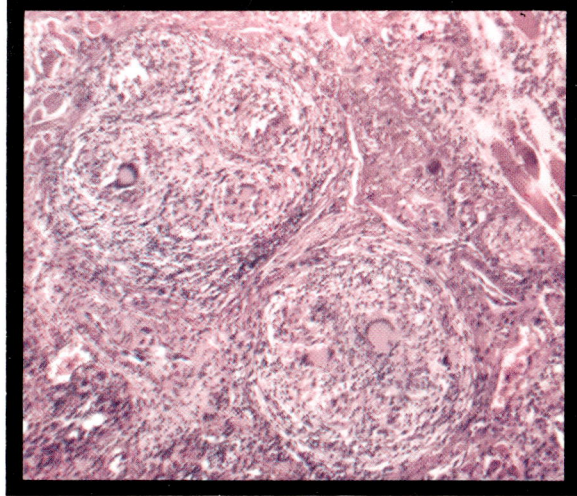

Tubercles   X 100

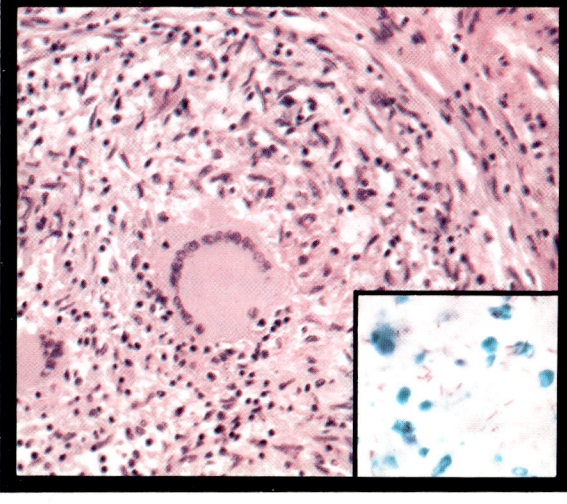

Langhans' Giant Cell X 300   **Tubercle Bacilli X 1000**

114   *Diseases of the Oral Mucosa and Jaws*

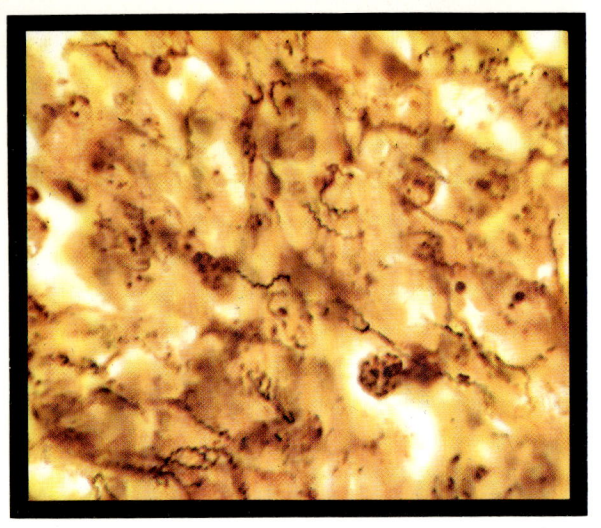

Spirochetes of Syphilis, Warthin-Starry-Kerr Stain   X 1480

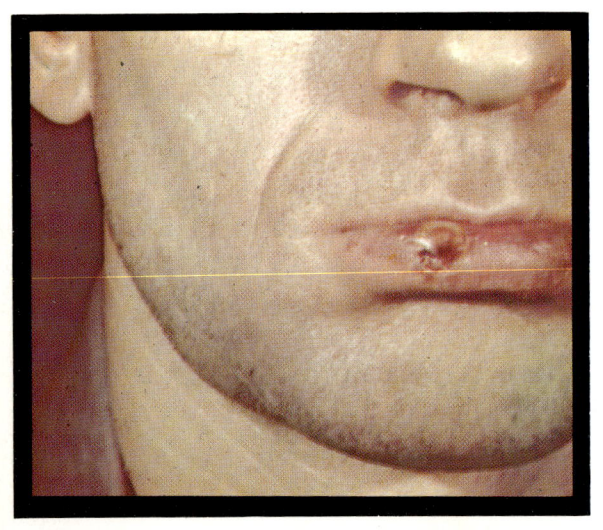

Chancre, Lip

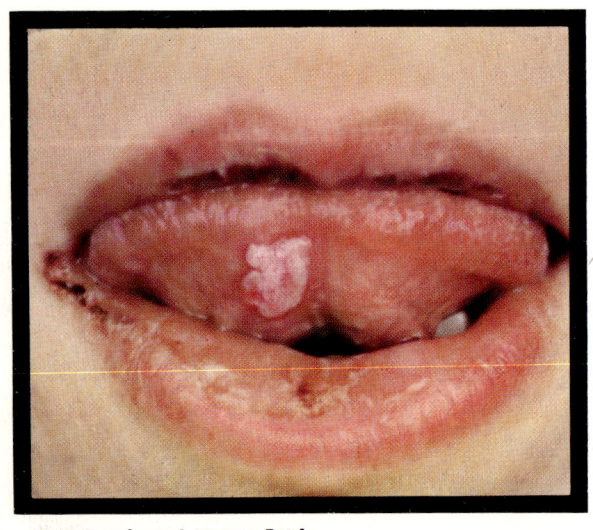

Split Papule and Mucous Patch

SYPHILIS

(Top) The causative organisms *(Treponema pallidum)* as they appear in tissue sections when specially stained with silver. The spirochetes of syphilis are tightly coiled (6 to 15 spirals) and are between 5 and 15 microns in length. They are highly motile and may penetrate intact tissue. These organisms die rapidly when not in living tissue.

(Center) The primary lesion, or chancre, appears at the site of invasion 2 to 6 weeks after inoculation. The chancre is raised and hard and usually measures less than 1/2 inch in diameter. After 2 or 3 days it ulcerates and is covered by a glazed crust. The base is very firm and, when palpated, feels like a rubber button under the tissue. Within a few days after the appearance of the primary lesion one or more regional lymph nodes enlarge (satellite bubo). The chancre will disappear, even without treatment, in 2 to 5 weeks, and the patient may not have a positive serology until this time. The lips and fingers are the most frequent sites of extragenital chancres. Clinically, a lip chancre, as shown in the picture, is difficult to differentiate from carcinoma (p. 155) and from a secondarily infected herpetic lesion. The diagnosis of an oral lesion as syphilis should be made with great caution on the basis of darkfield examination alone because of the morphologic similarity between *T. pallidum* and oral spirochetes.

(Bottom) Following the disappearance of the primary lesion there is a period of from 2 months to a year in which there are no clinical manifestations of the disease. The secondary stage often begins with symptoms similar to those of an attack of influenza—sore throat, neuralgic pains and headache. These are followed by a generalized lymphadenopathy and a mucocutaneous eruption. In the picture two types of secondary oral lesions are demonstrated. A split papule is seen at the corner of the mouth, half being on each lip. A mucous patch is apparent on the underside of the tongue. The latter lesion, which is usually slightly raised, begins as a macule, papule or vesicle; it rapidly ulcerates and becomes covered with a grayish-white membrane. It is highly infectious.

Syphilis (Cont.)

(Top) The skin lesions in the secondary stage of syphilis vary greatly in character but in general may be classified as being macular, papular or pustular. The eruption is usually generalized and symmetrical. The lesions often have a copper tinge and curved outlines. The cutaneous manifestations disappear in about 30 days, after which there may be a period of latency varying from 1 to 20 years before the appearance of tertiary lesions.

(Center) The gumma, a localized lesion of tertiary syphilis, is so named because it has the consistency of firm rubber. This lesion, which may occur anywhere in the body, is especially destructive to bone and cartilage. Gumma of the palate may perforate the bone; involvement of the vomer may result in a collapse of the bridge of the nose ("saddle nose"). This type of lesion gradually heals, with the formation of much scar tissue. Histologically, the gumma is somewhat similar to the lesions of tuberculosis, except that in the former, plasma cells predominate, the granulation tissue is quite vascular, and the endothelial cells are prominent. The primary and secondary lesions of syphilis are characterized by a marked vascularity and a preponderance of plasma cells, which are usually in perivascular arrangement.

(Bottom) A diffuse interstitial chronic inflammatory reaction in various tissues and organs is a more common manifestation of tertiary syphilis than the gumma. It is characterized by obliterative endarteritis and a gradual replacement of parenchymous structures by fibrous tissue. When this process occurs in the tongue, it is designated as atrophic, sclerosing, or interstitial luetic glossitis. Diffuse syphilitic inflammation in this organ is reflected on the dorsal surface by patchy areas of leukoplakia and smooth, shiny regions devoid of papillae. Carcinoma is much more frequent in individuals with luetic glossitis than in the general population.

Congenital syphilis is quite similar to the acquired form, except that there is no first stage, and the other stages proceed more rapidly. (See p. 48 for dental defects.)

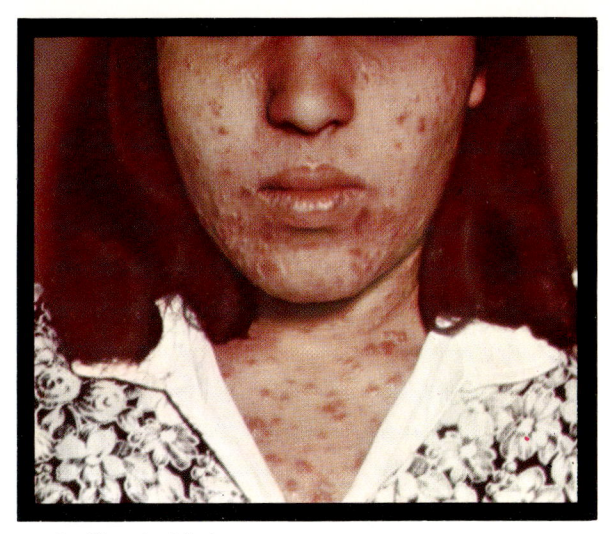

Papillary Syphiloderm

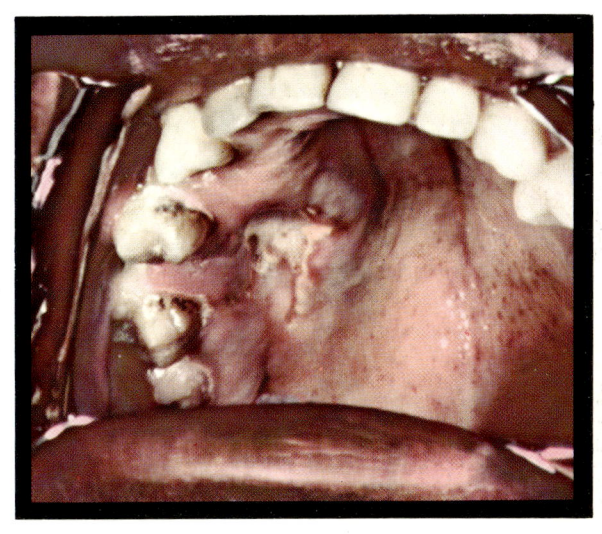

Gumma, Palate

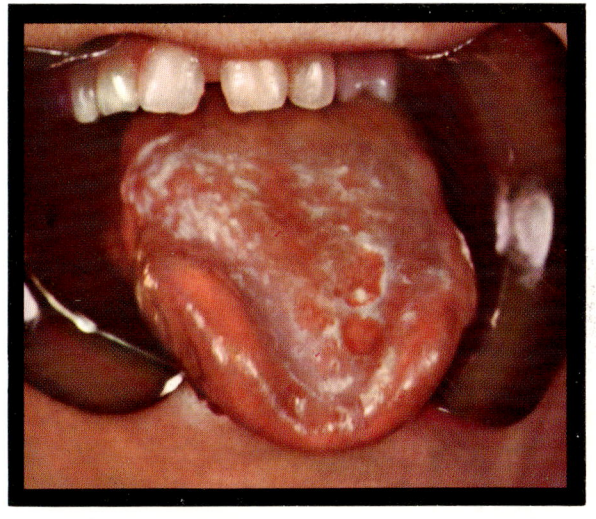

Atrophic Luetic Glossitis

HISTOPLASMOSIS

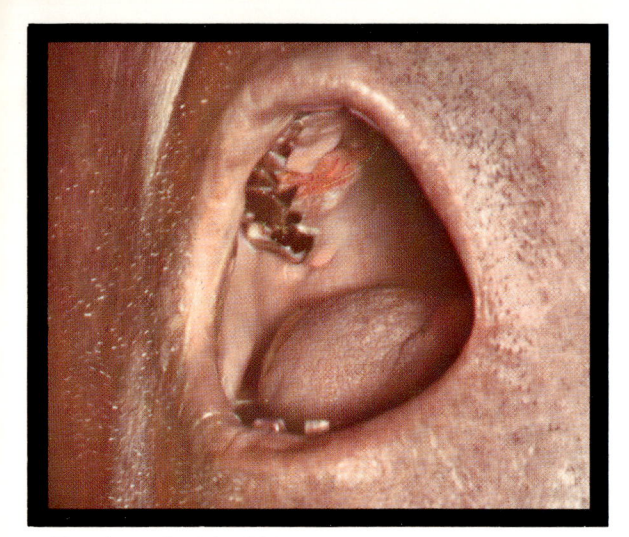

Histoplasmosis, Palatal Mucosa

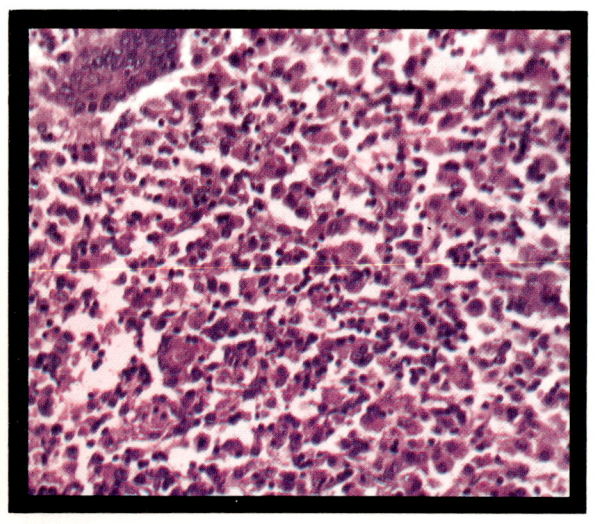

Histoplasmosis, Biopsy Specimen from Oral Lesion   X 215

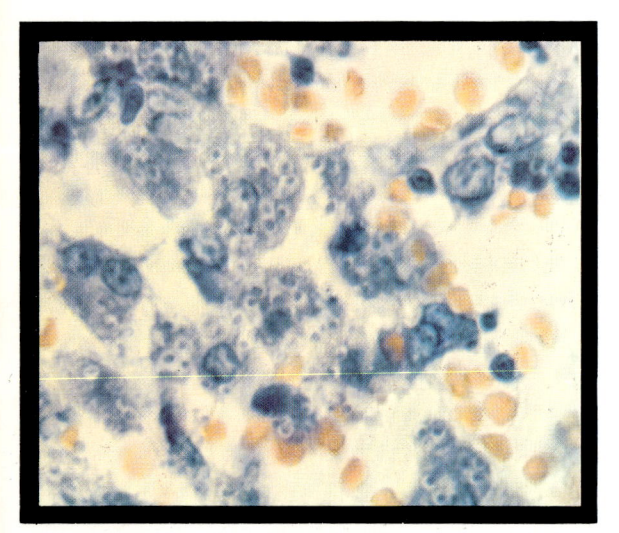

Histoplasma Capsulatum, Giemsa's Stain   X 970

Histoplasmosis, a specific infectious disease which affects mainly the reticuloendothelial system, is caused by the fungus *Histoplasma capsulatum*. At the site of entry (often the oral cavity) a slowly enlarging, indolent ulcer usually develops. The causative organisms may become widely disseminated, involving in particular the lungs, liver, spleen and bone marrow. As the disease progresses there is anemia, leukopenia, enlargement of liver and spleen, low-grade fever and continuing weight loss. This classical, disseminated form of the disease often runs a fatal course. If the disease remains localized, the prognosis is good. In certain areas of the United States nearly half of the adults give a positive reaction to the histoplasmin skin test. If a positive skin test is actually indicative of a previous infection, then a very mild, asymptomatic form of the disease is quite common. Dermal sensitivity apparently develops slowly, for individuals with the active disease are frequently negative reactors.

(Top) In this case of disseminated histoplasmosis, ulceration of the gingiva and palatal mucosa was the primary manifestation of the disease. The lesion was first noticed 2 months previously and had gradually increased in size. This patient's liver and spleen slowly enlarged, and there was radiographic evidence of lung involvement. He died of the disease 6 months after the appearance of the oral lesion.

(Center) Infection by *Histoplasma capsulatum* results in the formation of a granulomatous lesion characterized by moderate vascularity, epithelioid cells, caseation necrosis, and numerous macrophages containing the fungus. In the photomicrograph many large macrophages are apparent, but at this magnification the fungus cannot be visualized.

(Bottom) At higher magnification the organisms (round bodies 1 to 5 microns in diameter) can be seen packed in the macrophages. Each has a centrally placed nucleus and a clear, thick capsule. The organisms may easily be overlooked in routine hematoxylin and eosin preparations, especially if they are scarce.

Diseases of the Oral Mucosa and Jaws 117

ACTINOMYCOSIS

Actinomycosis, a deep fungus infection caused by the anaerobic *Actinomyces israeli* (*A. bovis*), is characterized by granulomatous lesions which eventually suppurrate. Abdominal, thoracic and cervicofacial forms of the disease occur; the last is by far the most frequent. In cervicofacial actinomycosis there is often a history of tooth extraction, and it is believed that the causative organisms, which are common inhabitants of the oral cavity, gain access to bone through the extraction wound. One or more months later the infection becomes apparent by the appearance of a slowly progressive, very firm swelling of the cheek or neck. Pus is evacuated externally from several sinuses when the lesion softens.

(Top) The cervicofacial swelling is of a typical light-purplish color, and at its superior and inferior aspects draining sinuses are apparent. The pus in this disease is scant but very thick. It contains tiny yellow granules (colonies of *A. israeli*) which may be seen grossly. As one sinus closes, others develop. Contiguous tissue gradually becomes involved, and more sinuses form. Cervicofacial actinomycosis has a good prognosis but often runs a protracted course.

(Center) Enlargement of a "sulfur granule" in a tissue section. The granule is surrounded by pus, at the periphery of which are numerous lipid-containing macrophages. One should suspect actinomycosis when examining granulation tissue which has numerous microabscesses and abundant foam cells, but the diagnosis should not be made unless the causative organisms are found. The granule is composed of numerous gram-positive, branching, filamentous organisms. At the edge of the granule the peripheral ends of the organisms may protrude slightly as eosinophilic, club-shaped enlargements.

CANDIDIASIS

(Bottom) Candidiasis (candidosis, thrush, moniliasis) on the tongue of a young child. The white covering appears like a mat of milk curds which leave, as seen in this picture, a red raw surface when scraped off. *Candida albicans,* a normal inhabitant of the mouth, is the cause. It produces disease in debilitated patients with low resistance and when long treatment with antibiotics has eliminated most of the competitive oral flora.

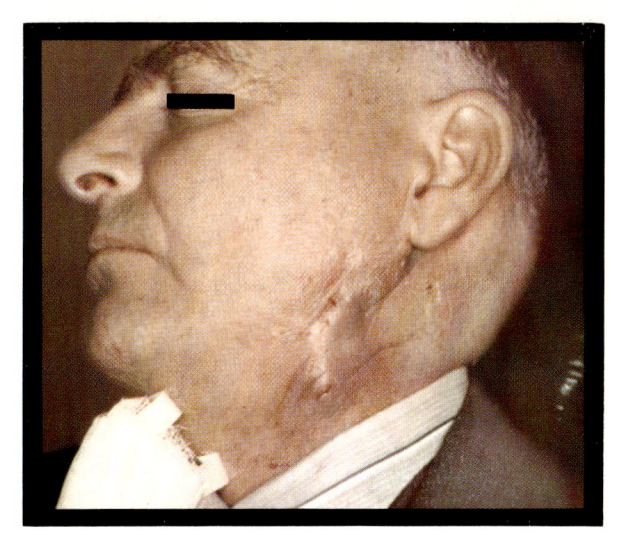

Cervicofacial Actinomycosis

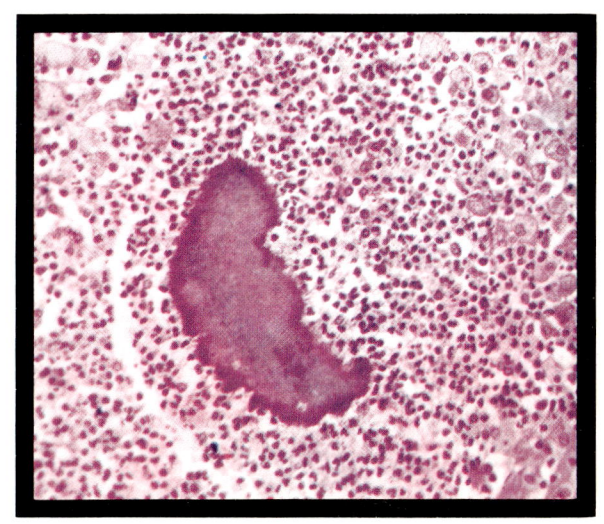

Colony of *Actinomyces Israeli*   X 220

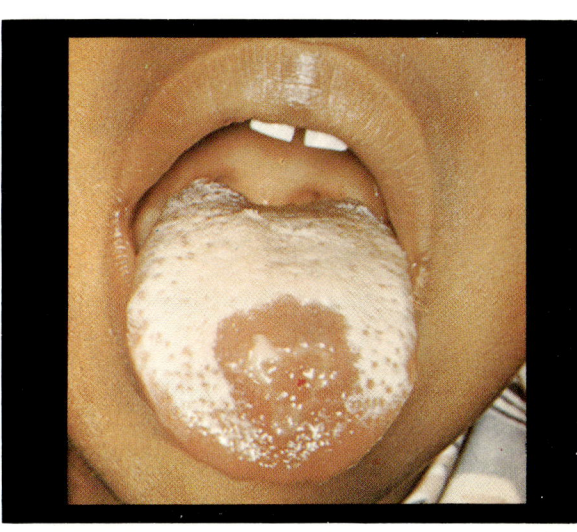

Candidiasis (Thrush)

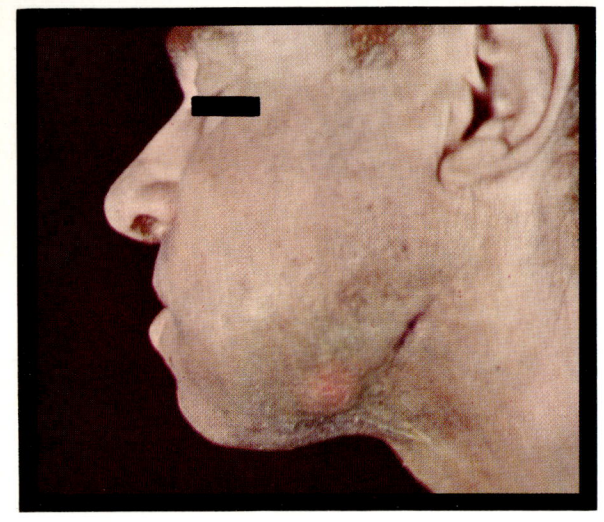

Chronic Osteomyelitis, Mandible

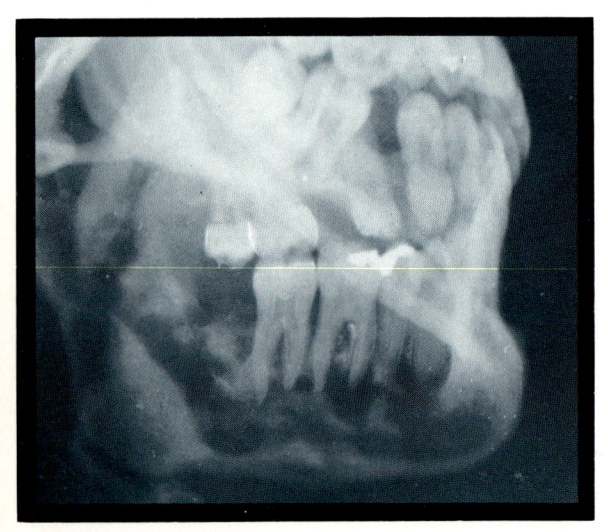

Osteomyelitis, Mandible

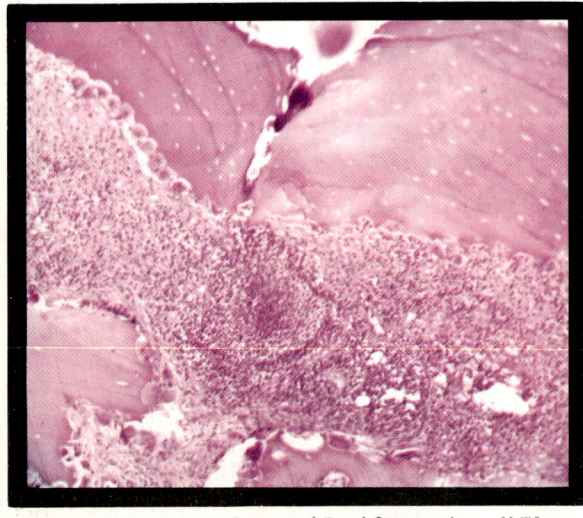

Osteomyelitis, Necrotic Bone, and Focal Suppuration   X 78

OSTEOMYELITIS

The term osteomyelitis (inflammation of bone marrow) is usually reserved for a fulminating suppurative inflammatory process involving a considerable portion of a bone. In the jaws the disease may be caused by extension of a periapical infection, by entrance of organisms through wounds or by blood-borne bacteria. Acute osteomyelitis is associated with a deep-seated, intense pain of the affected part and a rise in the patient's temperature. The inflammation, which spreads rapidly through the marrow and haversian spaces, results in the death of large amounts of bone. This bone necrosis may be in part the result of the direct effect of toxic products on the osteocytes but is caused mainly by loss of blood supply. The latter is due to thrombosis and the stripping of the periosteum from the bone by the formation of subperiosteal abscesses. Pieces of necrotic bone are separated from viable bone by osteoclastic action. These fragments of bone (sequestra), which are surrounded by pus, are eventually exfoliated. A sheath of new bone which forms at the periphery of the necrotic area is termed the involucrum.

(Top) Swelling of the cheek, a cutaneous abscess in the submandibular region, and a partially healed incision at the angle of the jaw are apparent. The abscess contained a fragment of necrotic bone. Several sequestra had previously been removed from an abscess which was in the region of the scar.

(Center) Extensive bone destruction in osteomyelitis of the mandible. Initially there is no x-ray evidence of this disease, for it is only after resorption or sequestration of bone has occurred that radiolucent areas can be seen. Radiographs taken after osteomyelitis has been arrested may suggest that the disease is still progressing, if the newly formed bone has not completely calcified and the necrotic bone is still being resorbed.

(Bottom) In the center of the photomicrograph is granulation tissue in which there is a small, localized collection of pus. The bone fragments are devital, for the lacunar spaces are empty. The edges of the bone are irregular, and numerous osteoclasts are lined up along the scalloped margins.

PYOGENIC GRANULOMA

(Top) Pyogenic granuloma is the name applied to a particular type of overgrowth of granulation tissue that occurs in some individuals in response to minor trauma. The granulomatous response, which is probably influenced by some intrinsic factor, is far out of proportion to the degree of injury. The small pyogenic granuloma shown here developed 3 days after the right side of the lower lip was pinched with forceps. This entity, which occurs in both skin and mucous membrane, may be sessile or pedunculated. It may vary in diameter from a few millimeters to 2 or 3 cm. The lesion is usually ulcerated but is sometimes covered by a very thin layer of epithelium. It may be red, purple or brown in color and have a smooth, granular or lobulated surface. These lesions occur equally in both sexes, tend to bleed easily when manipulated and will recur quickly if not adequately removed. Histologic examination of a lesion reveals an outgrowth of granulomatous tissue characterized by an extreme amount of endothelial proliferation. At the edge of the lesion the epithelium often tends to proliferate inward as if to separate the granulomatous mass from the underlying normal tissue. Near the surface of the overgrowth the connective tissue is young and delicate, and there are numerous small vascular spaces. If the lesion is ulcerated, there are many polymorphonuclear neutrophils in this area. In some regions there may be masses of endothelial cells not organized into vascular structures. Near the base of the lesion the vascular spaces are large and thin-walled and are surrounded by mature connective tissue stroma.

(Center) Topographic view of a pyogenic granuloma. It is covered by very thin epithelium, and the marked vascularity of the lesion is readily apparent. Pyogenic granuloma and granuloma gravidarum (pregnancy tumor) are identical histologically.

(Bottom) Higher magnification of the central portion of the above lesion. In the granulation tissue are a few lymphocytes and polymorphonuclear neutrophils, but most of the large cells are of the endothelial type. Some of these are forming very small vascular channels.

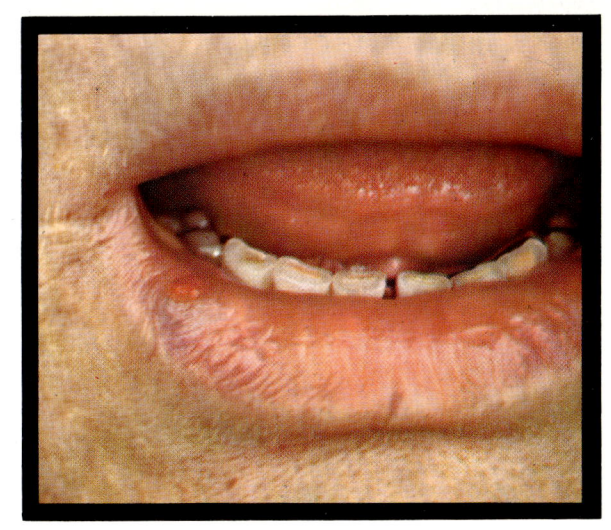

Pyogenic Granuloma (Granuloma Pyogenicum), Lip

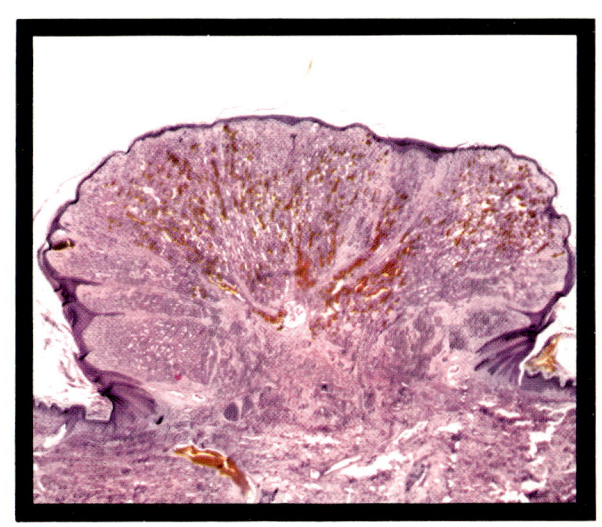

Pyogenic Granuloma   X 10

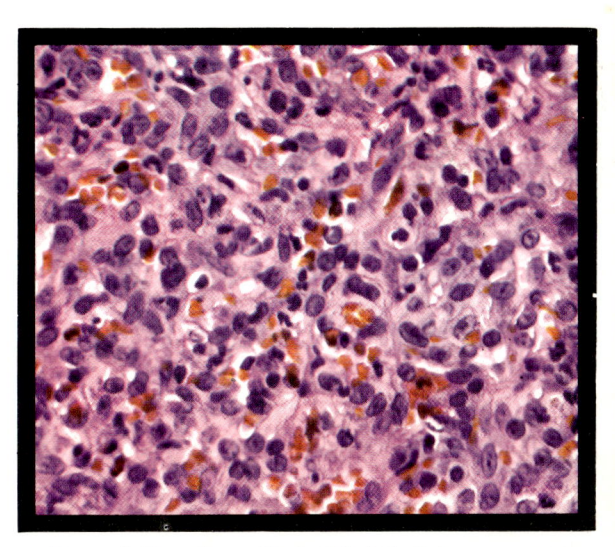

Pyogenic Granuloma, Marked Endothelial Proliferation   X 450

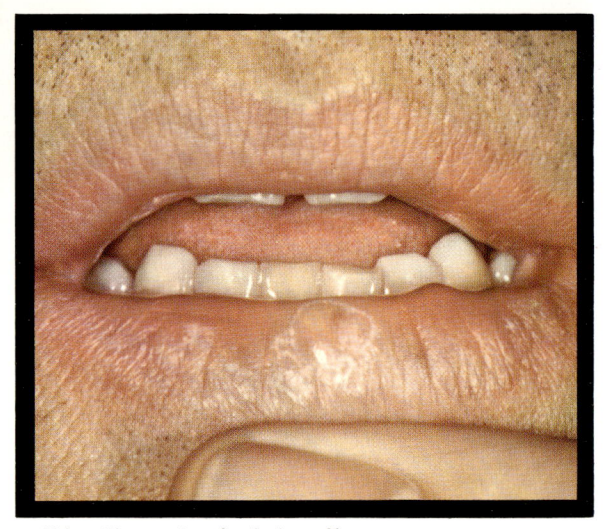

Lichen Planus, Annular Lesions, Lip

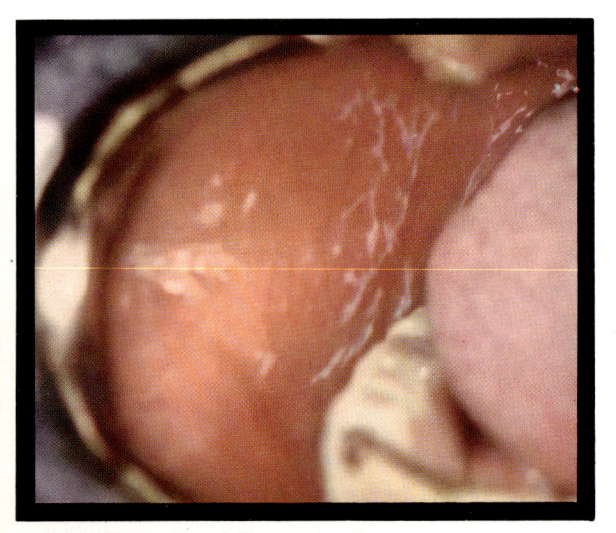

Lichen Planus, Buccal Mucosa, Lacelike Pattern

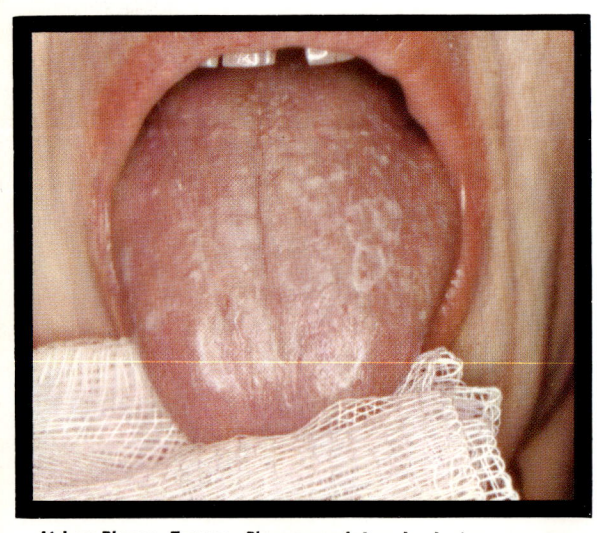

Lichen Planus, Tongue, Plaques and Annular Lesions

LICHEN PLANUS

Lichen planus is an inflammatory disease of the skin and mucous membrane characterized by keratotic lesions of various patterns. The etiology is not known, but the disease is often associated with some degree of emotional tension. Lichen planus is an annoying but not a serious affliction, and the lesions frequently regress when the emotional state of the patient improves. Oral manifestations may occur alone, or they may precede, accompany or follow cutaneous lesions.

(Top) The oral eruption, which occurs most frequently in the buccal mucosa, tongue and lower lip, is usually characterized by slightly raised, white, fine dots and thin lines (Wickham's striae). In the illustration, threadlike keratotic lines are evident on the lower lip. Near the midline is a large, ringlike lesion, and extending from its periphery are smaller lesions of annular configuration. On the right side of the lower lip is a small, white, keratotic plaque, which is also a manifestation of lichen planus, but it might not be recognized as such if it existed alone.

(Center) In the buccal mucosa are several interlacing fine white lines. Small raised dots mark the intersections of the lines. When lesions present a clinical appearance such as this, the diagnosis need not be presumptive, and a biopsy is unnecessary. Not all lesions of lichen planus are as typical as the ones shown here. There may be extensive white plaques, nodules and erosions. However, careful examination of the lesions may reveal Wickham's striae, which should suggest the diagnosis of lichen planus. The appearance of lesions is sometimes altered by cheek chewing, a habit not uncommon in individuals with this disease.

(Bottom) Extensive cornification on the dorsal surface of the tongue, simulating the clinical appearance of leukoplakia. On the left side of the tongue, however, there are annular lesions, posterior to which are discrete white dots, and in other areas a few thin, white lines may be seen. The presence of more characteristic lesions elsewhere in the oral cavity may help the differential diagnosis. In case of doubt, a biopsy is indicated.

Lichen Planus (Cont.)

(Top) Lichen planus of the gingiva is not common. The erosive type, as shown here, must be distinguished from desquamative gingivitis. The presence or absence of Wickham's striae should differentiate the two diseases. Erosive lesions occurring elsewhere in the oral cavity may at times closely resemble ulcerated lesions of lupus erythematosus, as fine white lines may also be associated with the latter. Erosive lesions of lichen planus are sometimes painful, but the nonerosive manifestations are symptomless. Lesions of this disease occurring in other mucous membranes are similar to those found in the oral cavity.

(Center) Cutaneous lesions of lichen planus may be generalized but are usually confined to a few areas, often symmetrically distributed. The flexor surfaces of the wrist, forearm and lower leg are the sites most frequently involved. The eruption, often pruritic, begins as very small, flat-topped, round or angulated papules covered by a thin, horny film. These enlarge and may coalesce. They have a glistening surface, and close inspection will reveal small white raised dots and linear streaks. The early lesions may be purplish red, while the older ones exhibit a light-violet hue. Brown macules, which are due to the presence of numerous melanophores in the upper dermis, often mark the site of healed lesions.

(Bottom) The histologic features of lichen planus, as shown in the accompanying biopsy specimen from the buccal mucosa, include: (1) an infiltration of lymphocytes in intimate relation to the epithelium and sharply limited to the upper corium; (2) liquefaction degeneration of the basal layer; (3) saw-toothed rete pegs; (4) prominent granular layer; and (5) a moderate degree of hyperkeratosis. Lesions in the oral mucosa often show no granular layer, and parakeratin may be formed rather than keratin. In the hypertrophic form of the disease there is considerable hyperplasia of the epithelium and an excessive amount of keratin. In the atrophic type the covering epithelium is thin, and the rete pegs are flattened.

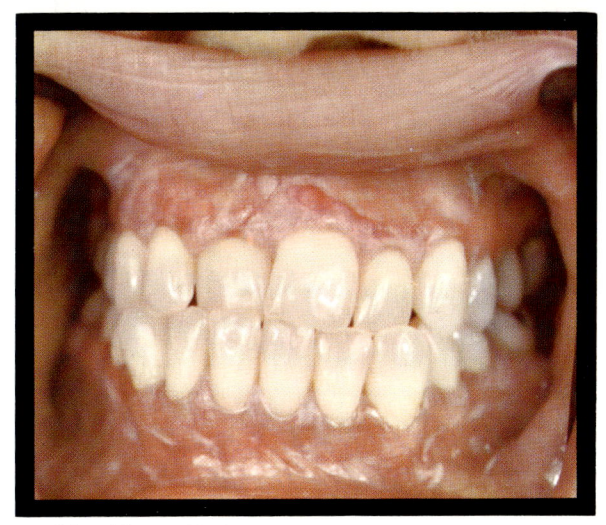

Lichen Planus, Gingiva, Erosive Lesions

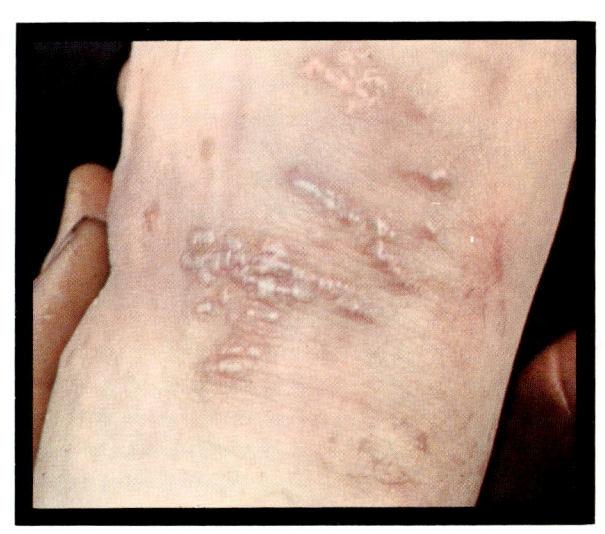

Lichen Planus, Cutaneous Lesions

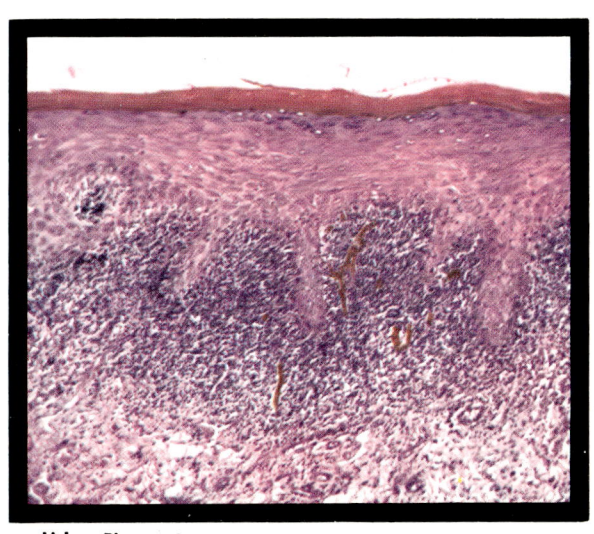

Lichen Planus, Oral Biopsy Specimen X 80

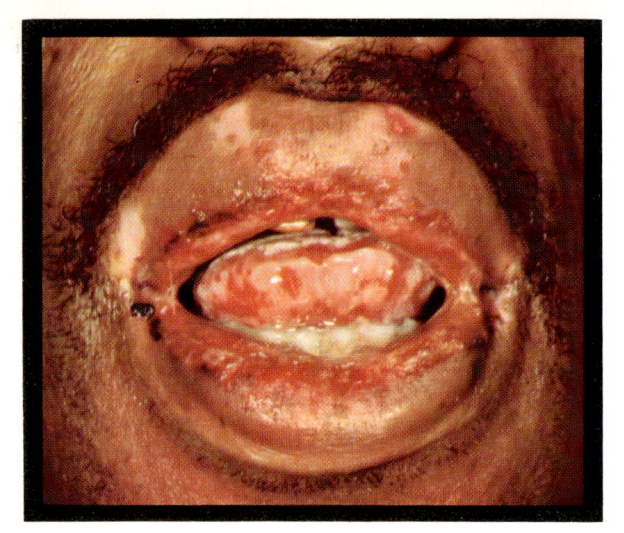

Erythema Multiforme, Tongue and Lip Lesions

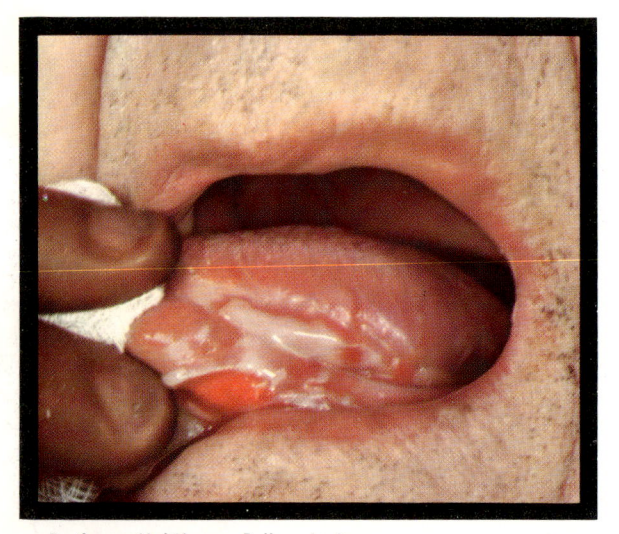

Erythema Multiforme, Bullous Lesions

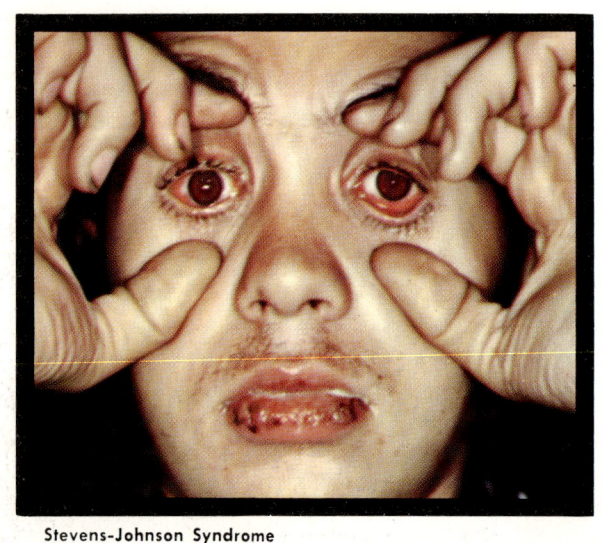

Stevens-Johnson Syndrome

ERYTHEMA MULTIFORME

Erythema multiforme is an acute inflammatory disease of unknown cause which is characterized by a variety of cutaneous and mucosal lesions. These lesions may be macular, papular, vesicular or bullous. The disease usually runs a course of from 10 to 20 days and tends to recur. In the oral cavity there are often extensive, superficially ulcerated, irregularly shaped red lesions which are sometimes covered by a grayish-yellow exudate. The whole oral and pharyngeal mucosa may be involved, making eating and swallowing most difficult. In severe cases there is often a sharp rise in temperature, headache and malaise, and the patient may be acutely ill for 3 or 4 days. Stevens-Johnson syndrome is a variety of erythema multiforme in which there are oral and ocular lesions, fever and severe constitutional symptoms. In some instances of erythema multiforme there may be a concomitant gynecomastia, and in these cases intensive vitamin B complex therapy appears to shorten the course of the disease and abort recurrences.

(Top) The entire tongue is raw and red, and a grayish pseudomembrane is apparent in several areas. The lip lesions, which are nearly healed here, tend to be covered with a hemorrhagic crust. The chief complaint, even in cases with extensive cutaneous manifestations, is usually related to the painful oral lesions. The treatment consists of relieving symptoms. A bland mouthwash is indicated, and systemic use of broad-spectrum antibiotics is useful in combating secondary infection. In some instances intravenous feeding is necessary.

(Center) In this early case of erythema multiforme a bullous lesion with a red areola is seen near the lateral margin of the tongue. In the floor of the mouth near the lip retractor a bulla has ruptured, leaving a raw, red surface.

(Bottom) Stevens-Johnson syndrome in a young adult. Conjunctivitis, sialorrhea and crusted lip lesions are apparent. The patient also had extensive intra-oral lesions, fever and leukopenia.

Diseases of the Oral Mucosa and Jaws

PEMPHIGUS VULGARIS

(Top) Pemphigus vulgaris, a rare, usually fatal disease of unknown etiology, is characterized by the formation of intra-epithelial bullae in the skin and mucous membrane. Oral lesions may be the first sign of the disease. Oral bullae are not commonly seen, for soon after formation they rupture, and much of the collapsed membranous covering is soon lost, leaving ulcerated areas around which there is little reaction. In this case an intact bulla is seen in the center of the palate, and 2 collapsed ones below and to the left. The diagnosis of pemphigus is difficult, and often it must be based at least partially on the clinical course of the disease. Exfoliated cytology may aid in diagnosis.

LUPUS ERYTHEMATOSUS

Numerous varieties of this disease are recognized, although in general it may be divided into two main forms—systemic and nonsystemic. In the nonsystemic form, which is relatively common and not serious, the lesions are limited to the skin and mucous membrane. The cutaneous eruption, which occurs most frequently over the bridge of the nose and malar eminences (butterfly pattern), consists of slightly raised, red patches covered by greasy keratin scales. In the central portion of oral patches there is often a superficial ulcer with slightly undermined edges. The main oral histologic findings are liquefaction degeneration of the basal layer of the epithelium and a patchy perivascular infiltration of lymphocytes. In the classical, systemic form of the disease, there is fibrinoid degeneration of collagen in numerous organs, as well as skin and mucosal lesions. While generally fatal, it may be controlled for many years by steroid therapy. The diagnosis of systemic lupus may be established by finding L.E. cells in peripheral blood or bone marrow.

(Center) Slightly raised, red, scaly lesions on the nose and one cheek. The eruption in this disease is usually aggravated by sunlight and may be progressive, fixed or transient.

(Bottom) The lower lip is swollen and somewhat everted, and there is a diffuse redness on the right side. Covering the involved area are peeling, grayish keratin scales.

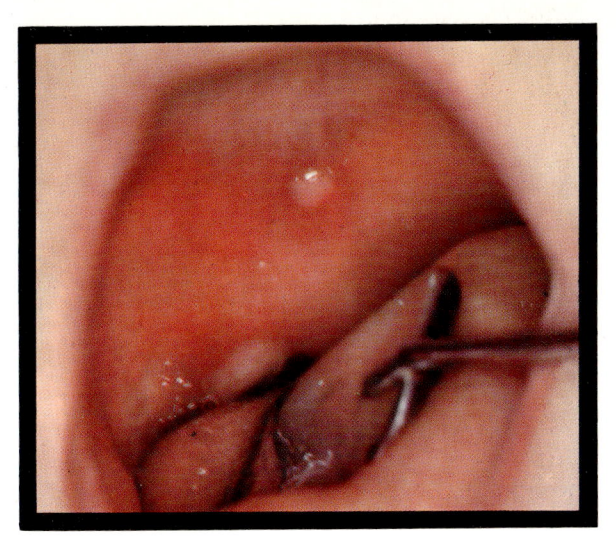

Pemphigus Vulgaris, Oral Lesions

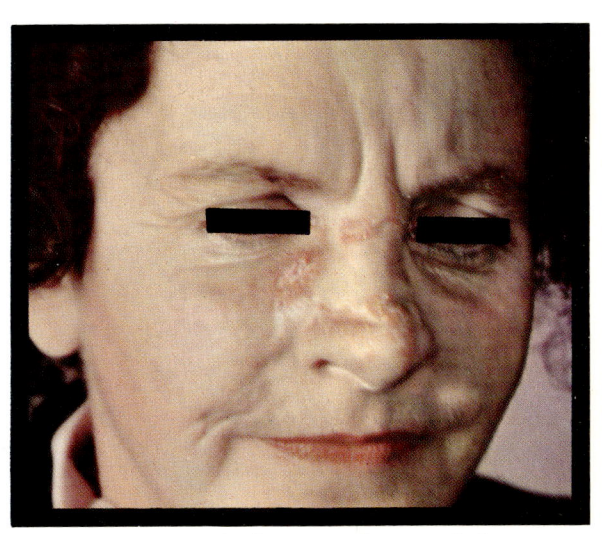

Nonsystemic Lupus Erythematosus, Cutaneous Lesions

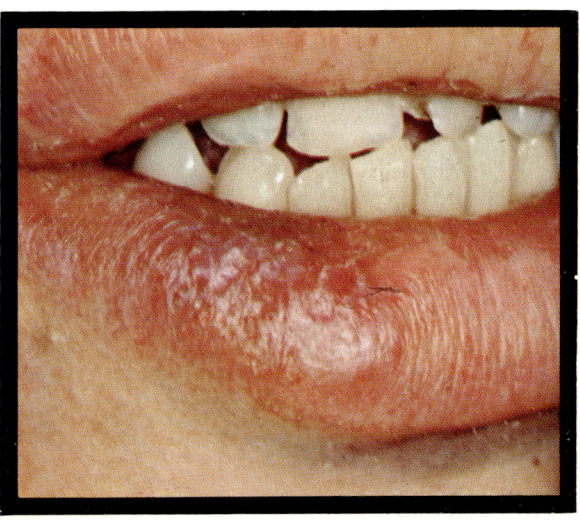

Nonsystemic Lupus Erythematosus, Lip Lesion

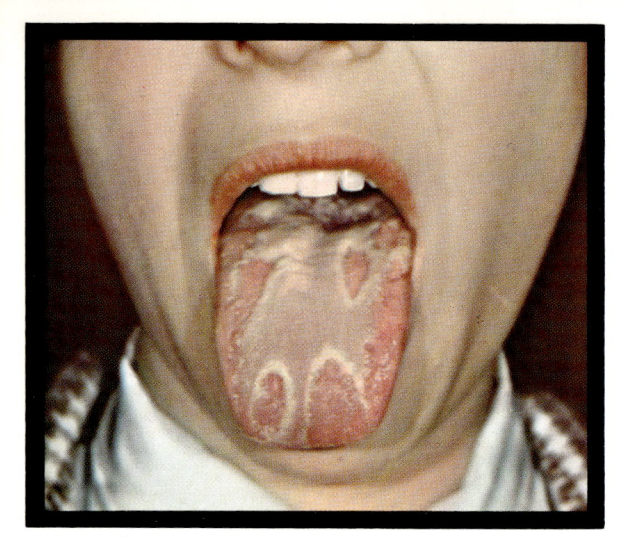

Geographic Tongue

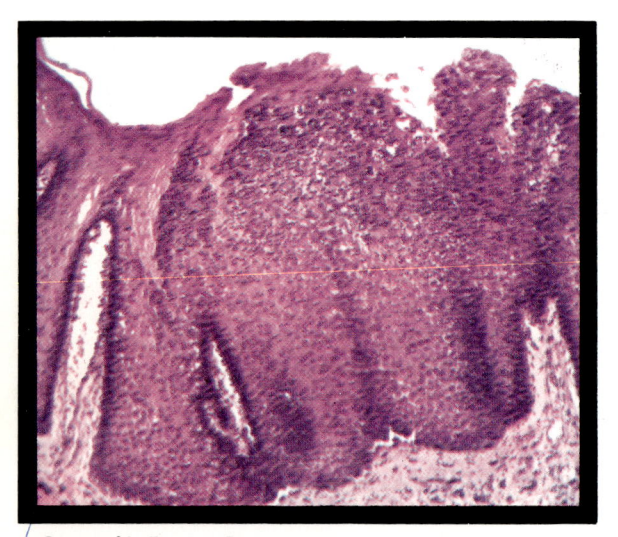

Geographic Tongue, Biopsy Specimen from Edge of Lesion   X 75

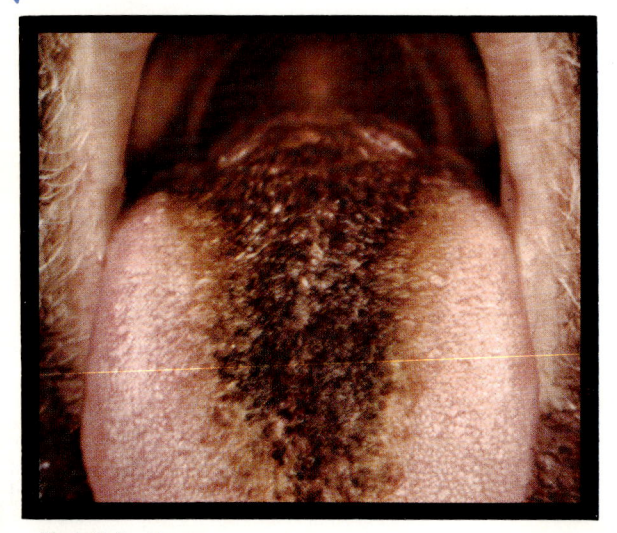

Black Hairy Tongue

GEOGRAPHIC TONGUE

(Benign Migratory Glossitis)

(Top) This disease is characterized by migrating circinate or ovoid inflammatory lesions on the dorsum of the tongue. These lesions, which arise without apparent cause, are red and slightly depressed and have a grayish-yellow border. The redness is related to loss of filiform papillae, desquamation of the superficial prickle cells, and hyperemia. Careful examination of a lesion will usually reveal that there is some regeneration of filiform papillae centrally, and that the redness is more intense near the periphery. Patients may complain of a slight burning sensation, but usually the lesions are painless. The degree of migration varies with the case; in some instances the lesions remain relatively static for weeks, while in others evidence of wandering is apparent every few days. There may be periods when the tongue is completely healed. This disease may persist for years, and satisfactory treatment is unknown. It is of no significance, but patients may need to be continually reassured of its innocuousness.

(Center) Near the center of the upper border is the raised periphery of a lesion. This area is characterized by parakeratosis; epithelial hyperplasia; long, broad, fused rete pegs; edema of the upper malpighian layer; and a heavy infiltration of polymorphonuclear neutrophils. To the left of this raised area is normal tongue mucosa, and to the right (red area clinically) there is desquamation of the epithelial cells. Further to the right, beyond the scope of this photomicrograph, was severe desquamation, with only thin epithelial plates remaining over the extremely vascular connective tissue papillae.

BLACK HAIRY TONGUE

(Bottom) Black hairy tongue (lingua nigra) is the name applied to a condition in which the filiform papillae are so greatly elongated that they somewhat resemble hairs. The "hairs" may become stained by food, tobacco or chromogenic microorganisms. Hairy tongue may develop following the use of various chemotherapeutic agents. (See p. 102.) It may also occur without apparent cause and in these cases tends to be persistent.

Diseases of the Oral Mucosa and Jaws

Black Hairy Tongue (Cont.)

(Top) Biopsy specimen from an individual with a persistent hairy tongue. At intervals along the upper surface are long projections of keratin which are hyperplastic filiform papillae. Desquamated keratin and other debris may be seen between the papillae. Compare with normal filiform papillae, page 5.

VARICOSE VEINS, TONGUE

(Center) Purplish-blue nodular areas on the ventral surface of the tongue. These varicosities (oral phlebectasia) are due to dilatation and increased tortuosity of the lingual veins. Dilated veins in this location are not uncommon in older individuals. They are probably of no clinical significance. In general, varicosities are related to increased venous pressure, weakness of the vein wall and lack of support by surrounding tissue. Complications such as ulceration, thrombosis and hemorrhage arising as a result of lingual varicosities are very rare. The patient should be advised of their innocuous nature.

HEREDITARY HEMORRHAGIC TELANGIECTASIA

(Osler-Rendu-Weber Disease)

(Bottom) This familial disease, which affects both sexes equally, is characterized by numerous dilated capillaries and venules in the skin and mucous membranes. The telangiectases may occur anywhere but are generally limited to the face, nasal mucosa, lips, tongue, floor of mouth, cheek, gastrointestinal tract and fingertips. They may be present in childhood but usually become more numerous and noticeable in the 3rd and 4th decades. The dilated vascular spaces appear clinically as red areas, often raised. Their vascular nature is apparent when they are compressed by a glass slide, for they can be seen to fade. They are usually small, as in the case pictured, but occasionally telangiectatic lesions as large as 0.5 cm. in diameter are seen. Epistaxis is a common symptom, but bleeding may occur from any of the lesions, arising spontaneously or as a result of minor trauma. Bleeding and coagulation time, clot retraction and platelet count are normal.

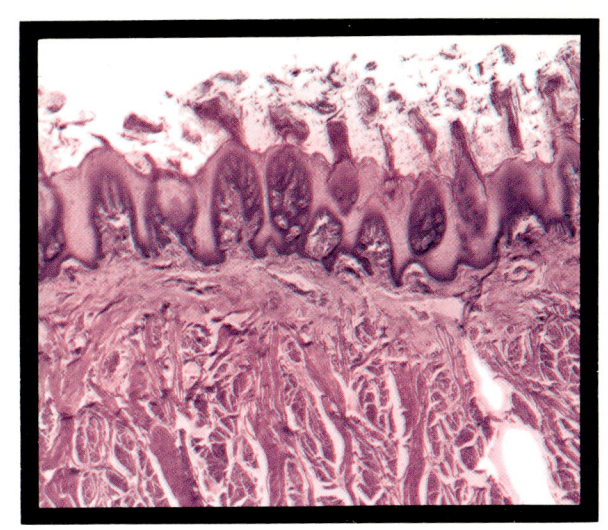

Black Hairy Tongue X 15

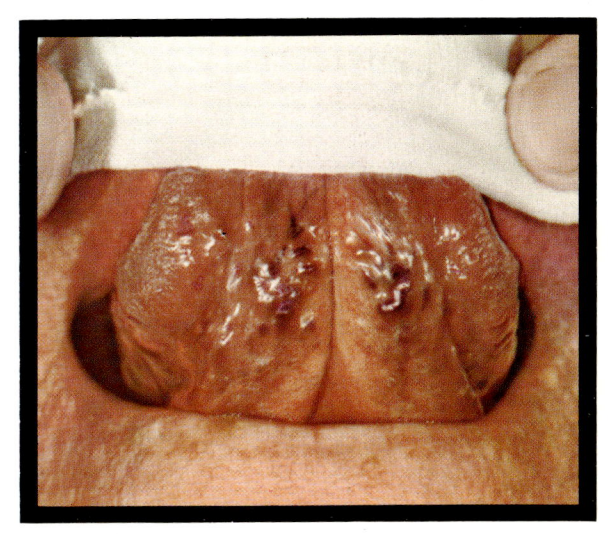

Lingual Varicosities

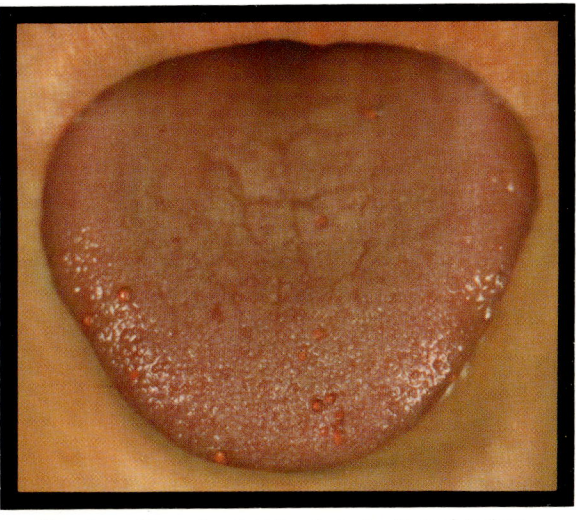

Hereditary Hemorrhagic Telangiectasia, Lingual Lesions

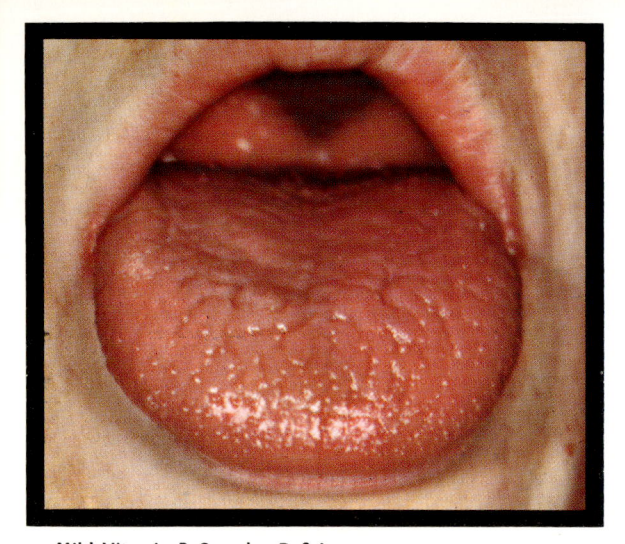

Mild Vitamin B Complex Deficiency

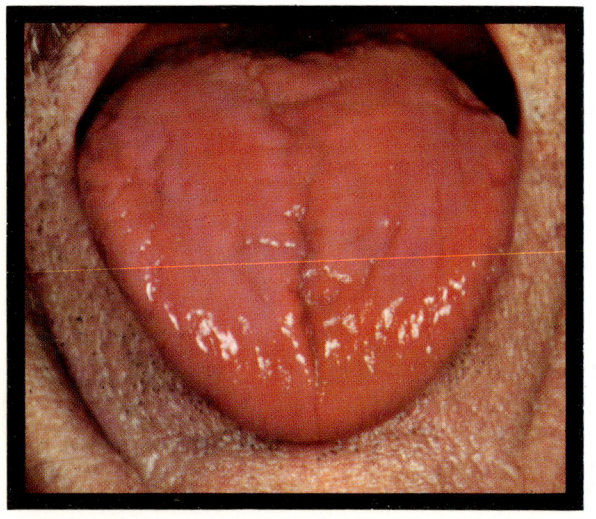

Vitamin B Complex Deficiency, Marked Papillary Atrophy

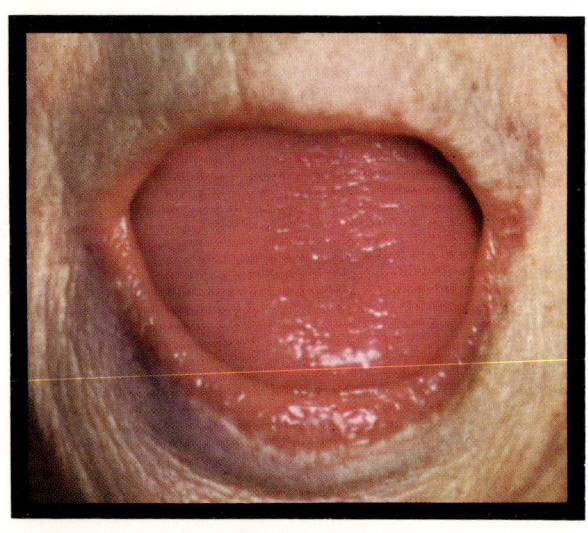

Vitamin B Complex Deficiency, Magenta Tongue

VITAMIN B COMPLEX MALNUTRITION

The most frequently occurring oral lesions related to nutritional disorders are those associated with vitamin B complex malnutrition. Among the factors constituting the B complex group are thiamine, nicotinic acid, riboflavin, B_{12}, folic acid, pyridoxine, choline, biotin and pantothenic acid. Seldom, if ever, is there a deficiency of only one of these substances, even in cases of beriberi and pellagra. Clinical manifestations of vitamin B complex deficiency include circumoral pallor, increased vertical markings of the lips, desquamation of the lips, angular cheilosis, seborrheic dermatitis in the nasolabial fold, magenta tongue, vascularization of the cornea, edema of the tongue, enlargement of fungiform papillae, fiery-red glossitis and stomatitis, and smooth tongue. A deficiency disease exists when an adequate amount of an essential substance does not reach tissues which need it for normal functioning. This may be due to failure of absorption or utilization as well as to dietary inadequacy. Diagnosis must usually be based on the presence of anatomic lesions, which do not appear until after the disease has been present for some time.

(Top) The fungiform papillae on the anterior portion of the tongue are enlarged. Bilateral angular cheilosis and an increase in the vertical markings on the left side of the upper lip are also apparent. The prominence of the fungiform papillae, a very early tongue change in vitamin B deficiency, is often overlooked. In this case the malnutrition was dietary, and there was a quick response to oral administration of vitamin B complex.

(Center) Malnutrition in this case is of long standing. There is a marked atrophy of both fungiform and filiform papillae, resulting in a very smooth dorsal surface. Intensive vitamin therapy for a period of months may be necessary in deficiencies of long duration before there is a remission of anatomic lesions. It is also important that a diet adequate in all essential nutrients be instituted.

(Bottom) Purplish-red (magenta) tongue with complete atrophy of the papillae, desquamation of the lower lip, and bilateral angular cheilosis. This is primarily a riboflavin deficiency.

Vitamin B Complex Malnutrition (Cont.)

(Top) Close-up of angular cheilosis in vitamin B complex deficiency. The lesion, which extends horizontally, involves both mucous membrane and skin. This patient was on an improperly fortified rice diet for the treatment of hypertension. Angular cheilosis may also result from a decrease in the vertical dimension, from licking the corners of the mouth (perlèche) or from drooling. With a marked loss of the vertical dimension, deep folds that slant downward are produced at the corners of the mouth. These become macerated because they are constantly bathed in saliva. It is not uncommon to find that a patient has angular cheilosis from both loss of vertical dimension and vitamin B complex deficiency.

CAROTENEMIA

(Center) The yellow skin color in the individual at right is the result of an excessive intake of carotene. This substance, a portion of which is converted into vitamin A in the liver, is found mainly in leafy, green, and yellow vegetables. Carotene is one of the pigments normally found in the epidermis and fat. An excess amount of it may be deposited in these tissues if the serum concentration exceeds a certain level. The pigmentation of the skin resulting from carotenemia is termed xanthosis cutis, aurantiasis cutis or carotenodermia. The patient shown is a strict vegetarian and for the last 18 months had eaten no meat, fish, fowl, or dairy products. He had been drinking the juice of 100 pounds of carrots a month.

(Bottom) Intra-oral view of above patient showing a carotenoid pigmentation, limited mainly to the soft palate. In xanthosis cutis the pigmentation is usually golden-yellow, the sclerae are rarely affected, and there is no pruritus. In jaundice the skin usually has a greenish-yellow tinge, pigmentation of the sclera occurs early, and pruritus is common. Appropriate laboratory tests for quality and quantity of serum bilirubin are important for differential diagnosis. Xanthosis cutis may occur in some diabetics and in a few rare conditions even when carotene intake is not high.

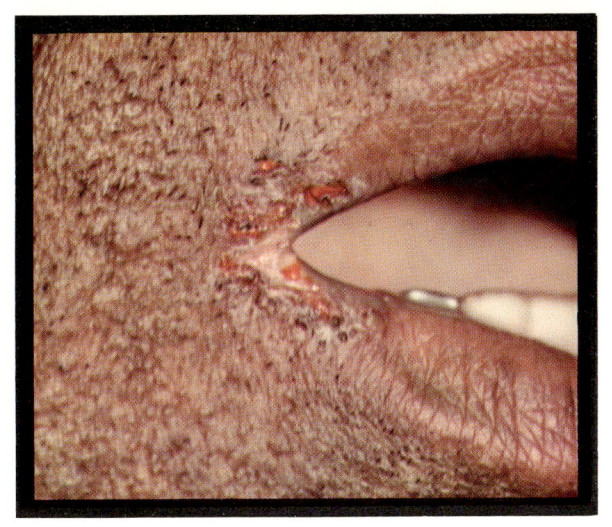

Vitamin B Complex Deficiency, Angular Cheilosis

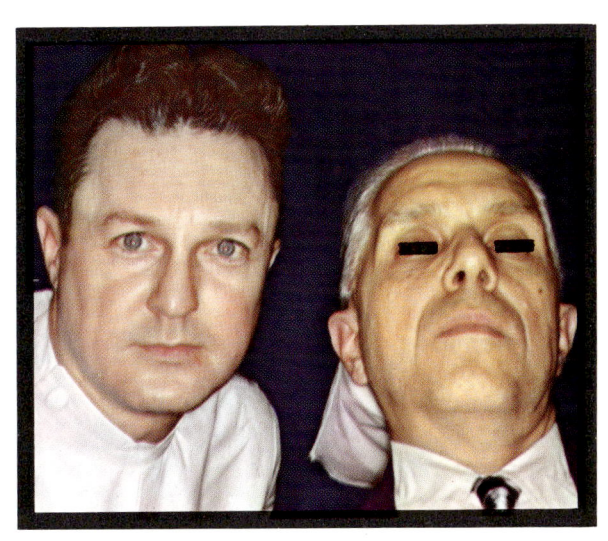

Xanthosis Cutis

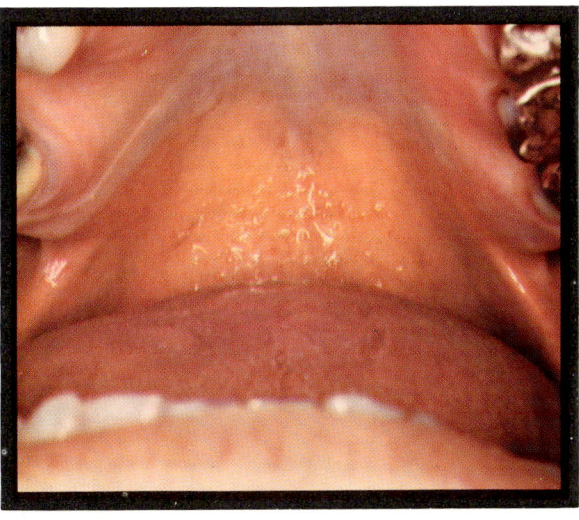

Oral Pigmentation Resulting from Carotenemia

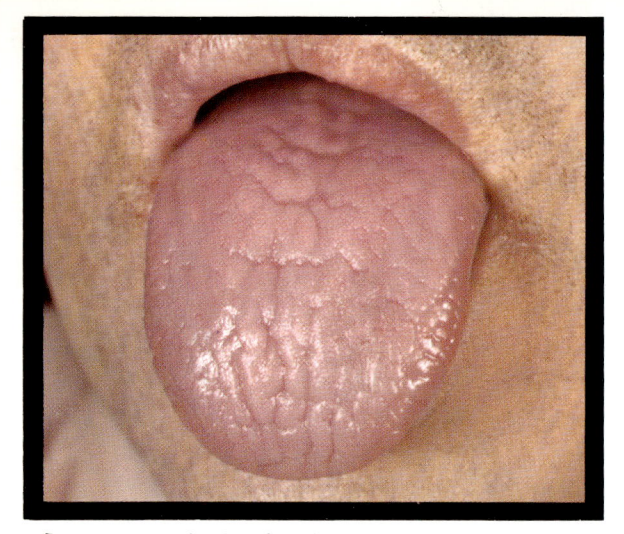

Pernicious Anemia, Atrophic Glossitis

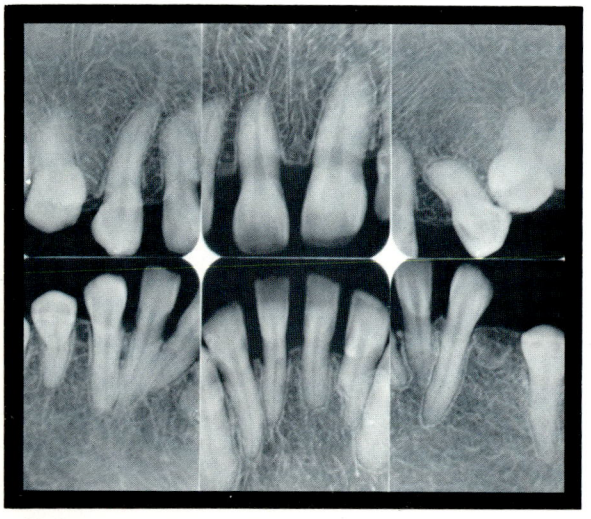

Mediterranean Anemia, "Hair-on-End" Trabeculae

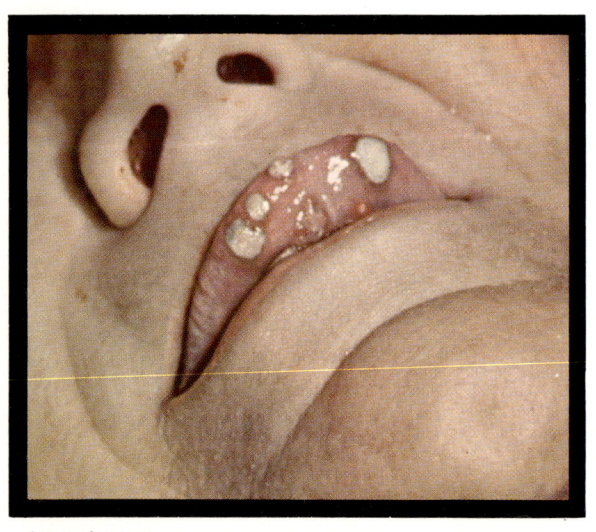

Agranulocytosis

PERNICIOUS ANEMIA

(Top) This disease is due to lack of an intrinsic factor in the gastric secretion without which absorption of the erythrocyte-maturing factor (vitamin B_{12}) is impaired. Laboratory findings: very low red cell count, macrocytosis, poikilocytosis, anisocytosis, normochromia, hypersegmented neutrophils, numerous megaloblasts in bone marrow, achlorhydria. Various signs and symptoms related to changes in hematologic, gastrointestinal and neurologic systems may be present. Among these, as shown in the illustration, are greenish-yellow skin color and glossitis. The dorsal surface of the tongue is atrophic, and the margins are red. In other cases the tongue may be painful and the lateral margins and tip fiery red.

MEDITERRANEAN ANEMIA

(Cooley's Anemia, Thalassemia)

(Center) This inherited disorder of defective hemoglobin synthesization, which is usually fatal, occurs mainly in people of Mediterranean ancestry. Laboratory findings: moderately low red cell count, hypochromia, microcytosis, anisocytosis, poikilocytosis, target cells, normoblasts. There may be icterus, splenomegaly, a mongoloid facies and a "hair-on-end" arrangement of the trabecular bone near the surface of the skull. In the accompanying radiographs this same trabecular change is seen in mandible and maxilla. Heterozygous individuals may have a mild, nonfatal form of the disease (thalassemia minor).

AGRANULOCYTOSIS

(Bottom) In agranulocytosis (malignant neutropenia) resistance to infection is very limited because of lack of circulating polymorphonuclear neutrophils. Often there are intra-oral ulcers, as shown here, with little reaction of the tissue. Drug idiosyncrasy and prolonged use of aminopyrine, sulfonamides, gold salts, barbiturates, thiouracil and excessive radiation are among the causes of repression of leukocyte formation. To prevent overwhelming infection and tissue destruction, the cause should be removed and antibiotics administered until the leukopoietic centers recover. Many cases have a fatal termination.

PRIMARY HYPERPARATHYROIDISM

This disease is due to an increased production of the parathyroid hormone, usually resulting from a functioning adenoma. The hormone (which regulates the renal excretion of phosphorus), when in excess, causes an immediate increase of phosphorus in the urine. This results in a fall of the serum phosphorus level, and as a consequence the serum calcium rises, which in turn leads to an increased excretion of calcium in the urine. Hyperparathyroidism is therefore characterized by hypercalcemia, hypercalciuria, hypophosphatemia and hyperphosphaturia. The most common complication of this disease is the formation of urinary calculi due to the high concentration of phosphorus and calcium in the urine. The most serious complication is the deposition of calcium in the kidney tubules (calcinosis), resulting in impaired renal function. The hypercalcemia is associated with a decrease in neuromuscular excitability which is manifested clinically by a generalized muscular weakness and constipation.

(Top) If the calcium excretion exceeds the intake, calcium is removed from bone. In advanced cases (von Recklinghausen's disease, osteitis fibrosa cystica) large regions of bone are replaced by connective tissue containing giant cells. In the case illustrated the cortex is expanded over 2 such giant cell lesions, one in the maxilla and one on the forehead.

(Center) The radiograph shown reveals a large region of radiolucency, resembling a cyst, transversed by a broad trabecula. The lamina dura (alveolar bone) is missing about the teeth, which resist resorption, and a smaller radiolucent lesion is adjacent to the 2nd bicuspid. Subperiosteal resorption along the margins of the middle phalanges and "cystic" lesions in the phalanges and long bones, as well as changes shown here in the jaws, are characteristic of osteitis fibrosa cystica.

(Bottom) Photomicrograph of a lesion removed from a patient with this disease. This lesion is called a "brown tumor" because of its gross appearance. The color is due to numerous hemosiderin-containing macrophages and extravascular red blood cells.

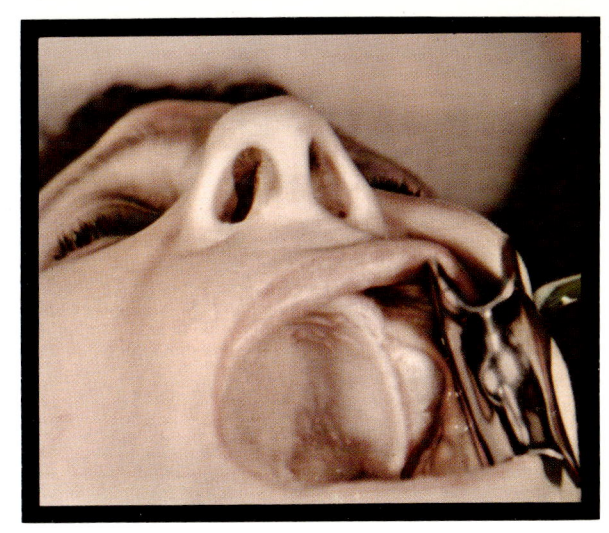

Hyperparathyroidism, Osteitis Fibrosa Cystica

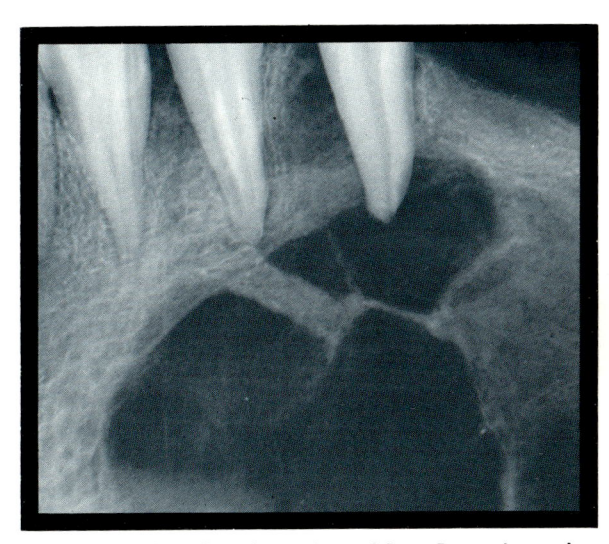

Hyperparathyroidism, Large Area of Bone Destruction and Loss of Lamina Dura

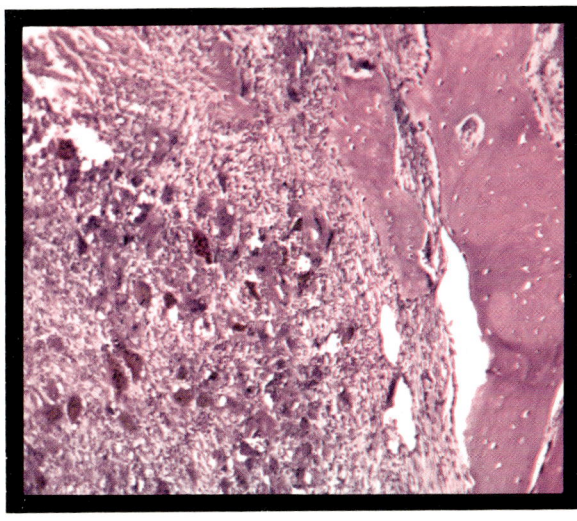

Hyperparathyroidism, Central Giant Cell Lesion X 80

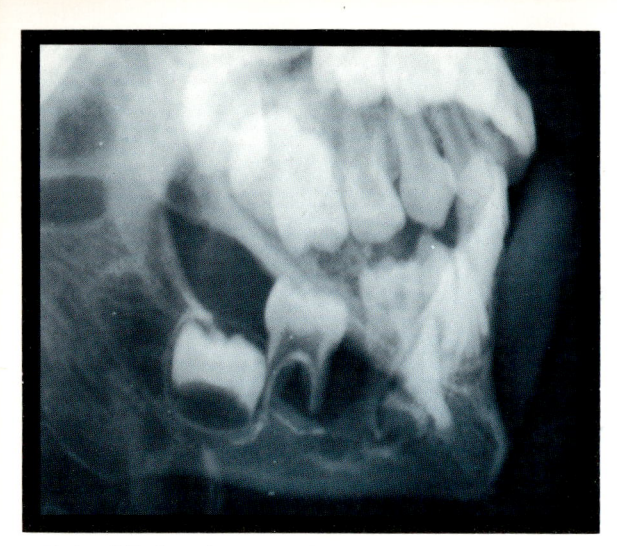

Eosinophilic Granuloma, Mandible

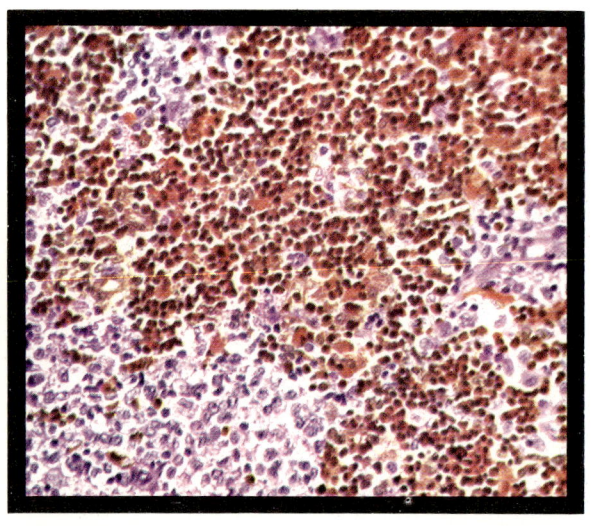

Eosinophilic Granuloma   X 220

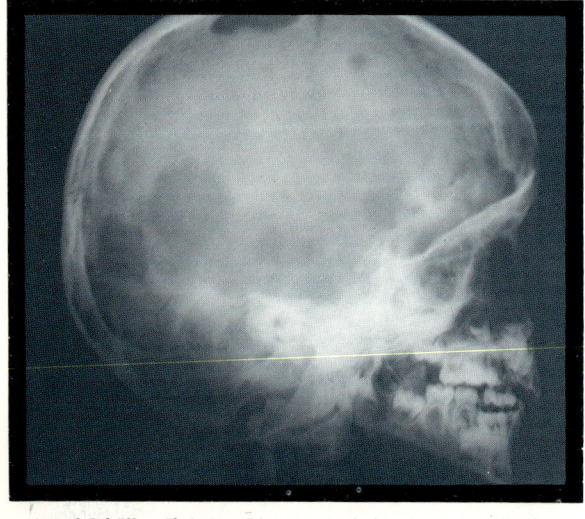

Hand-Schüller-Christian Disease, Radiolucent Areas, Skull

THE HISTIOCYTOSES

Eosinophilic Granuloma of Bone

(Top) Osseous destruction from an eosinophilic granuloma in the mandible of a young child. This granulomatous process, which may cause pain, begins in the medullary cavity and destroys bone quite rapidly. The lesion may expand the cortex, or it may perforate it and extend into soft tissue. An eosinophilic granuloma by its manner of growth may be mistaken clinically and radiographically for a malignant neoplasm. This entity, which occurs mainly in children and young adults, frequently affects only one bone. There are no extraskeletal foci or constitutional symptoms. A cure may be effected by curettement.

(Center) Biopsy specimen from the above case reveals granulation tissue in which there are masses of eosinophils and pale-lavender-staining vacuolated histiocytes.

Hand-Schüller-Christian Disease

(Bottom) This 4-year-old patient had multiple radiolucent areas in the skull, as shown here, as well as exophthalmos and diabetes insipidus (Christian's triad). The two latter manifestations are due to involvement of the orbit and the pituitary gland area. In this disease there may also be a limited number of other lesions in the skin, mucous membrane, bone and viscera.

The term histiocytosis has been applied to Hand-Schüller-Christian disease (chronic disseminated histiocytosis), Letterer-Siwe disease (acute disseminated histiocytosis) and eosinophilic granuloma (local histiocytosis), indicating that these are different manifestations of a single disease process. Letterer-Siwe disease rapidly involves almost all of the organs, and death occurs within a few months. Differentiation of these entities should not be based on histologic evidence alone, for the microscopic features may be quite similar. Other histiocytoses are Niemann-Pick disease (infants only, rapidly fatal, histiocytes contain sphingomyelin) and Gaucher's disease (familial, often chronic, histiocytes contain kerasin). Both of these diseases widely involve the reticuloendothelial system.

Diseases of the Oral Mucosa and Jaws

Hand-Schüller-Christian Disease (Cont.)

(Top) Microscopic appearance of a typical lesion in Hand-Schüller-Christian disease. Lipid-containing histiocytes, lymphocytes, plasma cells and eosinophils are embedded in a connective tissue stroma. The lipid is cholesterol. At this magnification the histiocytes appear as small, clear, circular structures with centrally placed dots. In Letterer-Siwe disease there are massive infiltrations of histiocytes, which usually do not contain lipid material.

SCLERODERMA

Diffuse scleroderma is a generalized collagen disease of unknown etiology. The most obvious clinical feature of this disease is stiffening of the skin, although symptoms may be variable and multiple. The collagenous fibers of the dermis swell and then atrophy, becoming packed together to form a dense connective tissue. The scarlike tissue limits motion and may gradually lead to inability to swallow. Skin appendages atrophy, the epidermis becomes thinned and may be hyperpigmented. Vascular lumina may be diminished due to intimal proliferation, and the kidneys, lungs, liver and muscles may become involved in the fibrosing process. A local form of the disease (circumscribed scleroderma) involves only limited regions of the skin and produces no visceral lesions.

(Center) This patient shows the typical picture of moderately advanced scleroderma. The natural lines of the face are nearly obliterated, she has a fixed expression giving her a Mona Lisa-like appearance, and her skin appears somewhat bronzed. The eyelids and fingers, particularly, show the atrophic, shiny appearance which overlies the collagenous changes in the connective tissue. Sclerosed tissue has produced discrete nodules on the eyelids. Because of the rigidity of her sclerosed skin she could not open her mouth wide, and the movement of her fingers was limited.

(Bottom) In some cases of scleroderma there is a uniform thickening of the periodontal membrane with disorientation of the periodontal fibers about one or more of the teeth—mainly the posteriors. An increase in the width of the lamina dura is often associated with this distinctive change.

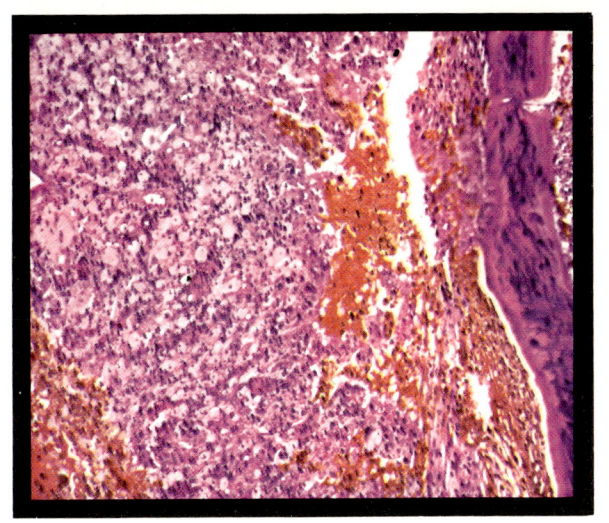

Hand-Schüller-Christian Disease   X 200

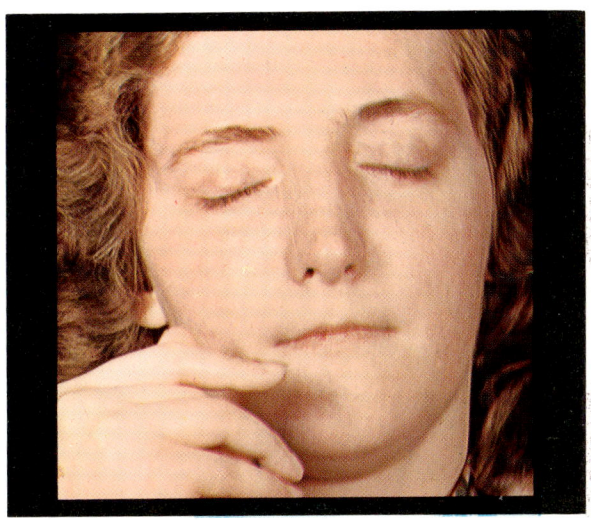

Scleroderma

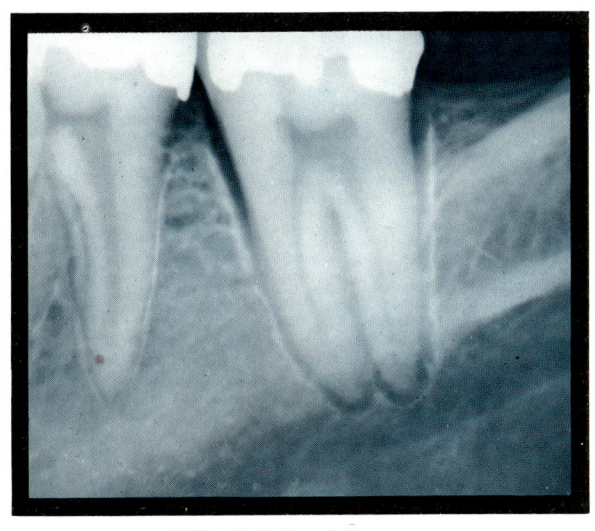

Scleroderma, Wide Periodontal Space About 2nd Molar

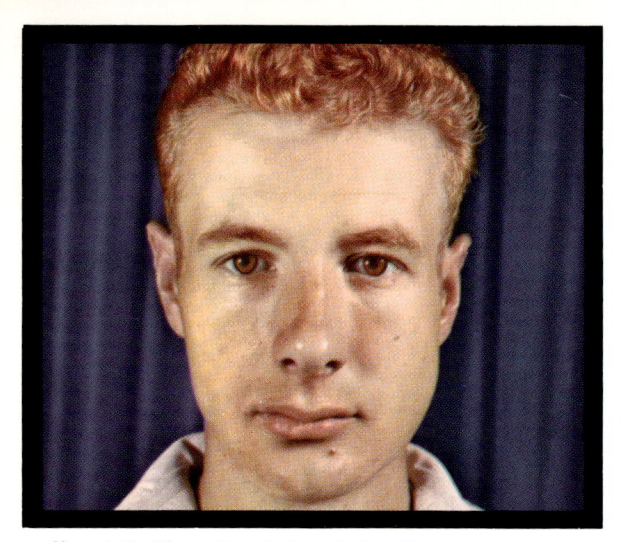

Monostotic Fibrous Dysplasia, Left Mandible

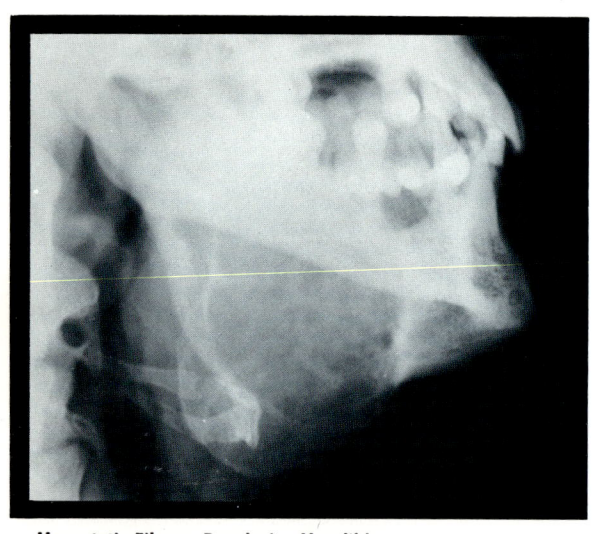

Monostotic Fibrous Dysplasia, Mandible

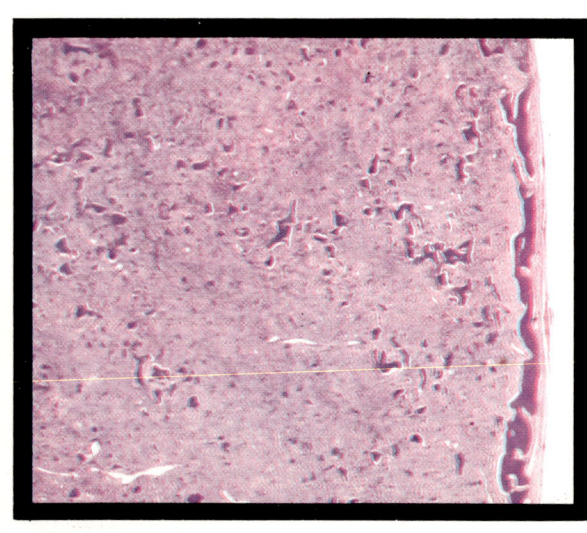

Fibrous Dysplasia   X 11

FIBROUS DYSPLASIA

Fibrous dysplasia is a skeletal disease characterized by replacement of the bone and bone marrow by a fibrous connective tissue. Numerous irregular and haphazardly arranged osseous spicules develop within the fibrous connective tissue. A polyostotic type of the disease is characterized by fibrous bone lesions that usually are unilateral, brown pigmentation of the skin, precocious puberty (in females) and other endocrine disturbances (Albright's syndrome). The monostotic type shows only the fibrous replacement of bone and bone marrow in one bone without related endocrine and dermal symptoms. Whether or not the two diseases are related is debatable. The terms osseous dysplasia and fibro-osseous dysplasia have been suggested for the monostotic type previously called ossifying fibroma (see p. 141).

(Top) Monostotic fibrous dysplasia in the mandible of a 24-year-old patient. The swelling of the left side of the face, which was asymptomatic, first became noticeable 4 years previously, following the extraction of 2 lower left molar teeth. Exploration of the lesion revealed that the cortex was very thin but intact, and the interior of the bone was filled with tough, brownish-white, resilient, gritty soft tissue.

(Center) Radiograph of patient shown above. The mandible shows a diffuse, poorly demarcated, multilocular expansile lesion that involves most of the body of the ramus on one side. The radiographic appearance varies with different stages of the disease, showing more radiolucency early and more radiopacity later. In this particular case the normal trabecular pattern has been lost, and the cortical layer is poorly defined. There is a ground-glass appearance, suggesting that there has been irregular calcification within the fibrous connective tissue.

(Bottom) Low-power view of a section of tissue from the case shown above. The lesion is composed largely of fibrous connective tissue with osteoblastic potential. There are numerous purple-stained spicules of bone scattered through the connective tissue and thin cortical bone at the right margin. The scattered osseous spicules absorb the x-rays to give the picture seen in the radiograph.

Fibrous Dysplasia (Cont.)

(Top) Higher magnification from one area of this case shows many calcified ovoid structures generally devoid of lacunae. Osteoblasts do not border these calcified masses. Viewing this one field, some might consider the calcified structures as cementum and diagnose this as a cementifying fibroma, a term which has aroused much debate.

ACROMEGALY

This disease of adults is caused by an overproduction of the growth hormone as a result of a functioning eosinophilic adenoma of the anterior lobe of the pituitary. Hyperfunction of eosinophilic cells occurring in young individuals (before epiphyses have closed) results in pituitary giantism. Acromegaly is characterized by an enlargement of the nose, ears, lips, tongue, mandible, hands and feet. It occurs with equal frequency in both sexes, and clinical manifestations usually first become apparent in the 3rd decade. In acromegaly numerous other glands of internal secretion are often indirectly involved. There may be a hyperplasia of the thymus, parathyroid, thyroid and adrenal glands and an atrophy of the ovaries or testes and the endocrine portion of the pancreas. Therefore, signs and symptoms related to multiple endocrine dysfunction may be associated with acromegaly. Headaches and impaired vision may result from enlargement of the adenoma.

(Center) A 65-year-old edentulous patient in whom the typical acromegalic characteristics (enlarged hands, lower jaw and lip) first became apparent 30 years previously. In physiologic-rest position the lower anterior alveolar ridge was 1-1/2 inches forward of the maxillary ridge. This fact, plus a marked macroglossia, made construction of satisfactory dentures most difficult.

(Bottom) Another patient, in whom separation of the teeth was the first observed clinical manifestation of acromegaly. During the active-growth period of this disease the correction of occlusion, the reconstruction of partial and full dentures, and the remaking of fixed bridges are continuing problems.

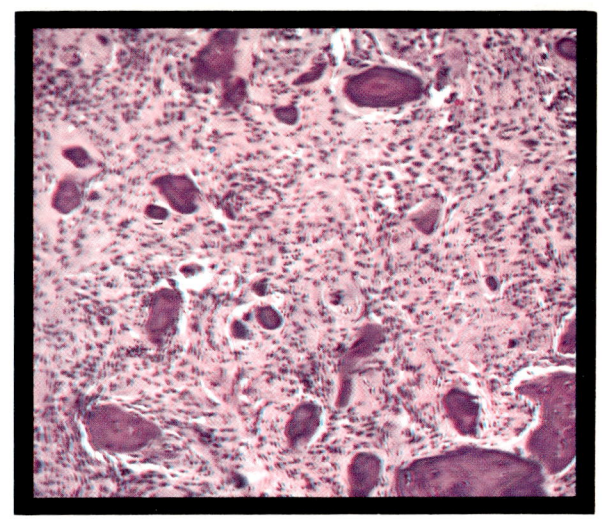

Fibrous Dysplasia   X 100

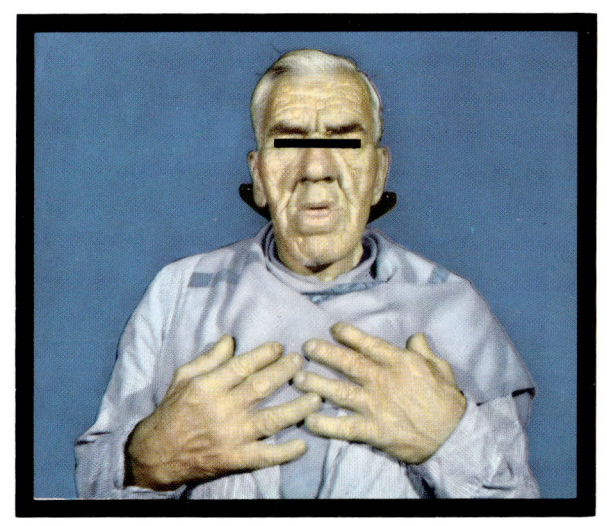

Acromegaly

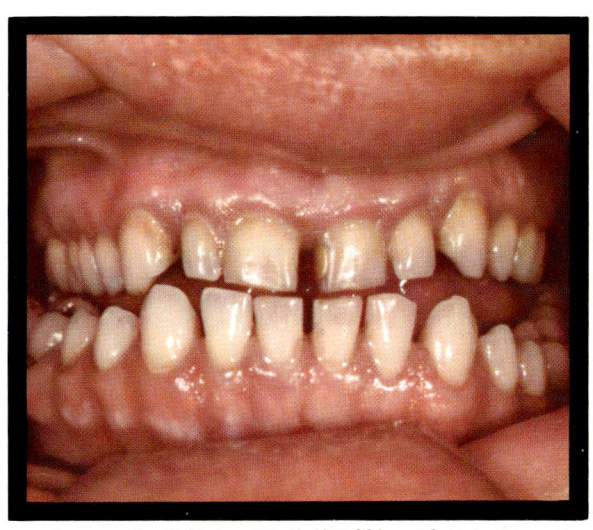

Acromegaly, Enlargement of Mandible and Separation of Teeth

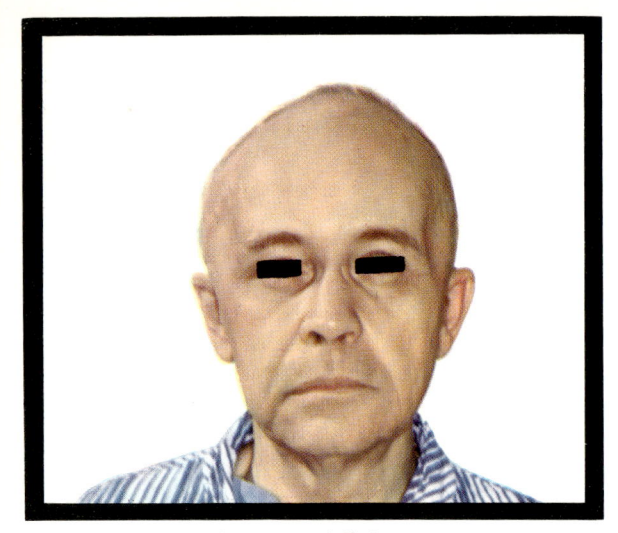

Paget's Disease, Enlargement of Skull

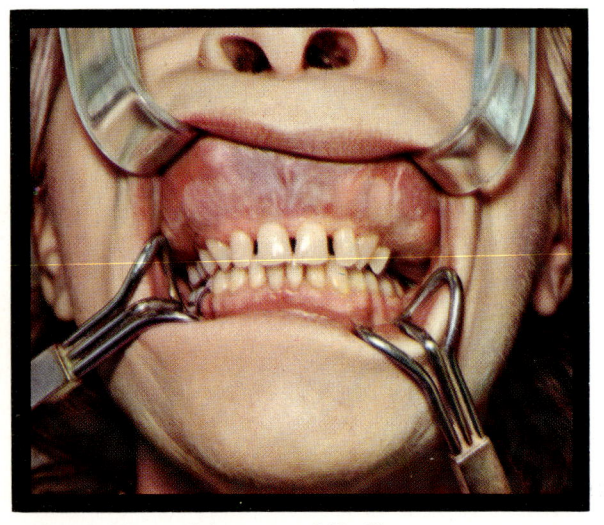

Paget's Disease, Enlargement of Maxilla

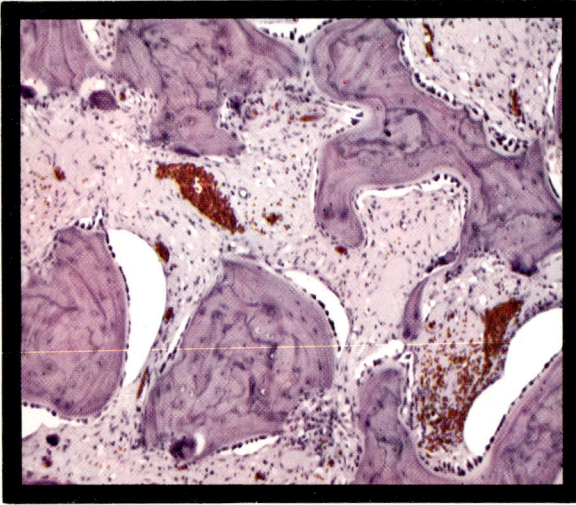

Paget's Disease, Mosaic Pattern of Bone   X 100

134   Diseases of the Oral Mucosa and Jaws

PAGET'S DISEASE OF BONE

(Osteitis Deformans)

This disease of adults is characterized by rapid resorption and extensive deposition of bone in a manner not related to functional needs. These two processes may go on simultaneously, or they may alternate. In the early stages resorption is more pronounced, but later osteogenesis becomes increasingly dominant, resulting in progressive enlargement of the affected bones. The newly formed bone will not stand stress; hence, if weight-bearing bones are involved, they may become compressed or bent. This is not a generalized disease of bone, although many bones may be affected. The serum calcium and phosphorus levels are usually normal; alkaline phosphatase is increased during the active phase of the disease. Sarcoma of the involved bones, arteriosclerosis and cardiac enlargement are apt to occur in individuals with extensive Paget's disease.

(Top) Nonsymmetrical enlargement of the skull, as in this case, is often the first indication of the disease. A rib, the pelvis, the left femur and the maxilla were also involved. Radiographic examination revealed the following: skull—"absorbent-cotton" appearance of the right parietal bone; maxilla—areas of osteoporosis adjacent to regions of sclerosis, trabeculae in other areas thin but close together, lamina dura almost completely obliterated. Hypercementosis (often present in Paget's disease of the jaws) was not evident in this case.

(Center) Marked enlargement of maxilla, with separation of the teeth. The antra were greatly diminished in size. Paget's disease, which is of unknown etiology, affects the maxilla more frequently than the mandible.

(Bottom) The dark-blue-staining, irregularly curved cement lines indicate where resorption ceased and osteoid was again deposited. These lines appear to separate various fragments, as in a mosaic or a jigsaw puzzle. The marrow is fibrous and quite vascular. Both apposition and resorption are evident on the margins of each bone spicule. The mosaic pattern is seen only in fully developed Paget's bone.

5
Neoplasms

INTRODUCTION

A neoplasm may be defined as an uncontrolled new growth (Ewing). Neoplasms arise spontaneously and exhibit independent unlimited growth, are usually nonfunctional, but if functional are independent of biological control. They always produce deleterious effect and may cause death of the host.

Neoplasms may be classified in numerous ways. The simplest way is to divide them into epithelial neoplasms and supporting tissue neoplasms. In each of these groups there are benign and malignant types. Benign epithelial neoplasms of stratified squamous epithelium are termed papillomas; of columnar epithelium, polyps (not to be confused with inflammatory polyps); and of glandular epithelium, adenomas. Malignant epithelial neoplasms are designated as carcinomas. The terms for most benign supporting tissue neoplasms are formed by adding the suffix "oma" to the histologic designation of the tissue of origin; e.g., fibroma, lipoma. Malignant supporting tissue neoplasms are called sarcomas, as fibrosarcoma, liposarcoma. Cancer is a general term applied to any type of malignant neoplasm. The term tumor is loosely used to indicate a neoplasm but is commonly used as a general term to designate a benign neoplasm or nonneoplastic overgrowth.

Benign neoplasms closely resemble their parent tissue, grow slowly by expansion, and remain localized. Malignant neoplasms are anaplastic, rapidly infiltrating growths which spread by metastasis. The individual cells exhibit hyperchromatism, abnormal division figures, altered polarity and variation in size, shape and proportion of nuclear mass. The aforementioned characteristics of benign and malignant tumors are applicable in general, but it is necessary to have specific knowledge about each neoplasm as histologic characteristics do not reflect a neoplasm's behavior. It is best to consider each type of neoplasm as a different disease.

Neoplasia is related to the inherent ability of cells to multiply. It seems probable that normally cell growth is regulated by an inhibitory factor; and further, that when this inhibiting influence is diminished or when stimulation to growth is too great to be controlled, a neoplasm results. The exact mechanism by which a cell becomes neoplastic is not known. Once the transformation has occurred, however, the trait of uncontrolled growth is transmitted to successive generations of cells.

Extrinsic factors that appear to be important in neoplastic transformation include coal tar and its products, chronic inflammation (from both trauma and infection), sunlight, heat, ionizing radiation and viral infections.

Neoplasia is not inherited, but it is evident that there is some intrinsic factor which conditions the neoplastic response to carcinogenic agents. The inherent factor in man is suggestive in many neoplasms but readily apparent in only a few, e.g., retinoblastoma. Neoplasms may develop from morphologic abnormalities which are themselves inheritable, e.g., carcinoma occurring in multiple polyps of the intestine.

Prevention is the ultimate goal of the cancer problem, but at present the mortality rate can be altered only by elimination of recognizable extrinsic factors, early diagnosis and early treatment. The treatment of neoplastic disease should be done by specially trained individuals, but early detection and verification of diagnosis by biopsy with immediate referral to the therapist is the responsibility of every practitioner. Any lesion which has existed for 2 weeks should be biopsied unless its exact nature is known.

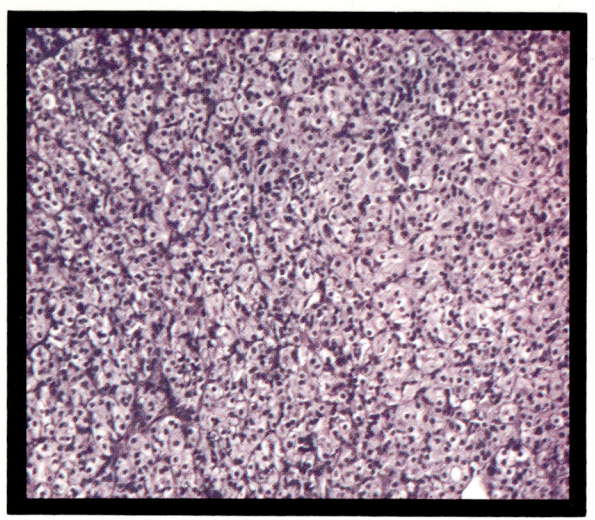

Serous Adenoma, Parotid Gland   X 100

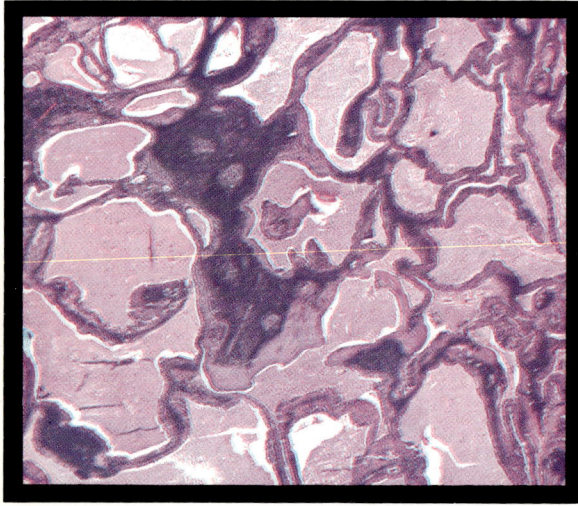

Papillary Cystadenoma Lymphomatosum   X 12

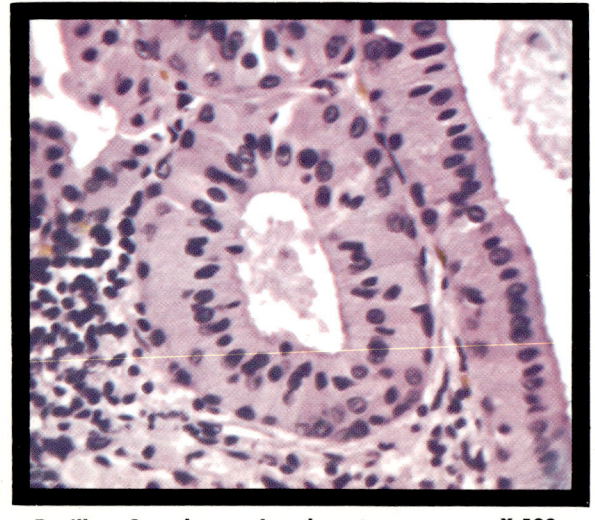

Papillary Cystadenoma Lymphomatosum   X 500

BENIGN NEOPLASMS

Adenoma

(Top) A benign neoplastic proliferation of acinar cells in the parotid gland. The cells, though not in normal acinar arrangement, closely resemble their histologic prototype and are relatively uniform in size, shape and staining quality. They may be slightly functional.

Papillary Cystadenoma Lymphomatosum

(Warthin's Tumor)

This benign neoplasm occurs in or near the parotid gland. It is probably always benign, although a few questionable exceptions have been reported. Clinically it appears as a slow-growing, hard, nontender lump over the angle or ramus of the mandible or behind the ear. This tumor, which sometimes occurs bilaterally, is much more frequent in males than in females, and its highest incidence is in the 5th decade. The designation "papillary cystadenoma lymphomatosum" is clearly descriptive of the histologic appearance of this entity. The neoplasm has a lymphoid stroma with germinal centers, and the epithelial parenchyma forms tubules and cystic spaces partitioned by numerous papillary projections.

(Center) In this topographic view the lymphoid stroma (dark-blue areas) and numerous large epithelial-lined cysts containing a pink-staining amorphous material are well demonstrated. Papillary projections are seen in a few of the cysts.

(Bottom) This photomicrograph illustrates the distinctive epithelium of this tumor. The tubule (center) and the microcyst (far right) are lined by large columnar cells with an eosinophilic cytoplasm and dark-staining peripherally located nuclei. Toward the basement membrane are 1 to 2 rows of cuboidal epithelial cells. The most widely accepted theory as to the histogenesis of this neoplasm is that it develops from salivary duct epithelium misplaced in lymph nodes located within or in the vicinity of the parotid. The characteristic epithelial cells in this neoplasm are quite similar to oxyphilic granular cells (oncocytes) found in nonneoplastic salivary gland tissue of individuals over 50 years of age.

Papilloma

Papillomas are benign neoplasms of squamous epithelium. The exophytic growth pattern forms varying numbers of projections. Papillomas may have a broad base firmly attached to the surface (sessile), or may arise from a slender stalk (pedunculated) and be freely movable. The surface of the lesion is white due to the high degree of keratinization and tendency for retention of keratin. Some papillomas consist of limp, white, threadlike projections which resemble somewhat the hyperplastic filiform papillae of hairy tongue; in others the projections are blunt, short and stiff; and in still others the surface has a cauliflowerlike appearance. A pedunculated papilloma may be readily diagnosed clinically, but without histologic examination the sessile, cauliflower type is difficult to distinguish from a papillomatous carcinoma.

(Top) Papilloma arising from floor of mouth in region of mandibular molar teeth. Papillomas are usually small in size and single, as in this case, but are sometimes large and multiple. Children occasionally have numerous lesions (juvenile papillomata) in the larynx, pharynx, and oral cavity which, until the age of puberty, tend to grow rapidly and to recur if removed.

(Center) This sessile type of papilloma has the clinical appearance of a wart (verruca vulgaris). Though a verruca is an epithelial overgrowth, it differs from a papilloma in being virus-induced and nonneoplastic. In addition it is always sessile, markedly hornified, and the rete pegs at its periphery bend in toward the center. Intranuclear inclusion bodies may occasionally be identified in verrucae.

(Bottom) Photomicrograph showing how the proliferating epithelium of a papilloma protrudes outward, forming numerous folds. Each fold is supported by a thin, vascular, fibrous connective tissue core. Cell detail cannot be seen at this magnification, but it is evident that the epithelium has a uniform character and the dark-staining basal layer is intact. Compare with papillomatous carcinoma (p. 159, top).

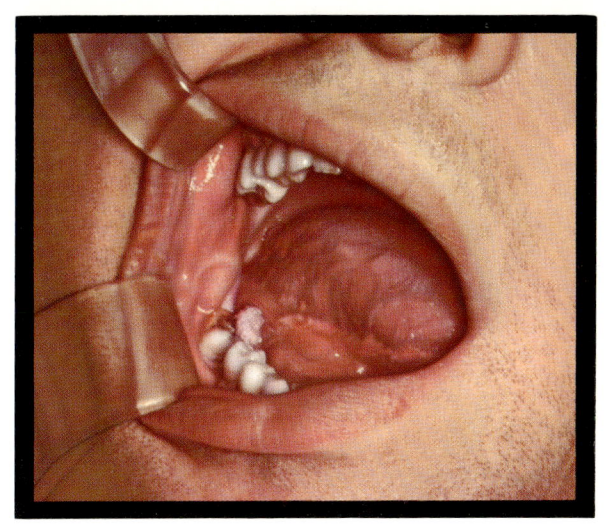

Papilloma, Floor of Mouth

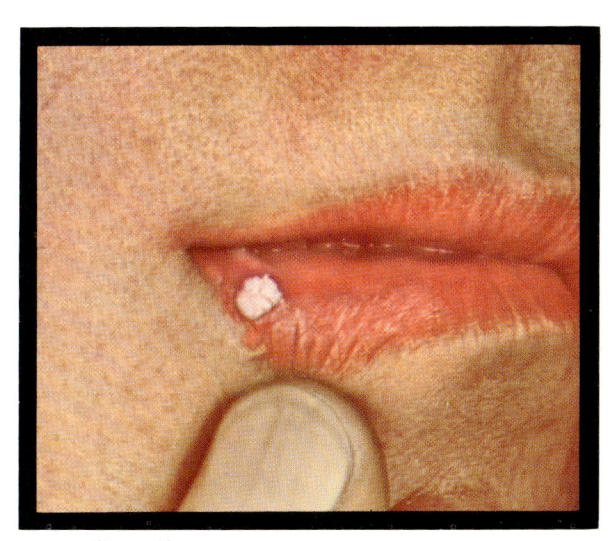

Papilloma, Lip

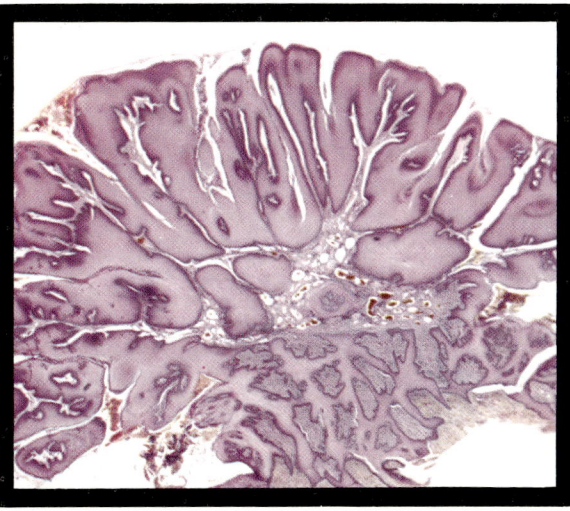

Papilloma X 6

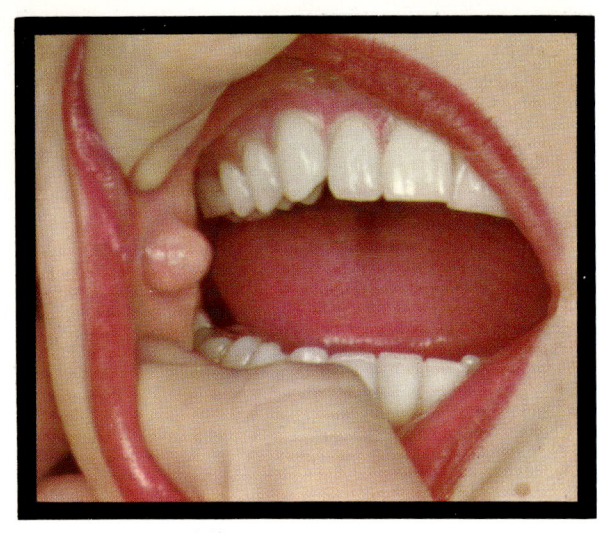

"Fibroma," Buccal Mucosa

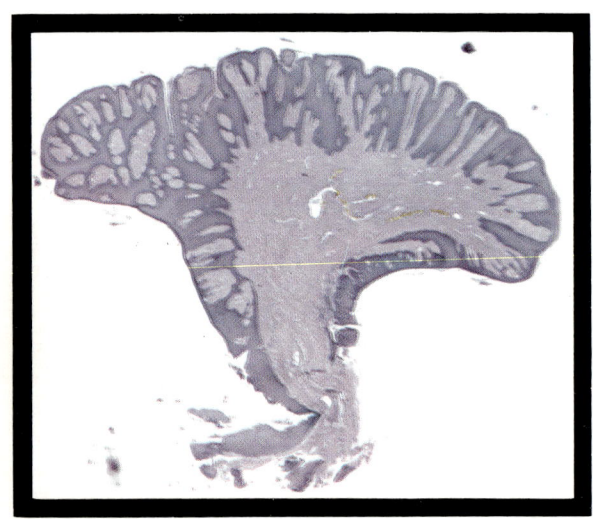

Fibroepithelial Polyp   X 10

Fibroma   X 100

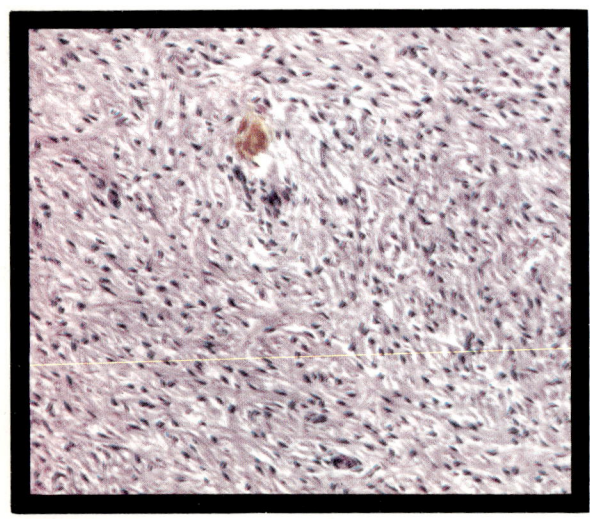

Fibroma

A true fibroma of the oral cavity is a rare entity. The term is often used, however, to designate localized proliferations of fibrous tissue which are hypertrophic scars or the result of long-standing irritation. Such nonneoplastic fibrous lesions are found in the buccal mucosa opposite the occlusal line, the lateral border of the tongue, the vestibular mucosa and the lip. They may be either sessile or pedunculated and are usually smooth-surfaced, firm and asymptomatic. These fibrous nodules are comparable to the hyperplasias from denture irritation (p. 94) and the fibrous epulides (p. 89). Rather than implying neoplasia by describing them as fibromas, it is more accurate to designate them as areas of subepithelial fibrosis, as fibrous hyperplasias, as irritation "fibromas" or as fibroepithelial polyps.

(Top) Histologic examination of this so-called fibroma in the buccal mucosa revealed compressed stratified squamous epithelium covering a core of dense, hyalinized fibrous connective tissue. Fibrous lesions in this location are usually the result of sucking and chewing on the cheek. They continue to grow slowly as long as they are traumatized, the increase in size being related to productive inflammation. If the irritation ceases, the lesion will stop enlarging and may decrease slightly in size.

(Center) The central portion of this pedunculated lesion is composed of dense fibrous connective tissue. The covering epithelium (blue) is markedly thickened, and broad, fused rete pegs extend deep into the underlying tissue. This enlargement is the result of an overgrowth of both epithelium and connective tissue. Such a lesion is sometimes designated as a fibroepithelial papilloma (fibropapilloma), the term being used to indicate the components and the configuration of the enlargement rather than to imply neoplasia.

(Bottom) A section from a continuously enlarging growth in the floor of the mouth. This is a true fibroma. There is a marked fibroblastic proliferation. The intensity of nuclear staining is uniform, and the nuclei vary little in size and shape. (Compare this lesion with its malignant counterpart, p. 165.)

Lipoma

(Top) A lipoma consists of adult fat cells which are grouped into lobules by vascular fibrous connective tissue septa. This type of neoplasm usually appears clinically as a light-yellow spherical enlargement which is soft to palpation. In the case illustrated the lesion is deeply situated, and therefore the characteristic yellow color is not apparent on the surface. Lipomas are common in the subcutaneous tissue of the trunk, upper extremities, and neck, but are less frequently encountered in the oral cavity. The most common locations in the oral regions are the buccal mucosa and the floor of the mouth. Lipomas grow slowly, and malignant transformation seldom occurs.

(Center) Supporting stroma is apparent at upper right. The clear circular structures are fat cells; those cut in the plane of their nuclei (which are compressed against the cell membrane) resemble signet rings. Lipid present is typical of that found in normal fat and is dissolved away in preparation, but may be demonstrated by special staining of frozen sections. It is generally believed that the fat in a lipoma is not available for nutritional purposes. Many fatty tumors contain fibrous connective tissue in excess of the usual quantity of supporting stroma in adipose tissue. These are termed fibrolipomas.

Myxoma

(Bottom) Myxomas are benign neoplasms representative of the embryonal stroma. They are composed of scattered stellate cells having delicate processes widely separated by mucoid material. Although benign, they are locally aggressive, nonencapsulated infiltrating lesions. They occur in joints and periarticular structures and often produce marked destruction of joints. They also may occur within bone. True myxomas are rare in the jaws, but some arise from the dental papilla. Although they have a similar histologic pattern, these odontogenic myxomas do not exhibit the aggressive behavior of the nonodontogenic myxomas, and cure may be accomplished by less radical surgery. The lesion in the jaw often is lobulated and radiographically may simulate the ameloblastoma, but, unlike that neoplasm, it does produce root resorption.

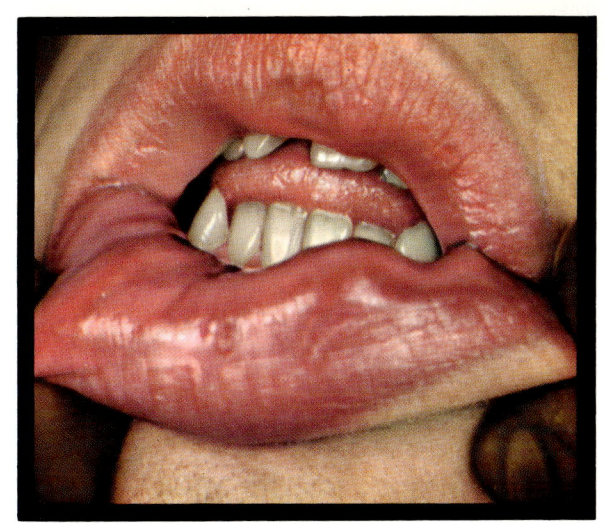

Lipoma, Lip

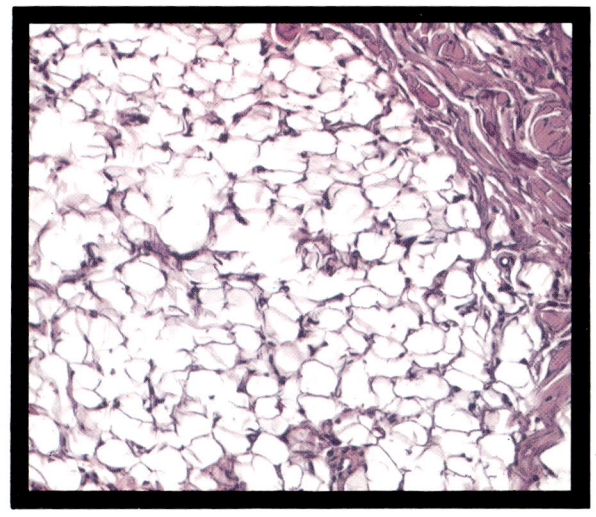

Lipoma   X 100

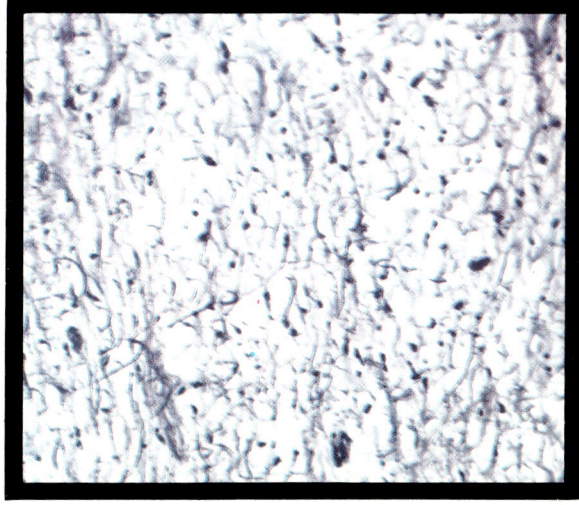

Myxoma   X 100

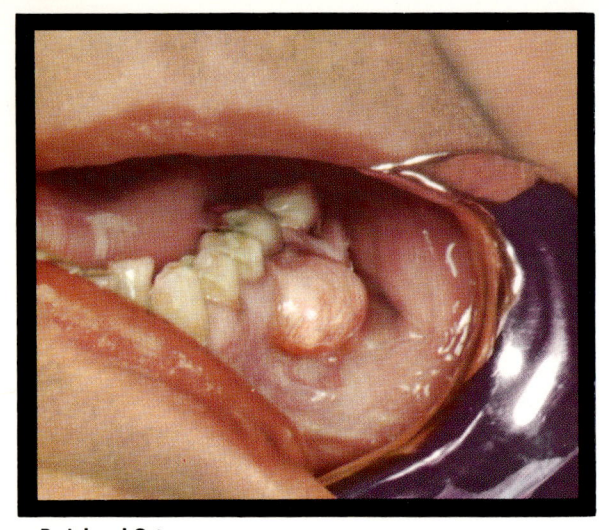

Benign Tumors of Osseous Origin

Neoplasms in this group are frequently an admixture of connective tissue, cartilage and bone. These osseous tumors vary greatly as to the proportion of each type of tissue as well as to the degree of organization of the component elements. For this reason there is much variation in the histologic appearance of these lesions, although basically they are closely related. The osteoma is composed almost entirely of well-differentiated mature bone; while others, like the osteochondromyxoma, are comprised of immature tissue of each type in varying proportions. Skeletal neoplasms arising from marrow, vessels or nerves are not usually considered to be of osseous origin.

(Top) Osteoma of moderate size on the lateral border of mandible near bicuspid region. The mucosa overlying this hard, bony enlargement is thin and blanched. Peripheral osseous nodules arise from the periosteum while central tumors arise from the endosteum. They increase in size slowly and generally are asymptomatic. Osteomas that are central in origin may cause some expansion of the cortical plates but do not produce the type of nodular mass seen here. It is sometimes difficult to differentiate between peripheral osteomas and hyperplasias of bone (exostoses) other than those commonly designated as tori. (See p. 23.) Generally the osteoma exhibits a greater capacity for growth and contains immature bone, while hyperostoses show laminated growth and mature compact bone.

(Center) Radiograph of the osteoma shown in the preceding picture. The sharply defined area of increased density can be observed superimposed over the 1st molar and 2nd bicuspid. The degree of radiopacity of the lesion indicates that the osseous structure is compact.

(Bottom) In this section of a dense osteoma of the type shown above, numerous heavy, irregular trabeculae are apparent. These are separated by small spaces containing vascular fibrous connective tissue. In older lesions fibrous connective tissue is nearly absent, while it is more plentiful in younger ones.

Peripheral Osteoma

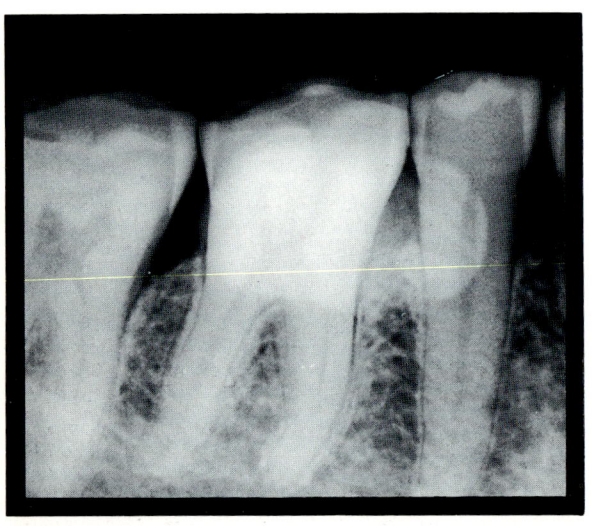

Peripheral Osteoma

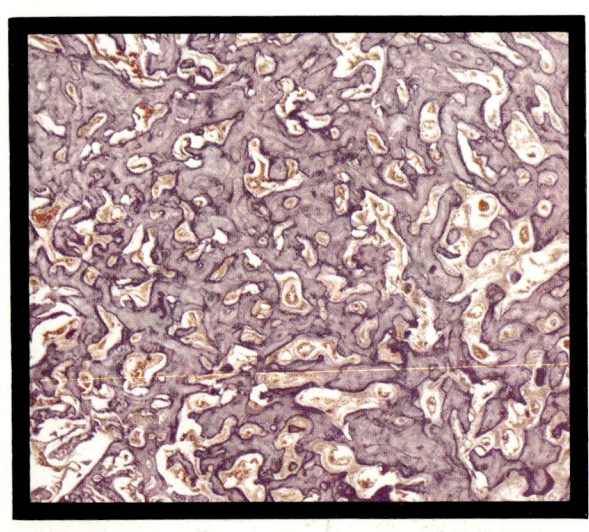

Osteoma   X 14

Benign Tumors of Osseous Origin (Cont.)

Benign tumors of osseous origin which contain more than one type of tissue are more frequently encountered than those of a single tissue type. Those with mixed elements are composed of varying amounts of myxomatous, fibrous, cartilaginous and osseous tissue and arise from less well differentiated cells than do the pure tumors. Varying degrees of mucopolysaccharide polymerization determine the character of the various components. The myxomatous components undergo transition to cartilage, and the fibrous tissue develops bone. These neoplasms are named by the types of tissue present in reverse order of predominance.

(Top) Large, sharply circumscribed lesion involving the body and angle of the mandible. It is radiolucent peripherally and radiopaque centrally. Histologic examination revealed that the tumor was composed of fibrous connective tissue and bone, with the latter tissue predominating (fibro-osteoma). At an earlier stage this neoplasm probably could have been designated as an osteofibroma or ossifying fibroma. Benign fibro-osseous neoplasms generally grow very slowly in adults. However, when they occur before puberty, they sometimes grow much more rapidly and produce a marked deformity. Ossifying fibrous tumors in some instances are difficult to distinguish from fibrous dysplasia (p. 132).

(Center) This photomicrograph demonstrates a cartilaginous area from an osteochondroma. The hyaline cartilage in this instance does not vary greatly from normal. (See p. 7.) Pure chondromas of the jaw are rare. Tumors containing cartilage should be examined thoroughly, for in some cases evidence of malignancy may be easily overlooked. See chondrosarcoma, page 165.

(Bottom) The photomicrograph depicts the histologic character of one portion of an osteochondromyxoma which occurred in the mandible. Near the top of the illustration there is an area in which the stroma has condensed, with the entrapment of cells, and represents bone. The large cells below this bone and in the homogeneous matrix represent cartilage. Bone also is evident in the lower left-hand corner.

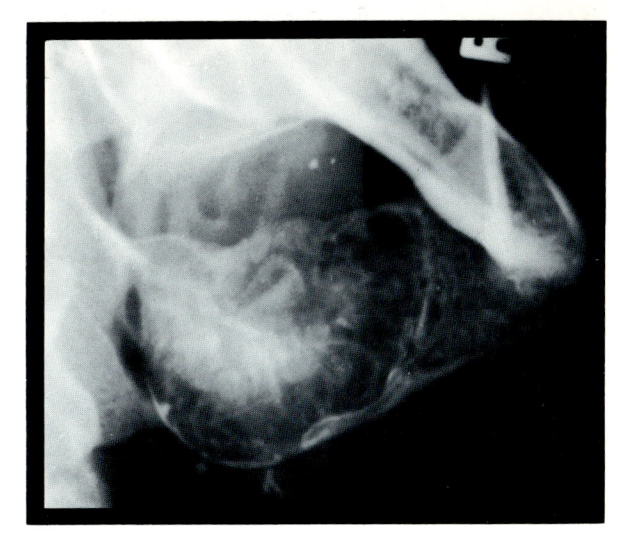

Fibro-osteoma, Mandible

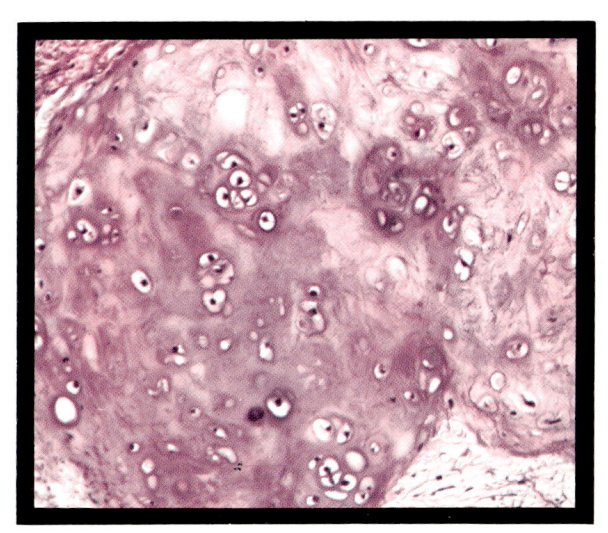

Osteochondroma   X 120

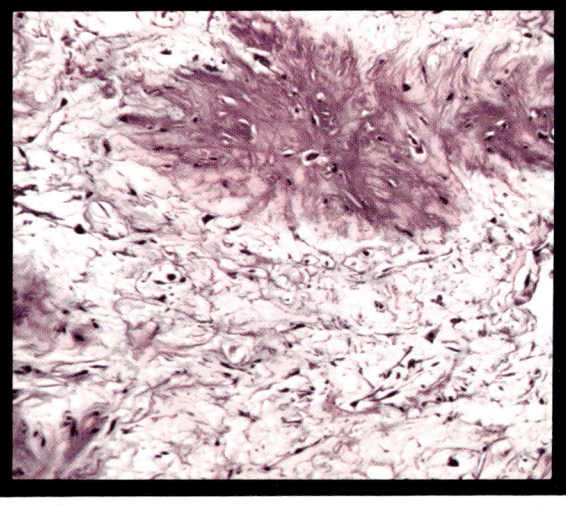

Osteochondromyxoma   X 100

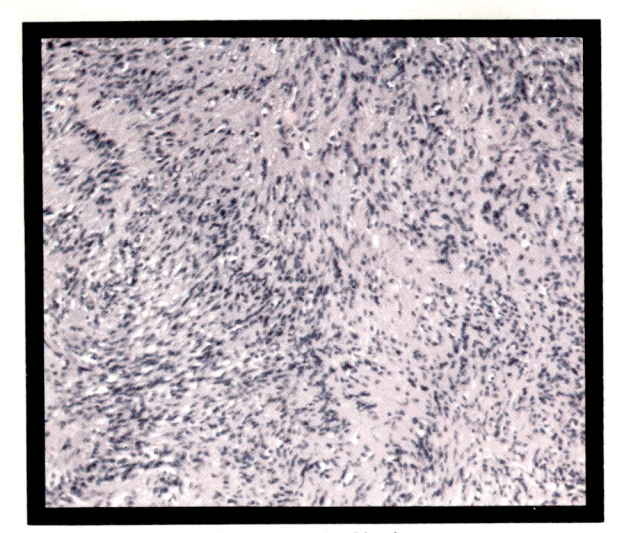

Neurilemoma (Schwannoma), Gingiva   X 100

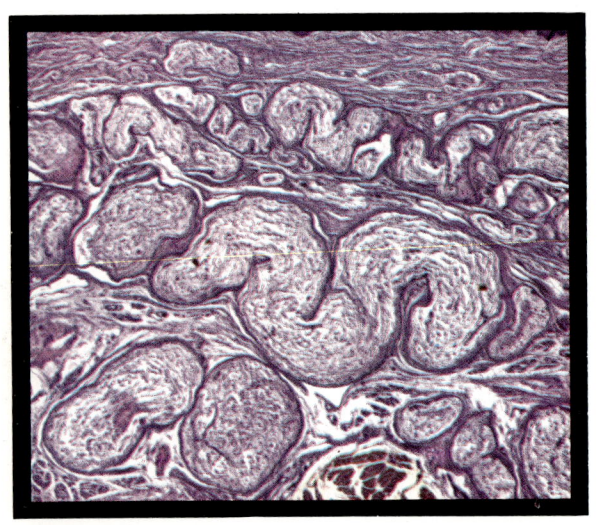

Neurofibroma, Tongue   X 70

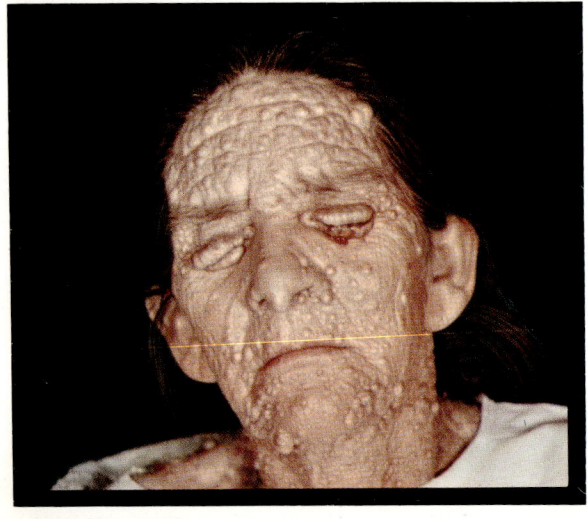

Neurofibromatosis

Neurilemoma

(Top) A neurilemoma (schwannoma) is a neoplastic overgrowth of Schwann cells, which normally constitute the neurilemma sheath of a peripheral nerve. (See p. 8.) These benign tumors are usually small, asymptomatic, well circumscribed and grow slowly. The photomicrograph demonstrates the typical histologic appearance of these lesions. In certain areas the long, narrow, spindle-shaped Schwann cell nuclei are parallel to each other (regimented). Adjacent to the palisaded nuclei are hyaline areas consisting of whorled cytoplasmic processes of the Schwann cells. These pinkish-staining areas are free of nuclei. This arrangement of tissue (best example at upper left) is called a Verocay body. Between the Verocay bodies are haphazardly arranged Schwann cells.

Neurofibroma

The neurofibroma is characterized by an overgrowth of all the elements of a peripheral nerve. These tissues (axon cylinders, Schwann cells and fibrous connective tissue) may be arranged in a variety of patterns in different lesions. Neurofibromas occur singly but often are multiple and constitute the main feature of neurofibromatosis (von Recklinghausen's disease). In this disease there may also be various developmental disturbances, *cafe au lait* spots on the skin, and nevi occurring alone or in association with neurofibromas.

(Center) A plexiform type of neurofibroma with proliferation within the nerve sheath, causing swollen, tortuous nerve fasciculi. The specimen was removed from the tongue of a 6-year-old boy because that organ was so large that it interfered with mastication, swallowing and enunciation. This is a developmental neoplasm not uncommon in the tongue.

(Bottom) Numerous cutaneous neurofibromas which had been present for several years. There is a tendency for neurofibromas to undergo sarcomatous change. Therefore it is generally agreed that once the diagnosis has been established by biopsy, further surgical procedures are undesirable unless there is clinical suspicion of malignant transformation.

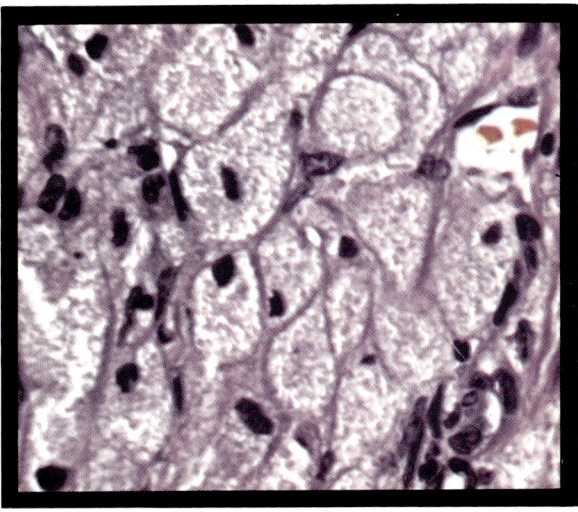

Myoblastoma

Myoblastoma (myoblastic myoma, granular cell myoblastoma) is a benign neoplasm consisting of large polyhedral cells with abundant granular cytoplasm. Agreement as to the histogenesis of this tumor has not been reached. It has been suggested that the constituent cells are (1) immature skeletal muscle cells (myoblasts), (2) giant granular fibroblasts, (3) derivatives of neural elements, or (4) degenerated adult skeletal muscle fibers. Electron microscope studies support origin from undifferentiated mesenchymal cells with leiomyogenic affinities. Myoblastomas may occur in sites other than skeletal muscle. They are most frequently found in the tongue, but may occur in the lip or gingiva. The gingival lesion when present at birth may be termed congenital epulis of the newborn. Only rarely does a patient have more than a single lesion, or one that exceeds 2 cm. in diameter. Pseudoepitheliomatous hyperplasia may be associated with some myoblastomas.

(Top) In this low-power view of a myoblastoma of the tongue, the neoplastic cells are confined to a triangular area which stains a light purple. The covering epithelium devoid of papillae appears clinically as a smooth red lesion. The long, narrow, reddish-staining strips of tissue in intimate relation to the neoplasm are skeletal muscle fibers.

(Center) At this magnification the character of the neoplastic cells is apparent. They are extremely large and of various shapes. The size of these cells and their dark-staining nuclei may be judged by comparing them with the red blood cells in the capillary at right. At a lower power the neoplastic cells might be mistaken for lipid-containing histiocytes (see p. 9), but in this photomicrograph it is apparent that these myoblastoma cells have granules in them rather than vacuoles.

(Bottom) This photomicrograph suggests early invasive carcinoma in the region overlying a myoblastoma, but the changes are typical of intense pseudoepitheliomatous hyperplasia stimulated by the underlying myoblastoma. Misinterpretation of the epithelial changes may result in unnecessary radical surgery.

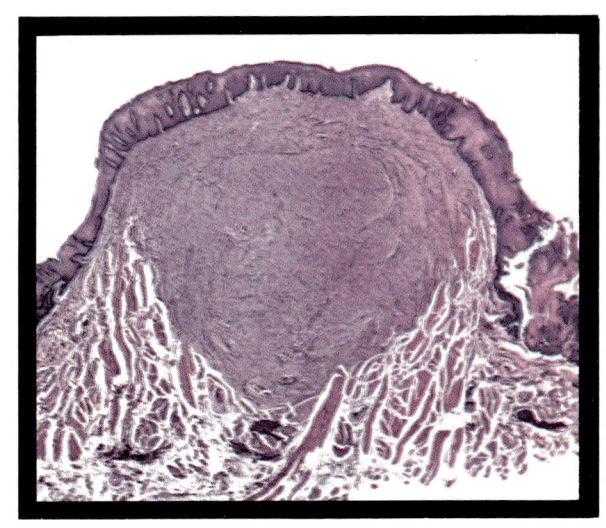

Myoblastoma, Tongue   X 6

Myoblastoma   X 500

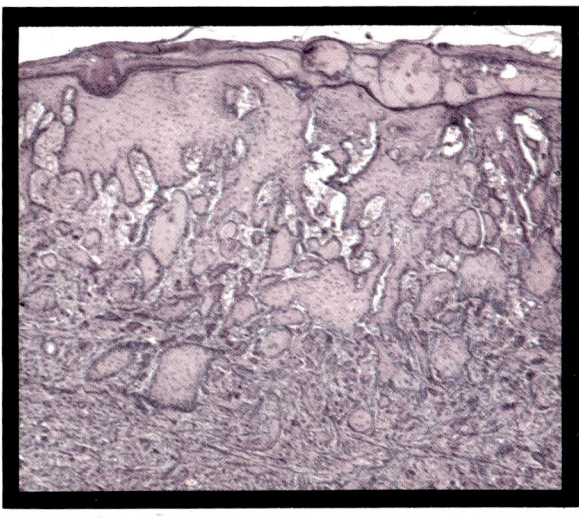

Myoblastoma, Pseudoepitheliomatous Hyperplasia   X 10

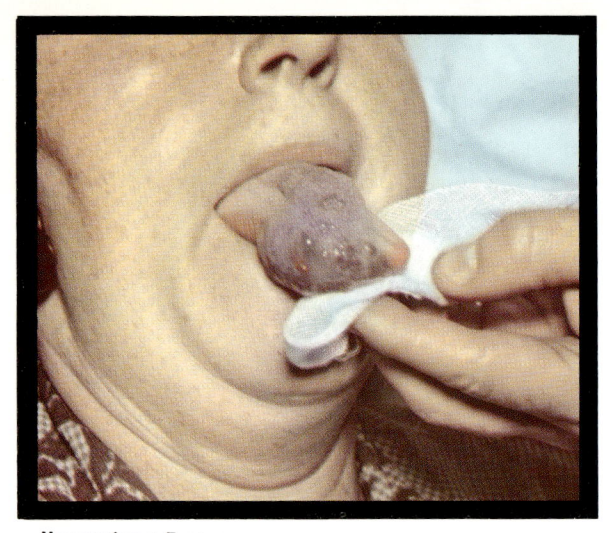

Hemangioma

Hemangiomas are benign tumors of blood vessels. They occur most frequently in the skin of the face and neck but are not rare in the tongue, buccal mucosa and lip. The bone, viscera and central nervous system may be involved. In Sturge-Weber syndrome flaming nevus of the face, central bone hemangioma, cranial involvement and contralateral convulsions are characteristic. The majority of skin lesions are present at birth and remain static. Some of the congenital lesions are considered developmental anomalies, not neoplasms. Varicosities and trauma-induced arteriovenous aneurysms (traumatic angioma) may show similar patterns. Hemangiomas may be divided into 3 types: capillary, cavernous and sclerosing. Hemangioma hypertrophicum (infantile hemangioma, hemangioendothelioma) is discussed on page 145.

(Top) Large cavernous hemangioma which had been present on the tongue since birth. Hemangiomas and lymphangiomas are the most common causes of macroglossia. Occasionally the whole tongue is involved and enlarges to such a size that it cannot be retained in the oral cavity.

(Center) Slightly lobulated hemangioma in the buccal mucosa. Hemangiomas are blue, purple or purplish-red in color and usually blanch when pressure is applied. Except for the port-wine stains, most of these lesions are elevated.

(Bottom) At the upper right-hand corner of the photomicrograph is a portion of the covering epithelium, which is compressed. In the underlying connective tissue there are several large, thin-walled endothelial-lined spaces containing numerous red blood cells. This lesion is classified as a cavernous hemangioma because the vascular spaces are of a large size. It is generally believed that these spaces intercommunicate. Hemangiomas are not encapsulated.

Hemangioma, Tongue

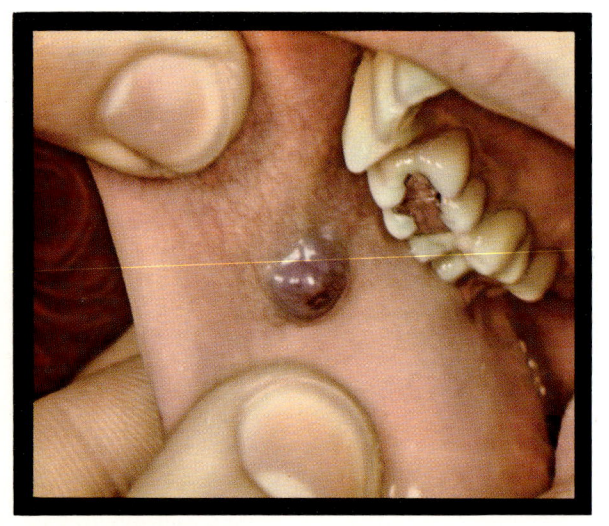

Hemangioma, Buccal Mucosa

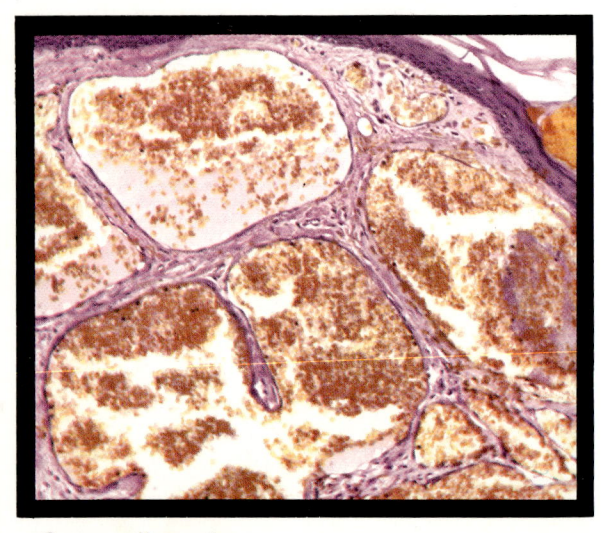

Cavernous Hemangioma

Hemangioendothelioma

(Top) Hemangioendothelioma (hemangioma hypertophicum), which was excised from the gingiva. At the top of the photomicrograph is slightly keratinized epithelium with flattened rete pegs. In the corium there are two very cellular areas which are separated by fibrous connective tissue. These areas consist mainly of endothelial cells. Many of these cells are packed together, while others have formed very small vessels which contain only one or two red blood cells.

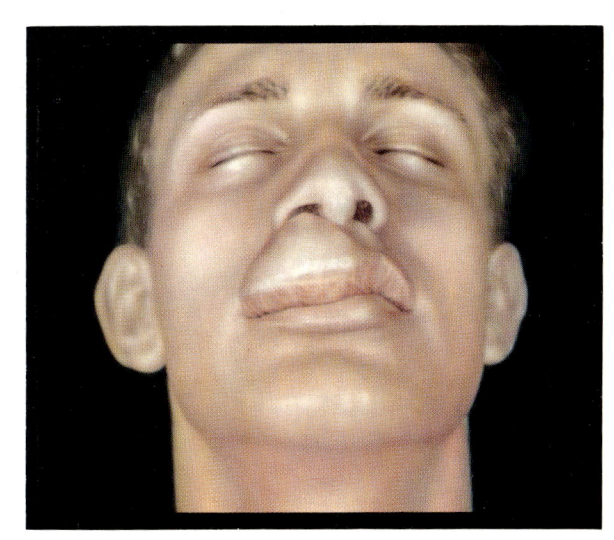

Lymphangioma

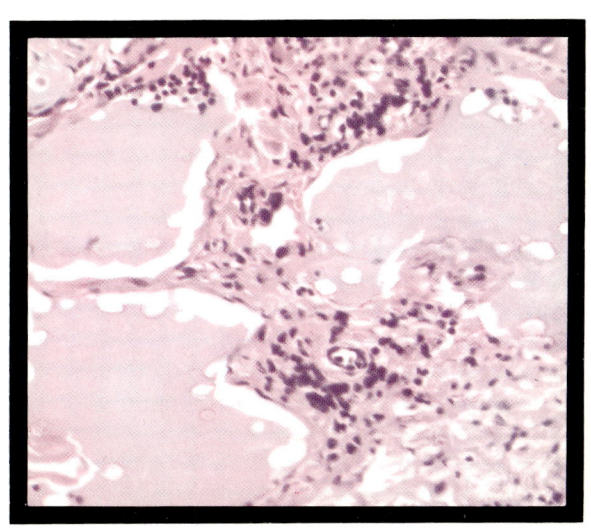

Lymphangiomas are composed of numerous lymph vessels, and most of them—like hemangiomas—are not true neoplasms. One form of this lesion, hygroma colli congenitum, has already been discussed under Developmental Disturbances on page 19. Lymphangiomas are not as common as hemangiomas. If they contain small lymph spaces they are termed "lymphangioma simplex"; if the spaces are large, the lesion is designated as lymphangioma cysticum. When lymphangiomas are very superficial, small lymph-filled vesicles may erupt on the surface (lymphangioma circumscriptum).

(Center) Marked enlargement of the upper lip from a large lymphangioma. This lesion, which was present at birth, has remained static for several years. Lymphangiomas are most frequently encountered in the tongue, lips, neck and inguinal regions. Clinically, the color of the skin overlying a lymphangioma is normal or slightly brownish.

(Bottom) This is a section from a patient's tongue which was markedly enlarged from a cystic lymphangioma. In 3 areas there are lakes of homogeneous light-lavender-staining material which is lymph. This material is contained in channels which are lined by a few flattened endothelial cells. In some instances macroglossia results from both hemangiomatous and lymphangiomatous elements. Histologically, a lymphangioma may be distinguished from a hemangioma only by the absence of red blood cells in the endothelial-lined spaces. If the tissue is fixed in alcohol, this criteria cannot be used.

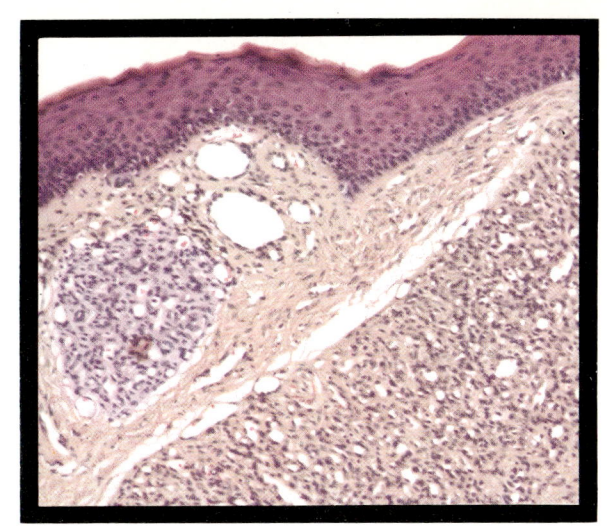

Hemangioendothelioma, Gingiva   X 100

Lymphangioma, Lip

Lymphangioma   X 100

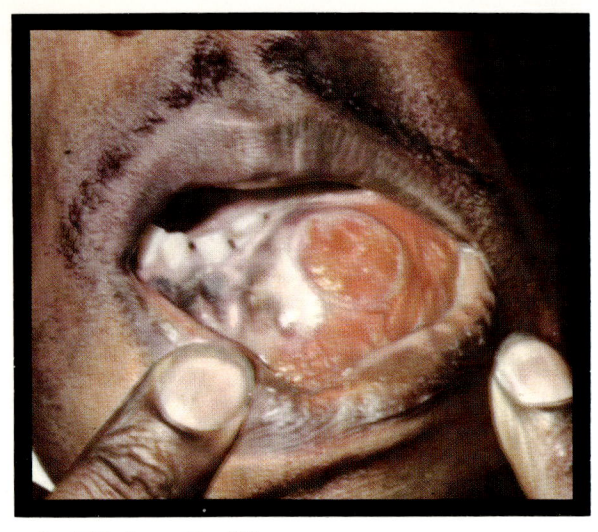

Ameloblastoma, Mandible

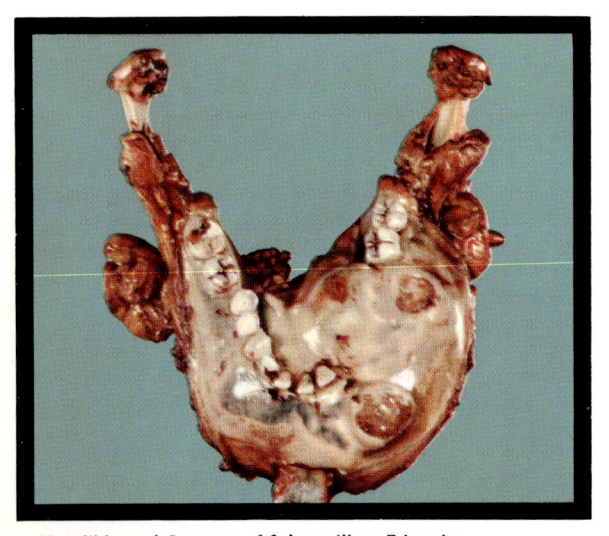

Mandible and Contents of Submaxillary Triangles from Above Case

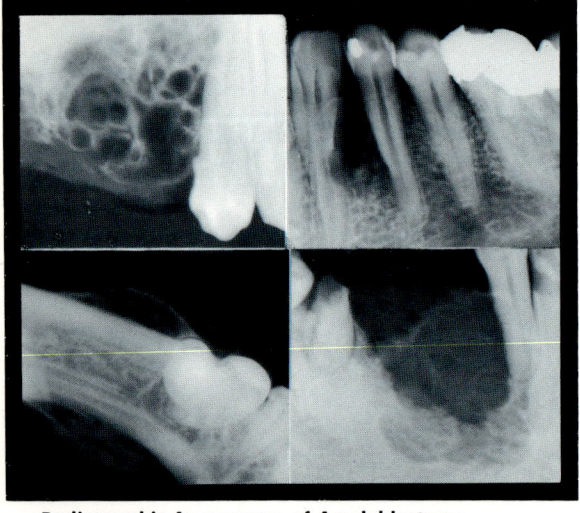

Radiographic Appearance of Ameloblastoma, Four Cases

Neoplasms of Odontogenic Origin

Three fundamental types of neoplasm arise from odontogenic tissue or from cells with a potential for forming dental tissues. They may be purely epithelial (ameloblastomas), purely mesenchymal (odontogenic fibromas, odontogenic myxomas), or mixtures of epithelial and mesenchymal elements in varying portions (mixed odontogenic tumors). The latter are identified by combinations of terms reflecting their histologic character, i.e., fibroameloblastoma, odontoameloblastoma (p. 149).

(Top) Large ameloblastoma (adamantinoma) of the mandible causing a marked deformity. This tumor, which is of 6 years' duration, had been inadequately removed 4 years before this photograph was taken. Ameloblastomas vary in aggressiveness but are usually slow-growing. They are about 5 times as frequent in the mandible as in the maxilla and are most commonly discovered during the 4th decade. Metastasis is extremely rare. Ameloblastomas occurring in the lungs are not necessarily metastatic; they may result from aspiration of neoplastic cells during surgical removal of an oral tumor.

(Center) Surgical specimens from above patient. Radiographs revealed bone destruction from the left 2nd molar to the right 2nd premolar. The anticipated extension into medullary spaces and involvement of a submandibular lymph node were demonstrated histologically. Infiltration into medullary spaces occurs because the tumor behaves as the proliferating dental lamina.

(Bottom) Small areas of bone destruction from ameloblastomas such as might be revealed by routine radiologic examination previous to clinical suspicion of the tumor. The radiolucent area in the upper right film between the cuspid and 1st bicuspid might be confused with a periodontal pocket. The occlusal view shows expansion of the cortex without perforation, which is typical, even in large lesions. Radiographic findings are not pathognomonic for ameloblastomas. Histologic examinations are required for definitive diagnosis.

Neoplasms of Odontogenic Origin (Cont.)

Ameloblastomas may vary greatly as to histologic pattern, but in each instance the tumor includes cells which resemble those seen in the enamel organ. Some of the component cells are often so arranged as to simulate structures seen in some early stage of tooth development. These neoplasms may be solid or cystic, but this is not a pertinent division, for the solid type is probably just a young tumor. The ameloblastoma is essentially benign but locally invasive and may kill by extension to vital structures. It is a central tumor that expands but usually does not perforate the cortical plates. Ameloblastoma may arise from remnants of the dental lamina, from the periodontal debris of Malassez and from the enamel organ. It also may arise from the wall of a dentigerous cyst.

(Top) In this solid type of ameloblastoma there is very little connective tissue stroma, and the numerous islands of epithelial cells closely approximate each other. These islands are bordered by palisaded columnar cells which resemble ameloblasts. In the central portion of each aggregation is a loose network of cells suggestive of stellate reticulum. Solid ameloblastomas often contain double rows of columnar cells quite like the dental lamina.

(Center) Typical pattern of ameloblastoma with epithelial islands having peripheral cells representative of ameloblasts surrounding delicate tissue of stellate reticulum type. A layer of cells suggesting stratum intermedium sometimes is present. Liquefaction, which can be responsible for the development of microcysts, is evident.

(Bottom) At the lower right a typical ameloblastoma with microcysts is replacing bone. The 3 large circular areas show tumor invasion into vascular spaces. All are cystic, and that at the upper left has an area of solid tumor adjacent. The cystic spaces are lined by flat, squamatoid epithelium typical of reduced enamel epithelium. If the biopsy specimen had been small and included only cystic elements of this type, it might have been misinterpreted as an odontogenic cyst.

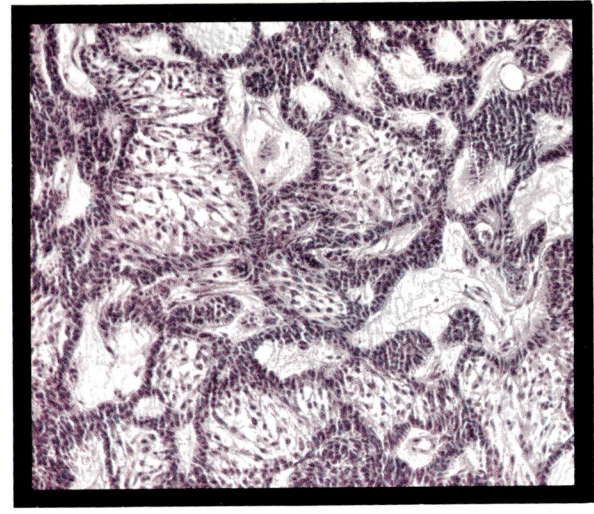

Amelobastoma, Plexiform Pattern   X 100

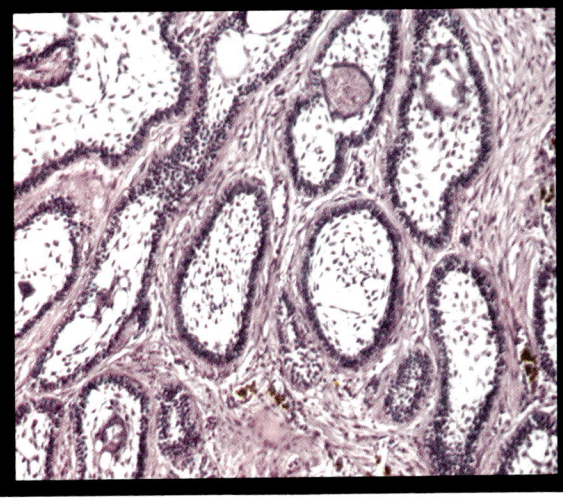

Ameloblastoma, Follicular Pattern   X 100

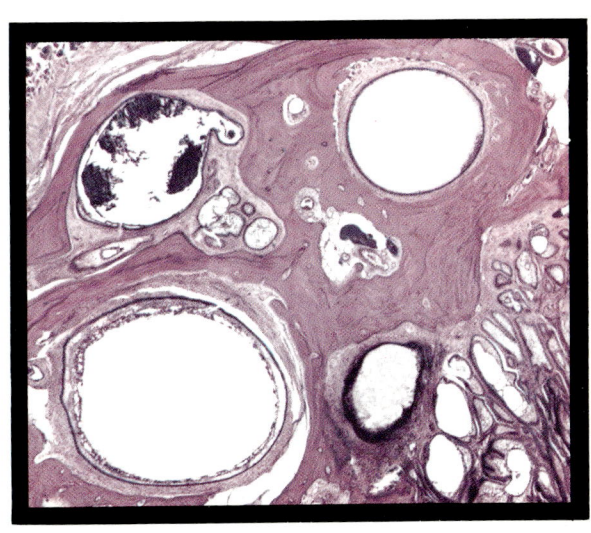

Ameloblastoma, Cystic   X 15

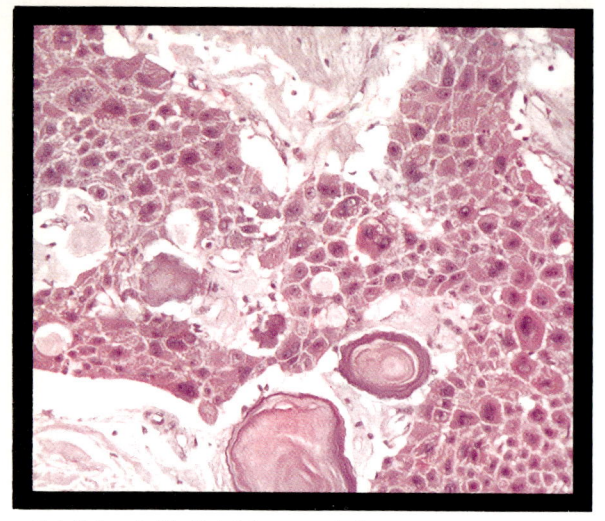

Calcifying Epithelial Odontogenic Tumor   X 100

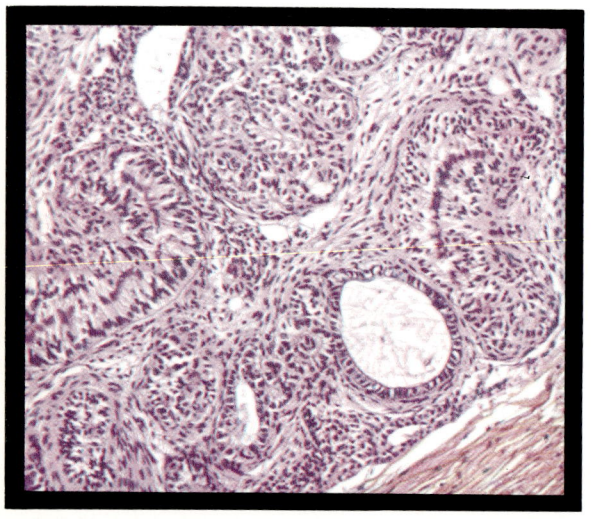

Adenomatoid Odontogenic Tumor   X 100

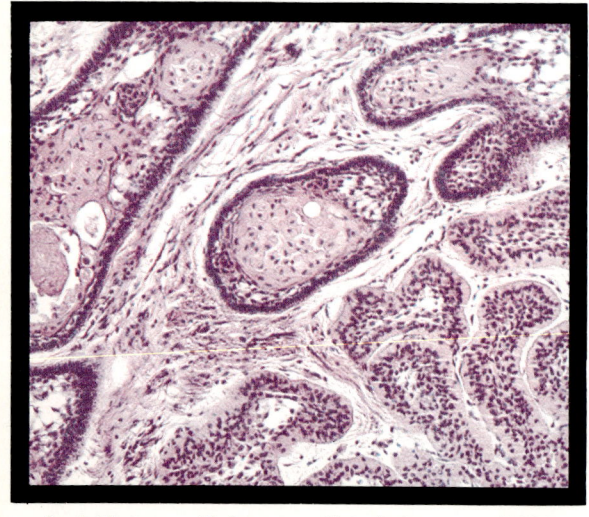

Ameloblastoma with Squamous Metaplasia   X 100

Neoplasms of Odontogenic Origin (Cont.)

(Top) Calcified epithelial odontogenic tumor (Pindborg) is composed of sheets of polyhedral epithelial cells in a connective tissue stroma. These closely packed cells sometimes are divided into islands or strands by the stroma. The nuclei, variable in size and shape, may be well differentiated or pleomorphic, as in this illustration. The slightly eosinophilic cytoplasm degenerates and tends to calcify, with the formation of Liesegang rings. Calcification may also occur in collagenous tissue. Amyloid had been described in the tumor cells and stroma. Most frequently this tumor is found in association with a nonerupted tooth although extra-osseous lesions have been reported. Radiographically, radiopaque flecks in the radiolucent lesion may result from the calcifications.

(Center) Several ductlike structures lined by a single row of columnar epithelial cells are apparent. Near the middle of the left and right borders are other structures typical of the adenomatoid odontogenic tumor (adenoameloblastoma). These structures consist of a double row of tall epithelial cells with basally placed nuclei. Between these 2 rows of cells is a dark-staining material which appears to have been secreted by these cells. The lesion most frequently appears as a cystlike radiolucency, associated with a nonerupted tooth in the maxillary canine region of a teen-ager. It grows slowly by expansion and is not aggressive. Conservative treatment is indicated, and recurrences have not been reported.

(Bottom) The epithelial islands in this section of ameloblastoma are surfaced by columnar cells. In the center are elements suggestive of stellate reticulum and nests of squamatoid cells. Ameloblastomas showing squamous metaplasia are designated acanthomatous ameloblastomas. This variety of lesion in a very few instances has undergone malignant change.

Two varieties not illustrated are granular cell ameloblastoma and granular cell fibroameloblastoma. In the former the epithelial cells, in the latter the connective tissue cells, are granular. The so-called pigmented ameloblastoma appears to be of neural crest origin and has been termed melanotic progonoma.

Neoplasms of Odontogenic Origin (Cont.)

(Top) A neoplasm of the mesenchymal portion of a tooth bud is often termed odontogenic fibroma or myxoma. It consists of delicate, loosely arranged fibrous tissue containing many stellate fibroblasts. It closely simulates pulp tissue. The odontogenic fibroma is a central fibroma of bone; its origin is suggested by its association with odontogenic epithelium, as seen here at the top of the picture. This epithelium is not neoplastic. Odontogenic fibromas do not often reach a large size.

(Center) There are 2 neoplastic components to this lesion, both arising from the tooth bud. Along the 2 lateral borders of the photomicrograph are portions of structures which resemble enamel organs. These constitute the epithelial portion of the neoplasm. The rest of the tissue is proliferating fibrous connective tissue in which the fibroblasts vary in staining reaction, size and shape. The proportion of fibrous and epithelial tissue varies from one tumor to another, as does the cellularity of the stroma.

(Bottom) The lesion exhibited here is an odontoameloblastoma, a type of mixed odontogenic tumor, with the soft-tissue elements to the left and the hard tissue to the right. The epithelium, proliferating in the connective tissue stroma, shows varying degrees of differentiation in an ameloblastomatous pattern. The purple-staining strip near the right border is enamel matrix which covers the red-staining dentin and lighter predentin.

Neoplasms histologically similar to ameloblastoma are found in the pituitary region. They arise from remnants of Rathke's pouch, an invagination of the primitive oral epithelium. Their histogenesis may be explained on the basis that the parent cells had the potentiality for forming an enamel organ. The "ameloblastomas" of the tibia probably are basal cell carcinomas or epithelial implants which simulate the pattern of the ameloblastoma.

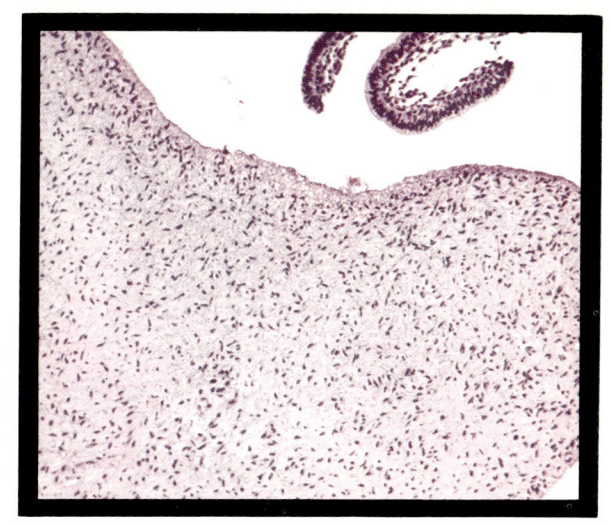

Odontogenic Fibroma — X 100

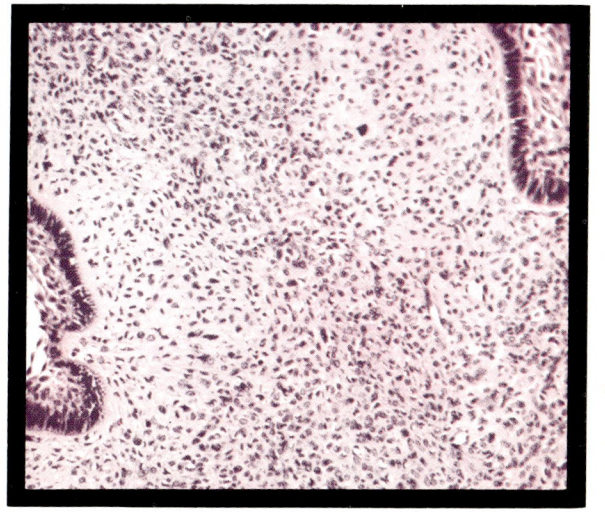

Fibroameloblastoma — X 100

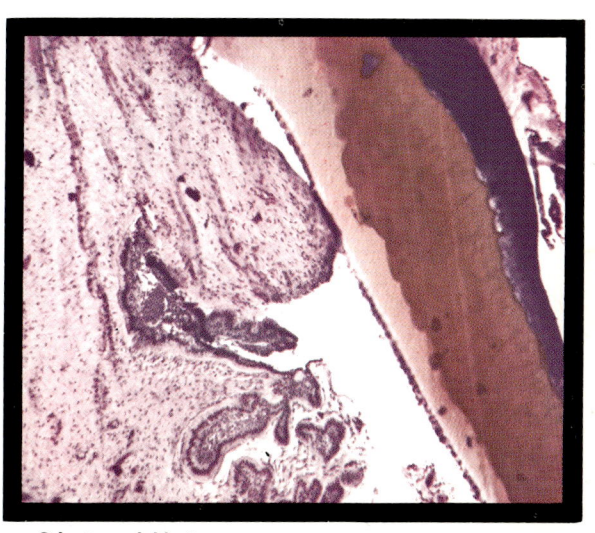

Odontoameloblastoma — X 50

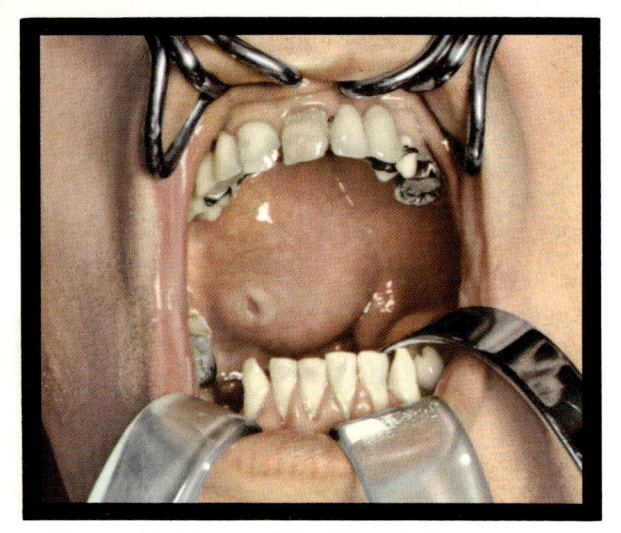

Pleomorphic Adenoma (Mixed Tumor), Palate

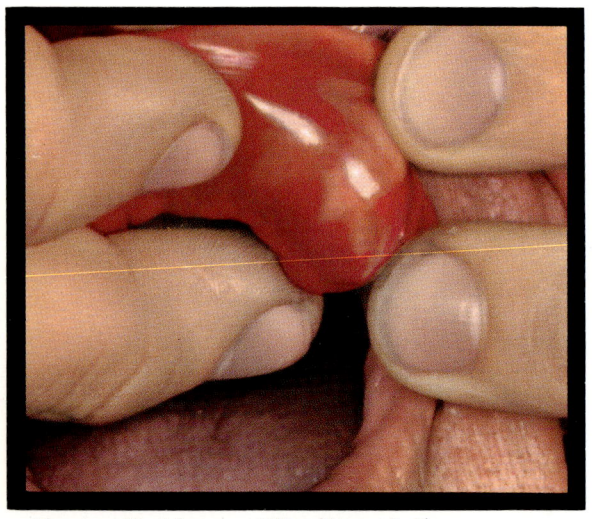

Pleomorphic Adenoma (Mixed Tumor), Lip

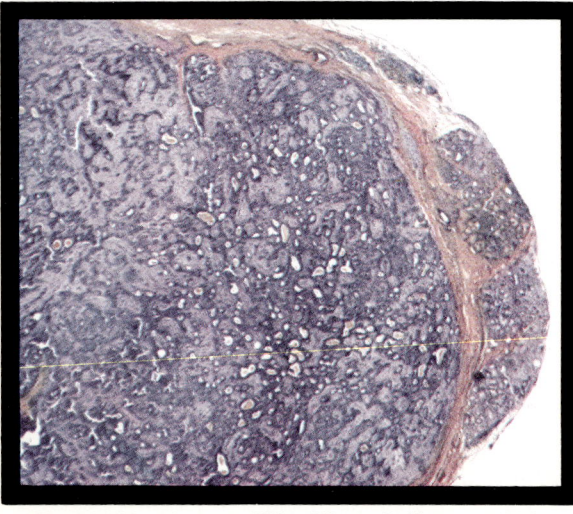

Pleomorphic Adenoma (Mixed Tumor), Lip   X 12

Benign Mixed Tumors of Salivary Gland Origin

(Pleomorphic Adenoma)

Mixed tumors of the major or accessory salivary glands are predominantly benign (exception, p. 153) neoplasms containing both epithelial and mesenchymal elements. Many investigators consider only the epithelial portion to be neoplastic and prefer the term pleomorphic adenoma to mixed tumor. The epithelial component of the tumor may consist of round, polyhedral, elongated or stellate cells which stain uniformly and are relatively small. These cells may be arranged in strands, islands, duct-like structures or large masses. The mesenchymal portion of the neoplasm may be composed of fibrous tissue (dense, hyalinized, loosely arranged or myxomatoid), pseudocartilage or bone. Either epithelial or connective tissue may predominate, and the tissue pattern may vary greatly in different lesions and in different areas of the same tumor. Mixed tumors are most frequently encountered in the parotid. The most common oral sites are the lips and palate. Mixed tumors usually grow very slowly and appear clinically as smooth, spherical enlargements which are asymptomatic and firm to palpation. They tend to recur as the result of incomplete excision or, in some instances, because of multicentric origin.

(Top) Large benign mixed tumor involving both the hard and the soft palate. It enlarged slowly to its present size in 6 years. The lesion was of bony hardness and interfered with swallowing, breathing and enunciation.

(Center) The spherical enlargement on the left side of the upper lip might be mistaken for a lipoma or mucocele. This lesion, however, was extremely firm, which should make one suspect a mixed tumor. Because of their accessibility to surgery, mixed tumors of the lip are readily cured. They grow very slowly and usually do not reach a large size.

(Bottom) In this low-power view of a pleomorphic adenoma arising from accessory salivary gland tissue in the lip, a portion of the capsule (reddish-staining) may be seen. To the right of this capsule is normal salivary gland tissue and to the left, the tumor.

Benign Mixed Tumors of Salivary Gland Origin

(Pleomorphic Adenoma) (Cont.)

(Top) This is a higher magnification of the tumor shown in the last picture on the preceding page. At right is a vertical strip of reddish-staining connective tissue, the tumor capsule. To the right of this capsule several normal mucous acini are apparent. (Compare with those on p. 4.) To the left of the capsule the histologic character of this tumor is demonstrated. It is composed of uniformly dark-staining cuboidal epithelial cells in some areas arranged in a ductal pattern. The epithelial cells in other areas are extending from the ducts in strands and in other regions are clumped in irregular masses. The stroma in this portion of the tumor consists of loosely arranged cellular connective tissue which stains a light blue, due to its myxomatous character.

(Center) It is apparent that this mixed tumor is quite different histologically from the one in the preceding picture. Here the epithelial component predominates, and the epithelial cells are not in strands, ducts or islands but are in one large mass. The clinical course of such cellular tumors does not appear to be different from that of the other varieties.

(Bottom) At far left are small, round epithelial cells arranged in islands and ductlike structures. In the remainder of the section is a light-lavender homogeneous substance in which a few cells are entrapped. The tissue in this area simulates hyaline cartilage, especially in regions where an occasional cell has a clear halo about its nucleus. This pseudocartilage is a common finding in mixed tumors and in some instances may be the predominating feature. Some believe that the hyaline matrix is extravasated epithelial mucin which has widely separated the epithelial cells; others consider it to be of mesenchymal origin.

Other benign neoplasms of salivary gland origin are acinic cell adenoma, Warthin's tumor and oxyphilic cell adenoma (oncocytoma). The first two are discussed on page 136. The latter consists of large cells with pinkish-staining cytoplasm.

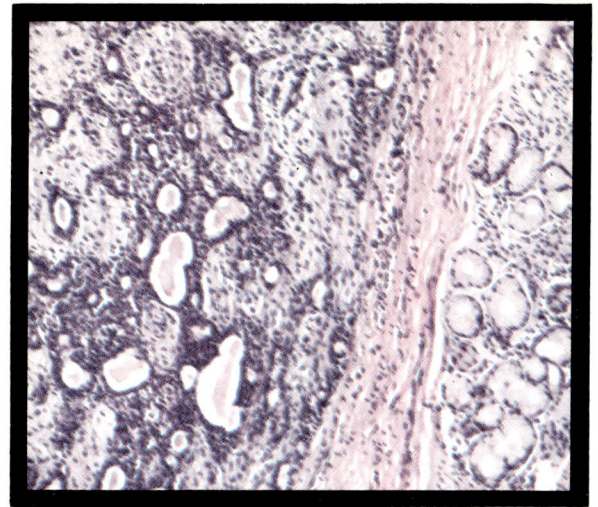

Pleomorphic Adenoma (Mixed Tumor), Lip   X 90

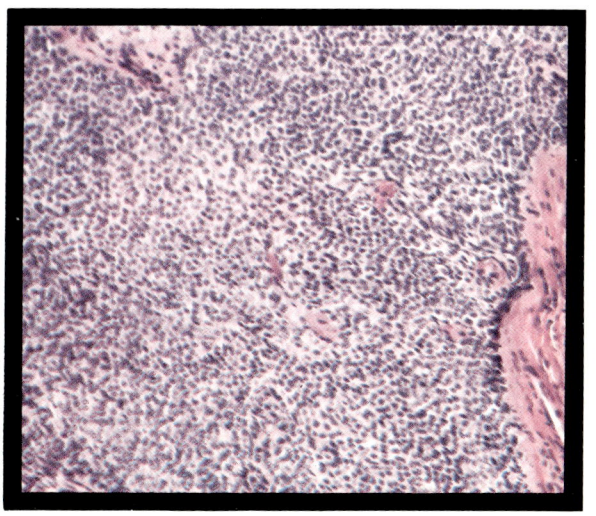

Pleomorphic Adenoma (Mixed Tumor), Cellular Area   X 100

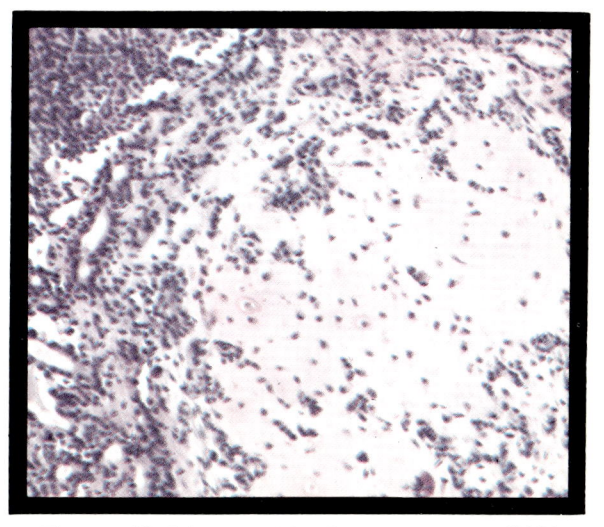

Pleomorphic Adenoma (Mixed Tumor), Pseudocartilaginous Area   X 100

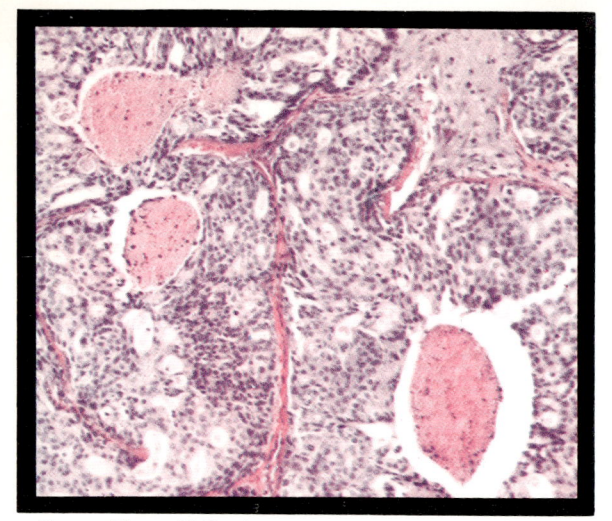

Mucoepidermoid Carcinoma   X 100

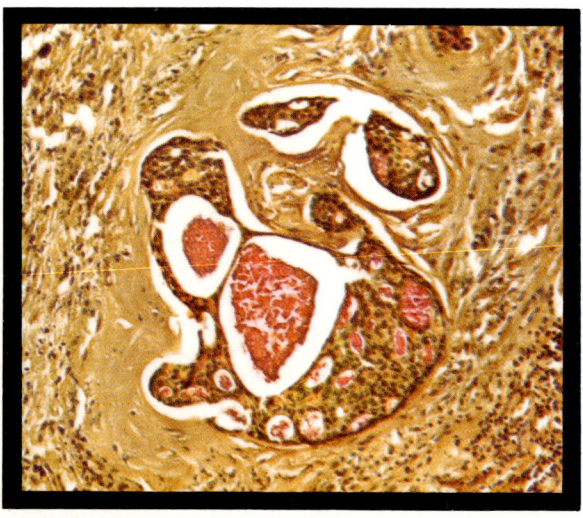

Mucoepidermoid Carcinoma, Mucicarmine Stain   X 100

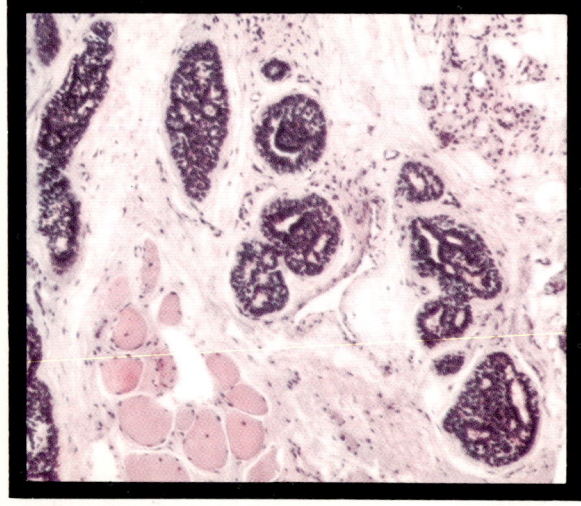

Adenoid Cystic Carcinoma   X 90

MALIGNANT NEOPLASMS

Malignant Salivary Gland Neoplasms

Malignant neoplasms originating from salivary gland epithelium include the mucoepidermoid carcinoma, the adenoid cystic carcinoma, squamous cell carcinoma, papillary adenocarcinoma, acinic cell carcinoma, acidophilic cell adenocarcinoma and the so-called malignant mixed tumor (carcinoma in pleomorphic adenoma).

(Top) The mucoepidermoid carcinoma consists of mucous cells, epidermoid cells and small cuboidal cells. These neoplastic cells may be arranged in sheets or islands. They may also form thick-walled, ductlike structures, as seen in this photomicrograph. Mucoepidermoid carcinoma may be subclassified according to degree of malignancy. Those of low-grade malignancy are considered by some to be benign lesions and may be designated as mucous cyst adenomas to emphasize their benign character. When considering the diagnosis of mucoepidermoid carcinoma, care must be exercised not to interpret ductal changes due to inflammation (squamous metaplasia and mucous cell proliferation) as being neoplastic.

(Center) A portion of a mucoepidermoid carcinoma which has been stained to show mucin (red). The cells staining red are similar to those which appear colorless in the top picture. It is apparent that the material in the lumenlike spaces also has a high mucin content. Inflammation, resulting from spillage of mucin into the stroma, is a common finding in these tumors.

(Bottom) This tumor consists of small, dark-staining cells arranged in groups. In each group are clear areas of various sizes ("swiss cheese effect"). In other instances there may be anastomosing cords of cells which surround various-sized spaces, dense cords of hyaline stroma separating groups of epithelial cells, or a histologic pattern identical with that of some skin tumors. Adenoid cystic carcinoma (pseudoadenomatous basal cell carcinoma, cylindroma, basaloid mixed tumor) is frequently misjudged as being benign. It is a nonencapsulated, slow-growing tumor which is difficult to eradicate. Often there is a history of numerous recurrences with extensive destruction locally. Distant metastases generally occur only late in the disease.

Malignant Salivary Gland Neoplasms (Cont.)

(Top) Except for the 2 ducts seen near the lower left border, the normal parotid tissue has been completely replaced by malignant squamous cells. These vary in size and shape, and many contain large hyperchromatic nuclei. Squamous cell carcinoma may develop in a mixed or mucoepidermoid tumor, or directly from metaplastic ductal epithelium.

(Center) This malignant epithelial tumor originated from accessory salivary gland tissue in the floor of the mouth. It is characterized by vascular papillary projections which are bordered by a single row of epithelial cells. These cells vary in size and shape. In some the hyperchromatic nuclei are at one end of the cell, and in others at the opposite end. In certain instances the nuclei are so large that they nearly fill the cells.

(Bottom) Radiographic appearance of a maxilla which was invaded by an adenocarcinoma of salivary gland origin. It is apparent that, in addition to the extensive bone destruction, the mesial and lingual roots of the 1st molar have been irregularly resorbed, leaving spikelike projections. Whenever "spiking" of the roots is seen, the diagnostician should suspect a malignant lesion.

The acinic cell adenocarcinoma may be composed of either serous cells (serous cell adenocarcinoma) or mucous cells (mucous or clear cell adenocarcinoma). Both varieties appear quite similar to the salivary gland adenoma appearing at the top of page 136, except that their component cells are not of such uniform character. The acidophilic cell adenocarcinoma (malignant oncocytoma or oxyphilic cell carcinoma) is composed of large cells with reddish-staining cytoplasm somewhat like cells in Warthin's tumor, although not as regularly shaped. The term "malignant mixed tumor" is applied by some individuals to a cancerous growth of salivary gland tissue which in some areas exhibits qualities of a conventional mixed tumor. Others prefer to designate such a lesion according to its malignant component (e.g., adenocarcinoma or squamous cell carcinoma) and limit the use of "mixed tumor" to benign lesions.

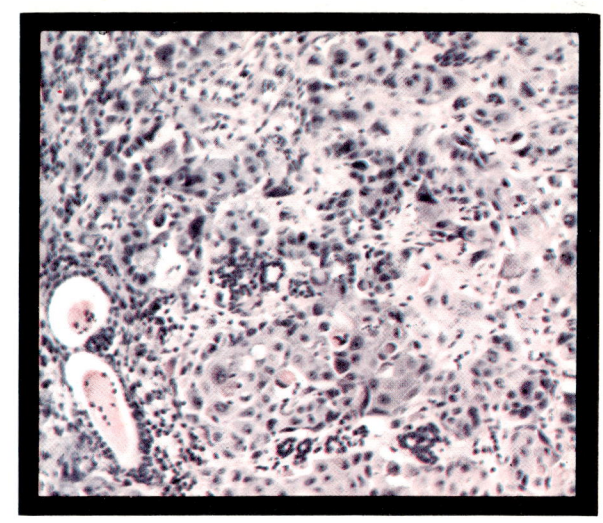

Squamous Cell Carcinoma, Parotid Gland X 100

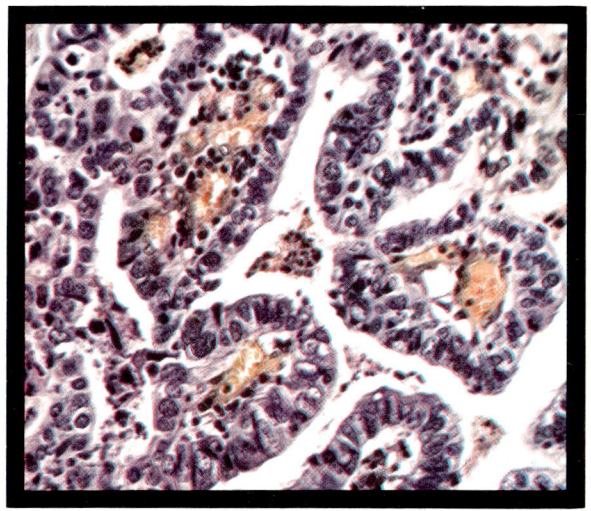

Papillary Adenocarcinoma X 220

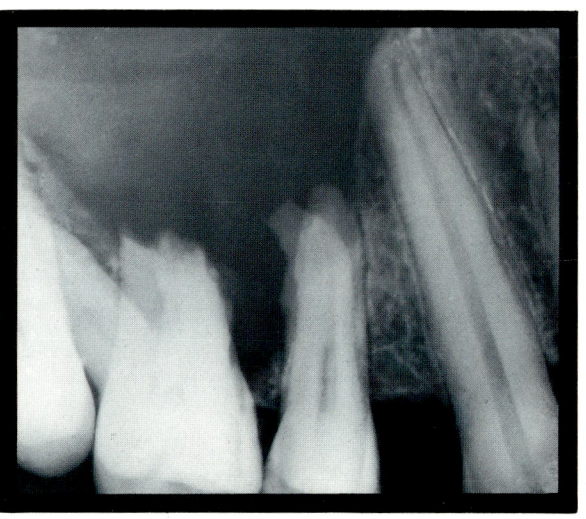

Adenocarcinoma, Maxilla

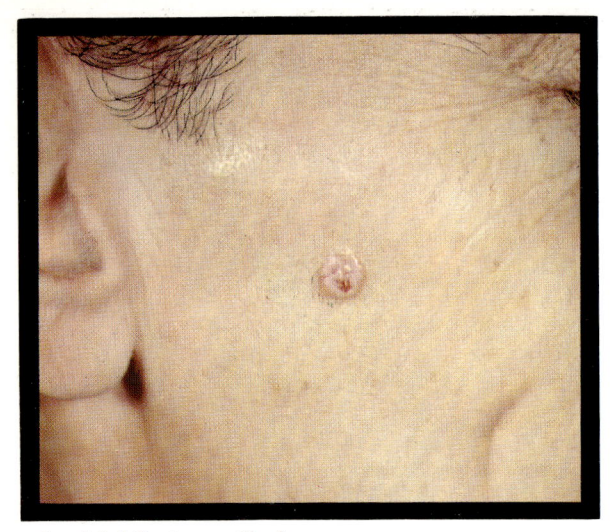

Basal Cell Carcinoma, Cheek

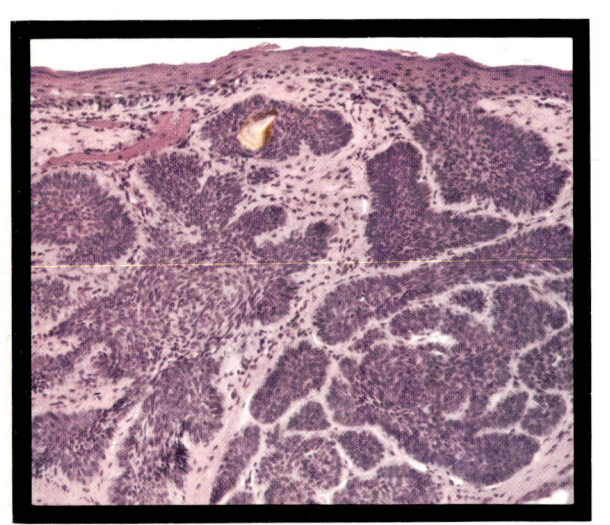

Basal Cell Carcinoma   X 100

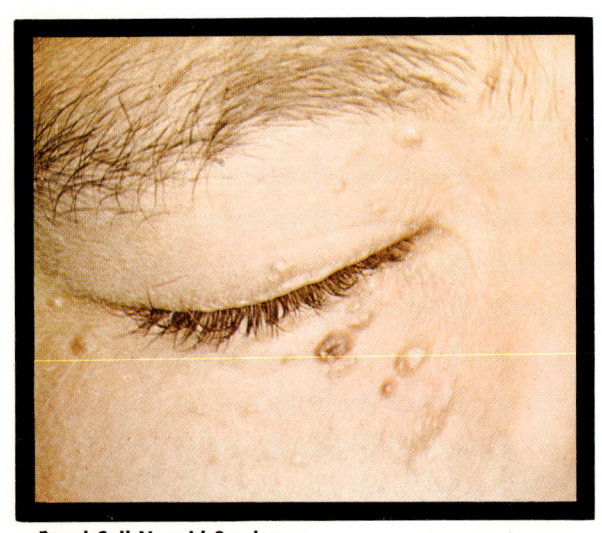

Basal Cell Nevoid Syndrome

Basal Cell Carcinoma

Basal cell carcinoma usually arises from the basal cells of the epidermis, but it may originate from the outermost cells of hair follicles or sebaceous glands. It may occur anywhere in skin but is most common on the upper part of the face. It grows very slowly and rarely metastasizes. It may be readily cured by excision or by radiant energy. If left untreated, it may destroy the whole face and invade the underlying bone and cartilage. This neoplasm may extend into the oral or ocular mucous membranes but rarely originates in these areas. This lesion is the least malignant of all the cancerous growths, and—except in very advanced cases—the prognosis is excellent. It is most common in males with light-colored skin which has become dry and atrophic from exposure to wind and sunlight.

(Top) This basal cell carcinoma is a raised, waxy, slightly ulcerated lesion which reached its present size in 2 years. It usually begins as a small papule with a scaly surface. The patient may believe it is a "pimple" which is slow to heal because the scab continually comes off. Basal cell carcinoma at this early stage may be differentiated clinically from an inflammatory lesion by its very thin, threadlike, raised, pearly border with central necrosis.

(Center) Typical microscopic appearance of basal cell carcinoma. The malignant epithelial cells are oval or cylindrical and have deeply staining nuclei. These cells are arranged in islands of various sizes and shapes. At the periphery of each island there is a single row of radially oriented cells. This regimented arrangement is best seen at upper left. At upper right the origin is evident.

Basal Cell Nevoid Syndrome

(Bottom) This 13-year-old boy had basal cell lesions about both eyes. Microscopically, they were similar to the lesion in the center picture. Keratin-filled cysts in the jaws were enucleated on several occasions. Removal of carcinomas and cysts as they occur is a continuing but essential treatment. Bifid ribs, pitted palms and other defects may be associated with the syndrome, as well as basal cell carcinomas and keratocysts.

Squamous Cell Carcinoma

Squamous cell carcinomas of the oral cavity are usually moderately well differentiated neoplasms. In general, they are more frequent in men than women. The prognosis varies according to the location, but the cure rate for each area is dependent on how early in the disease proper treatment is instituted. Oral carcinoma may appear as a keratotic plaque; a crusted ulcer; a noncrusted ulcer, either superficial or deep; a slightly raised lesion with central ulceration and a rolled border; a slightly raised red lesion; or a verruciform growth.

(Top) The most frequent site of oral carcinoma is the lower lip—generally on the vermilion border about halfway between the commissure and the midline. It may begin as a keratotic plaque, as shown here, or as a crusted ulcer which might be mistaken for herpes labialis. Metastasis, which is usually to the submaxillary lymph nodes, does not occur early. The prognosis is very good unless the lesion is extensive.

(Center) The carcinoma in this instance is a sharply circumscribed, crusted ulcer which might be confused with a syphilitic chancre. On each side of the lesion atrophic changes similar to those seen in solar cheilosis are evident (p. 106); the surgical treatment of such a case should include vermilionectomy as a prophylactic measure. Carcinoma so situated in the midline may metastasize to the submental lymph nodes.

(Bottom) This lesion is slightly elevated above the surface, and it has a characteristic firm, rolled border. Unless a carcinoma is in an extremely early stage, it is not possible to get the fingers under it when attempting to lift it up. Carcinoma of the lower lip is principally a disease of men. It is rare in Negroes. It usually occurs during the 6th decade but is not uncommon in much younger individuals. Solar cheilosis is often a predisposing change, as is demonstrated here.

Carcinoma in the upper lip has a low incidence. It may metastasize to the upper cervical, preauricular or submaxillary lymph nodes. It grows more rapidly than carcinoma of the lower lip, and its prognosis is not as good.

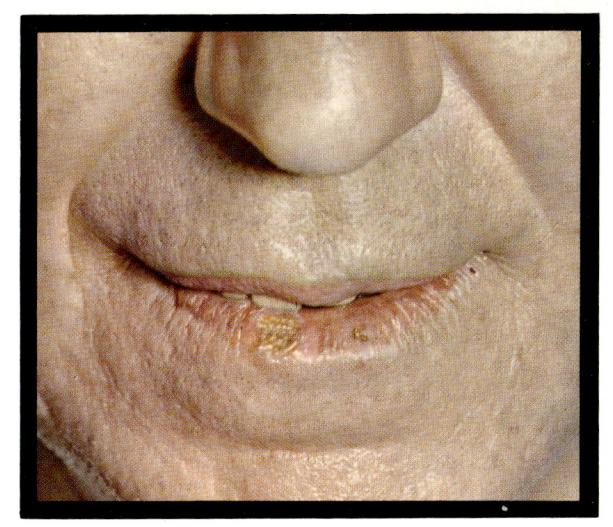

Carcinoma, Lip

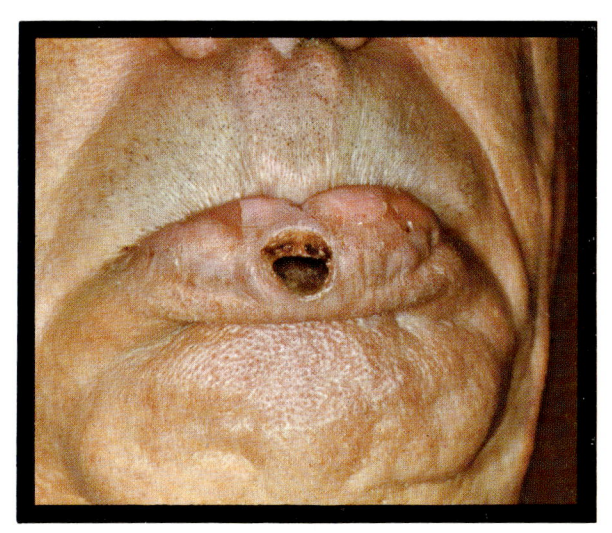

Carcinoma, Lip

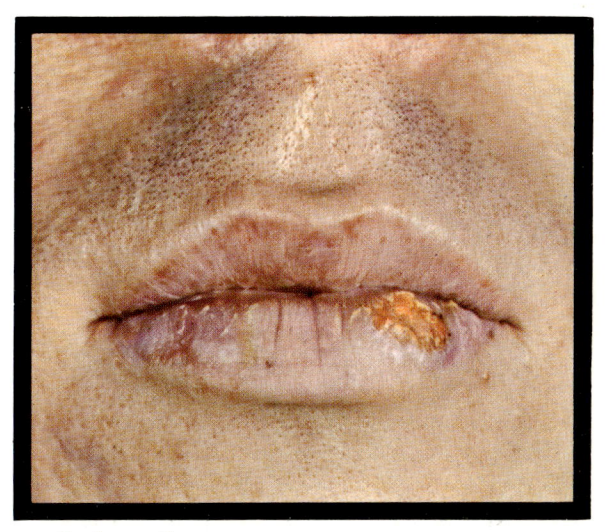

Carcinoma, Lip

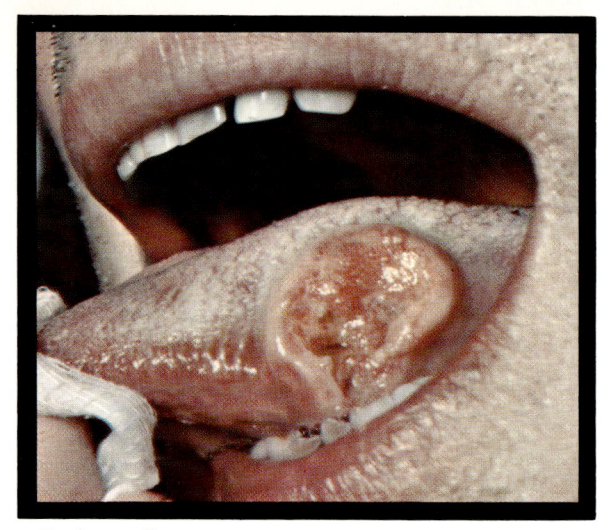

Carcinoma, Tongue

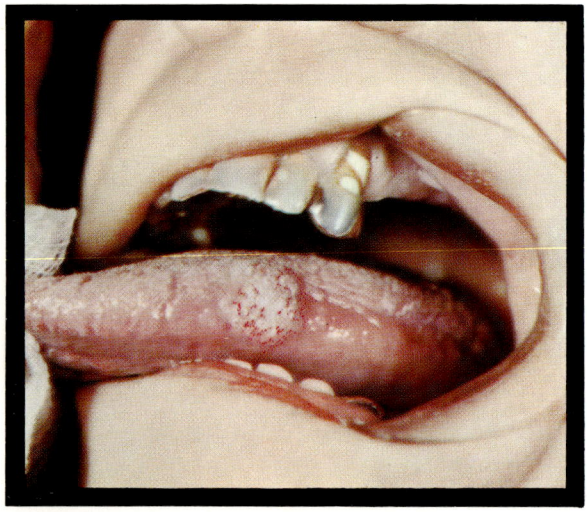

Carcinoma, Tongue, Early Lesion

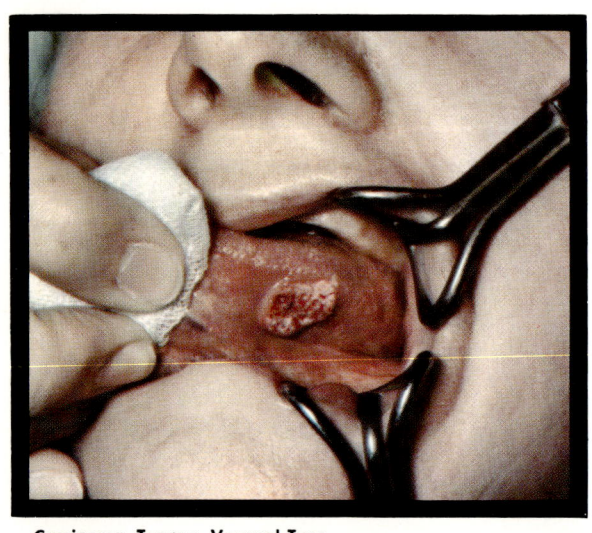

Carcinoma, Tongue, Verrucal Type

Squamous Cell Carcinoma (Cont.)

The second most frequent site of oral carcinoma is the tongue. Squamous cell carcinoma involving the tongue usually arises in the middle third of the lateral border or on the ventral surface. It is relatively rare on the tip and dorsum except in those cases which are associated with luetic glossitis (p. 115). Carcinomas of the tongue metastasize very early, usually to the subdigastric group of lymph nodes. Proper treatment must be instituted while the lesion is still small if a long survival period is to be anticipated. Procrastination in biopsying a suspicious lesion may result in a needless fatality.

(Top) Typical appearance of a moderately advanced squamous cell carcinoma on the lateral border of the tongue. The periphery of the lesion is raised, rolled and firm. The central portion is ulcerated and has a granular appearance.

(Center) This very early carcinoma is seen as a slightly elevated keratotic lesion on the lateral border of the tongue just forward of the maxillary cuspid tooth, which has a gold restoration. When first discovered, it appeared that the lesion might be inflammatory—the result of irritation from a broken partial-denture clasp. Upon elimination of this possible causative factor, however, the lesion did not regress, and a biopsy was done, which revealed the true nature of the growth. Because cancer in its early stages is not painful, many lesions which are not readily visible to the patient are not detected by him until they are fairly extensive. Therefore the best opportunity to detect intra-oral cancer early is afforded to practitioners making routine oral examinations.

(Bottom) A broad, elevated, slightly ulcerated, verruciform lesion on the undersurface of the tongue. This might be misdiagnosed clinically as a sessile papilloma. Palpation, however, would reveal marked induration, which should leave little doubt as to the serious nature of the lesion. Carcinomas of the verrucous type may offer a better prognosis than deeply ulcerated ones of similar size.

Squamous Cell Carcinoma (Cont.)

(Top) This carcinomatous lesion involving the alveolar ridge and the vestibular mucosa is bisected by a groove. This groove was produced by pressure from a denture flange. Inflammatory lesions which are fissured and ulcerated are frequently observed in patients wearing ill-fitting dentures. Such lesions may appear somewhat similar to the carcinoma shown here, but they will quickly disappear after the denture is trimmed.

(Center) Squamous cell carcinoma of the palate appearing as an ulcer with slightly raised, rolled edges. Such a lesion may be preceded by nicotinic stomatitis (p. 97). Palatal carcinoma is relatively common in countries where cigars and cigarettes frequently are smoked by putting the lighted end in the mouth. Carcinoma of the floor of the mouth (which must be suspected early and treated adequately) often appears as a shallow but extensive ulcer not unlike this palatal lesion. Some carcinomas of the palate and buccal mucosa are papillomatous and well differentiated.

(Bottom) A large carcinoma in the retromolar region and buccal mucosa appears as an ulcer with a heavy distinct rolled border. The patient did not notice it until it was large enough to impinge on the upper jaw when occluding.

Oral carcinoma may simulate other disease processes and vice versa. Therefore, if too much reliance is placed on the clinical characteristics, many incipient carcinomatous lesions will be overlooked. Some mucous membrane carcinomas are not ulcerated but appear as red, raised innocent-looking lesions. It is good practice to take a biopsy of every lesion of over 2 weeks' duration, the exact nature of which is not known. There is no harm in biopsying a lesion which proves to be noncancerous. Any disadvantage associated with biopsy of a cancerous lesion is far outweighed by the advantage of establishing the diagnosis. The time between microscopic diagnosis and definitive treatment should be minimal. Oral cytology may serve as a useful adjunct to biopsy but is not a substitute for the biopsy.

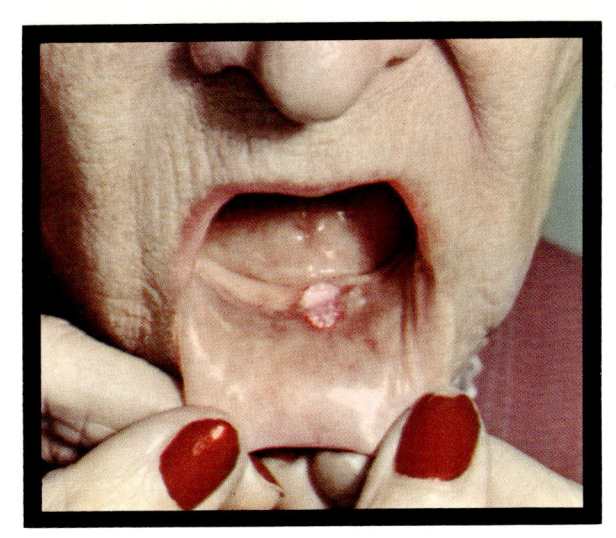

Carcinoma, Alveolar Mucosa

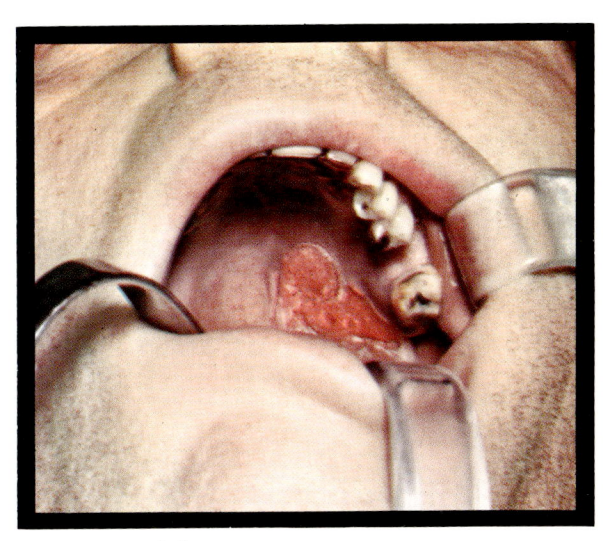

Carcinoma, Palate

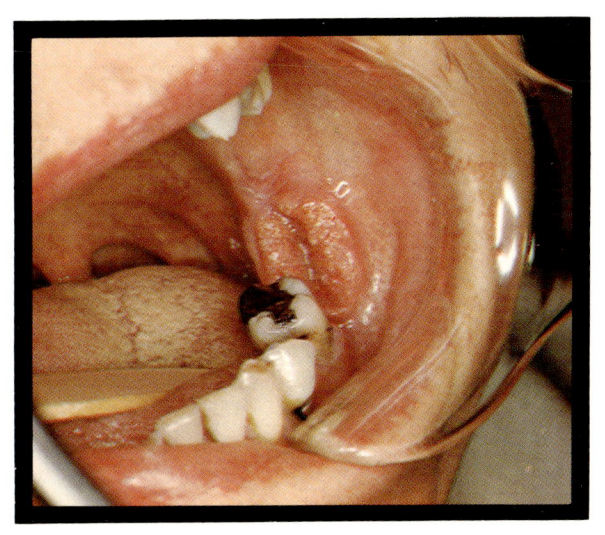

Carcinoma, Retromolar Region

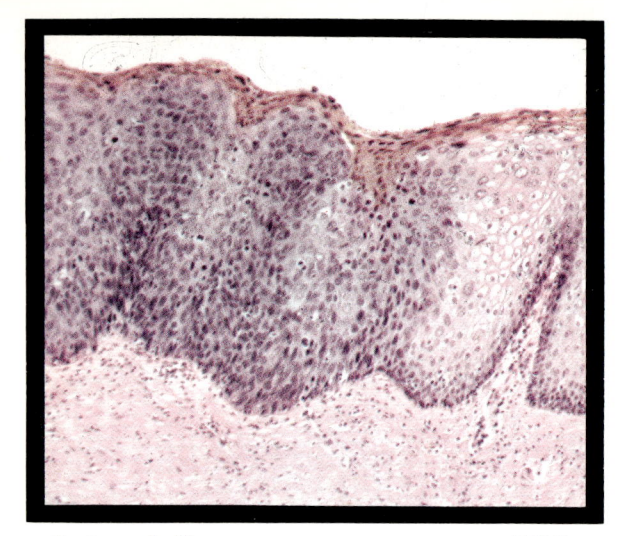

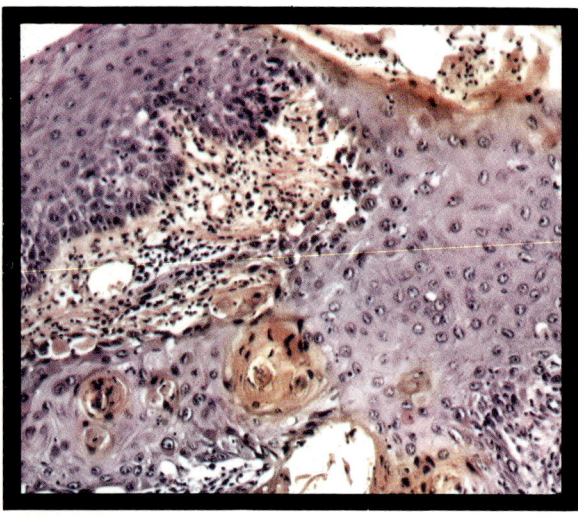

Squamous Cell Carcinoma (Cont.)

(Top) Carcinoma in situ (intra-epithelial carcinoma) may appear at the edge of an infiltrating carcinoma or may be the only mucosal change in the area. It is characterized by malignant changes which are limited to the epithelium. It eventually becomes invasive. The photomicrograph includes the junction between normal epithelium (far right) and carcinoma in situ. To the right of center there is an abrupt change in the character of the epithelium. To the left of this area the cells are not in normal arrangement. There is an increased number of cells as well as alteration in their character. The nuclei are variable in size and hyperchromatic. The basal layer, however, is intact. The epithelial changes in carcinoma in situ are somewhat similar to those in premalignant leukoplakia, except that they are more extensive.

(Center) Relatively well differentiated squamous cell carcinoma is demonstrated in this photomicrograph. In the upper left-hand corner there is a segment of surface epithelium which is relatively normal. The squamous epithelium in the rest of the photomicrograph is carcinomatous. It shows loss of organization. The cells are large, with abundant light-blue-staining cytoplasm. Properly oriented basal cells are not evident at the periphery. At lower left is a strand of epithelium containing circumscribed nests of cells which have abundant eosinophilic cytoplasm and pyknotic nuclei.

(Bottom) At top center the covering epithelium is thin, nonpapillated and hyperkeratotic. The subepithelial connective tissue is heavily infiltrated with inflammatory cells. In the center of the photomicrograph is a large, circular, laminated hyaline structure surrounded by epithelial cells. This is a so-called epithelial pearl. Such structures are commonly found in moderately well differentiated squamous cell carcinoma. To the right of this central mass and at the far left are nests of atypical epithelial cells. Below the pearl are other malignant cells which are somwhat difficult to recognize because of the heavy inflammatory infiltrate.

Carcinoma in Situ   X 100

Squamous Cell Carcinoma   X 150

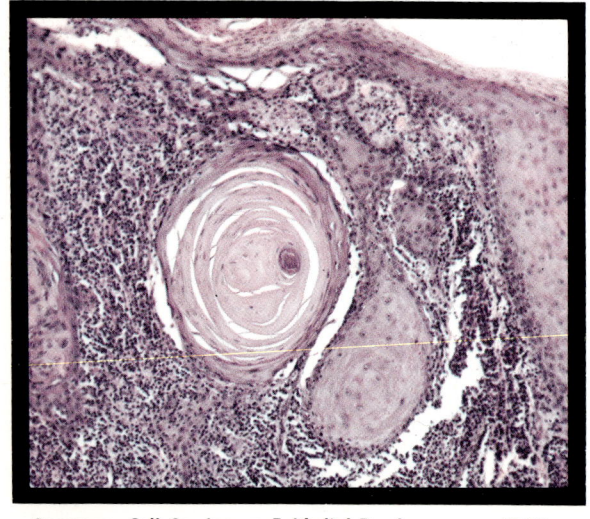

Squamous Cell Carcinoma, Epithelial Pearl   X 80

Squamous Cell Carcinoma (Cont.)

(Top) Low-power view of a verrucous or papillomatous squamous cell carcinoma of 1 year's duration. At far left is normal surface epithelium. The numerous projecting structures are composed of atypical epithelial cells (not apparent at this magnification). Keratohyalin and cellular debris are entrapped between the fingerlike projections. It is apparent that this carcinoma has not invaded deeply; much of it extends above the normal mucosal level. Clinically it might have been confused with a papilloma, wart or keratoacanthoma. Carcinomas growing in a verrucal pattern tend to be fairly well differentiated lesions. In some instances the diagnosis may be missed microscopically if the pathologist is not given sufficient material to examine. Verruciform carcinomas generally have a better prognosis than other types, but this advantage may be somewhat offset by the fact that their true nature is not always suspected clinically until they have reached a large size.

(Center) Some of the characteristic alterations observed in squamous cell carcinoma are demonstrated in this photomicrograph. Nearly all of the cells are large, with abundant, light-staining cytoplasm. There is much variation in nuclear form and in staining characteristics. Many nuclei are vesicular and have distinct nucleoli. In some cells the chromatin material is compact and stains intensely. There are numerous mitotic figures, some of which are abnormal. Several typical division figures can be seen near the upper right-hand corner. To the left and above these are a few cells with vesicular nuclei and prominent nucleoli. Large, bizarre cells are apparent at the lower right and left.

(Bottom) A portion of a poorly differentiated (highly malignant) squamous cell carcinoma. It is apparent that there is a marked variation in nuclear size and pattern. Near the right border are several large, bizarre nuclear masses. A similar mass is seen at lower left. Three pyknotic chromatin masses are seen near upper right. The nuclei in some of the cells are pale-staining but have prominent nucleoli. The cell boundaries in many instances are indistinct.

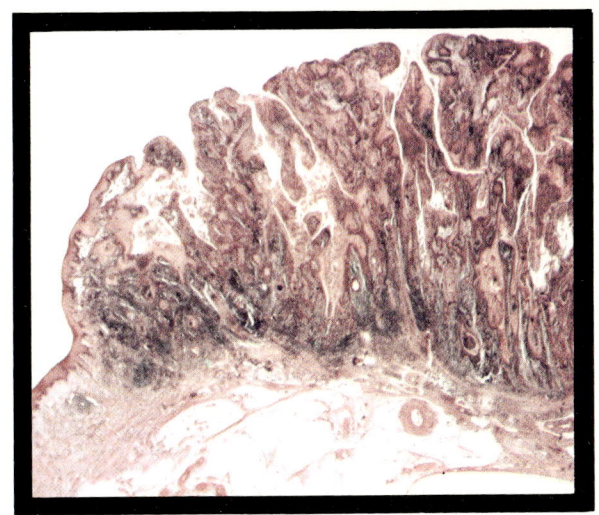

Squamous Cell Carcinoma, Verrucous Type   X 7

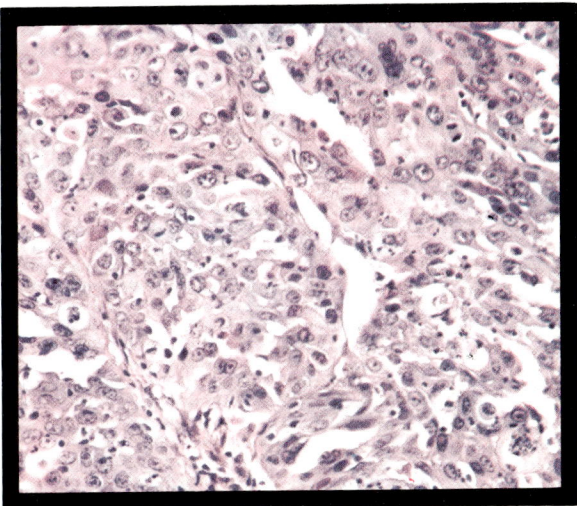

Squamous Cell Carcinoma   X 180

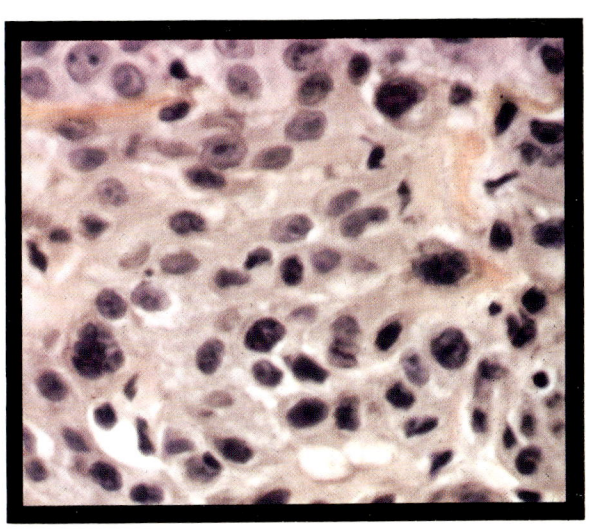

Squamous Cell Carcinoma   X 450

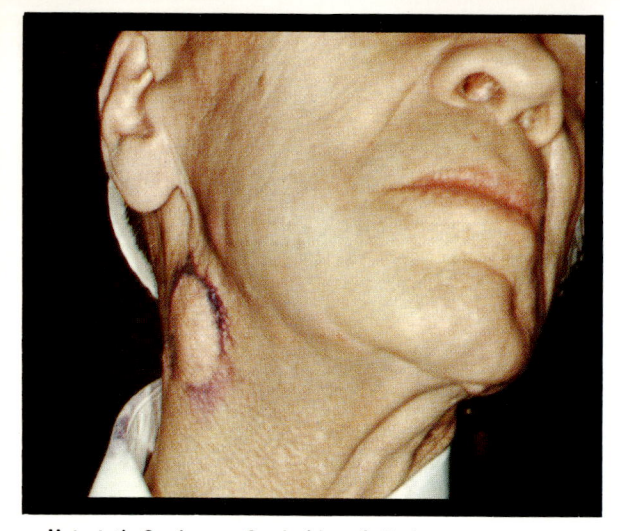

Metastatic Carcinoma, Cervical Lymph Node

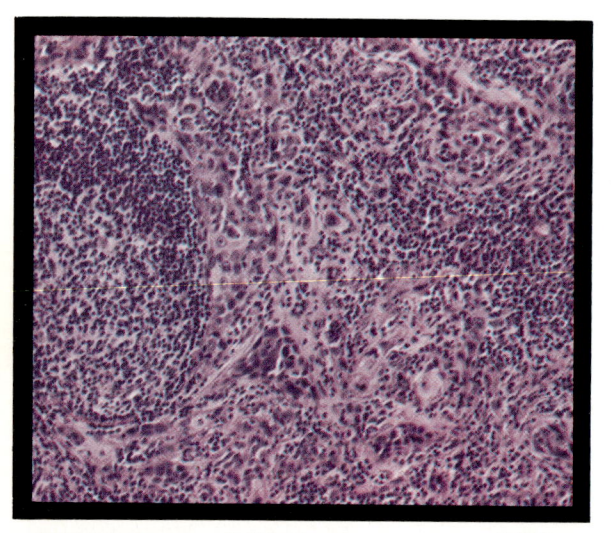

Metastatic Squamous Cell Carcinoma   X 100

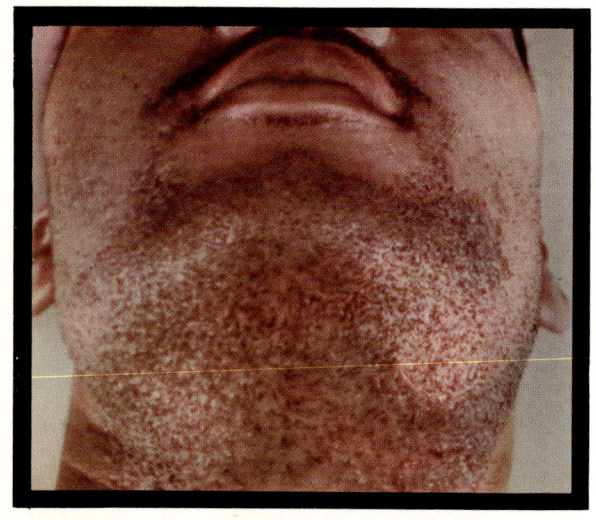

Metastatic Lympho-epithelioma, Left Cervical Nodes

Squamous Cell Carcinoma (Cont.)

(*Top*) The nodular enlargement of the lateral neck, outlined with indelible pencil, is a lymph node invaded by carcinoma metastatic from the oral cavity. Squamous cell carcinoma almost always metastasizes by the lymphogenous route. Knowledge of the lymph drainage of the tumor site will enable one to anticipate which lymph nodes may become involved. Enlargement of lymph nodes in adults, unless obviously related to inflammatory disease, should be considered the result of metastatic cancer until proved otherwise.

(*Center*) Squamous cell carcinoma which has metastasized to a lymph node. Some of the lymph node architecture is still discernible. At far left is a circular mass of lymphocytes which is a germinal center (lymphoid follicle). In the rest of the photomicrograph are neoplastic epithelial cells which are characterized by moderately abundant cytoplasm and large pleomorphic nuclei. Lymphocytes are scattered among the malignant cells. In some instances an entire node will be replaced by neoplastic tissue.

Carcinoma of the Nasopharynx

(*Bottom*) Carcinomas arising in the nasopharynx have a tendency to remain small and symptomless at their primary site. Frequently the first obvious manifestation of the disease is metastatic lymphadenopathy, as shown here. This patient, who was referred for dental examination, had no complaints except for the asymptomatic swelling near the angle of the mandible. This had been present for 3 months and had not responded to penicillin therapy. Clinical and radiographic examination did not reveal any disease process in the oral cavity which might be related to the enlarged lymph nodes. The oral diagnostician, being cognizant of the peculiarities of cancer of the nasopharynx, suggested that this region be examined for neoplastic disease. A very small lesion was discovered which proved to be a lympho-epithelioma, one of the nasopharyngeal carcinomas. Despite intensive x-ray therapy, the disease proved fatal in 12 months, with widespread metastasis.

Carcinoma of the Nasopharynx (Cont.)

(Top) Histologic appearance of a lympho-epithelioma. Near the center and the lower border are several large oval or circular structures. These are nuclei of malignant epithelial cells. They contain at least one large nucleolus. Such nucleoli have some affinity for eosin and may stain slightly red. The borders of the epithelial cells are very indistinct. Scattered among these cells, and also in the adjacent tissue, are several lymphocytes. Lympho-epitheliomas, transitional cell carcinomas, and other poorly differentiated tumors of the nasopharynx are sometimes designated as anaplastic epidermoid carcinomas. A few nasopharyngeal neoplasms are moderately well differentiated squamous cell carcinomas.

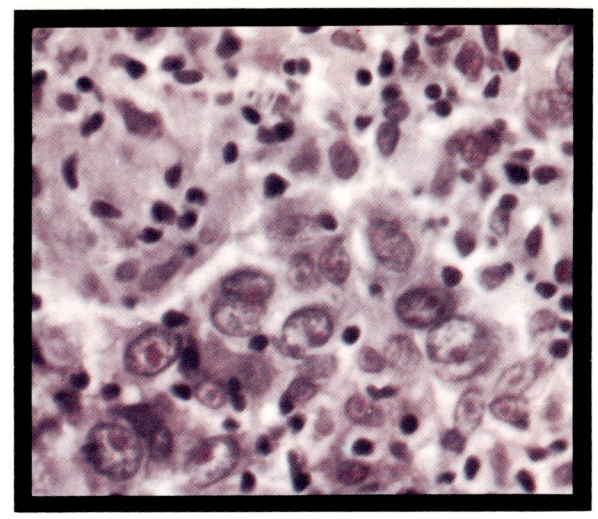

Lympho-epithelioma (Schmincke Tumor)   X 500

Multiple Myeloma

Multiple myeloma, an invariably fatal neoplasm arising in the bone marrow, is characterized by a slow but progressive destruction of skeletal parts. Its highest incidence is after the 4th decade, and it occurs in men more frequently than in women. The bone lesions, which are sharply outlined, contain closely packed cells of the plasma cell type. Most, but not all, cases are characterized by Bence-Jones protein in the urine and an increase in the serum protein with a reversal of the albumin-globulin ratio.

(Center) The radiolucent areas in the molar regions were discovered when radiographs were taken to determine the cause of pain in the mandible. A skeletal survey revealed "punched-out" lesions in many of the bones, one of which appears at the top of this illustration. Occasionally, a spontaneous fracture of an involved weight-bearing bone may be the first indication of this disease.

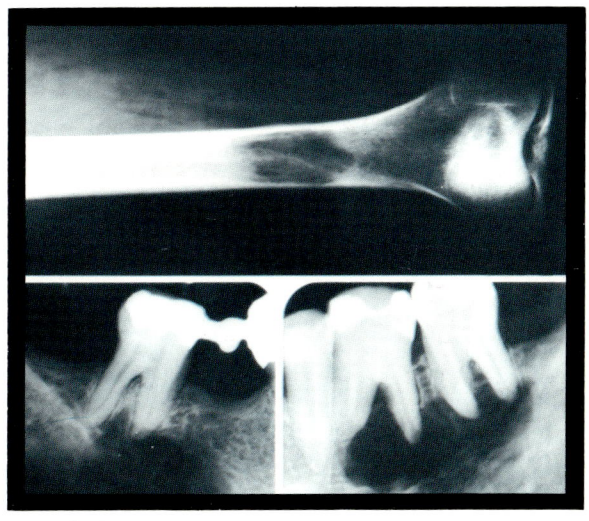

(Bottom) Moderately compact mass of cells, many of which closely resemble plasma cells. (See p. 8.) Care must be exercised not to make the diagnosis of myeloma based on the presence of a mass of plasma cells in granulation tissue. In multiple myeloma there is some degree of pleomorphism, the cells are closely packed, and stroma is very scant.

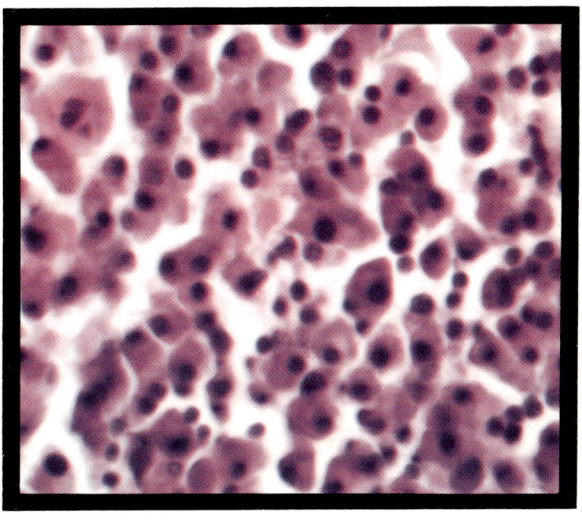

Multiple Myeloma, Mandible and Femur

Multiple Myeloma, Biopsy Specimen   X 500

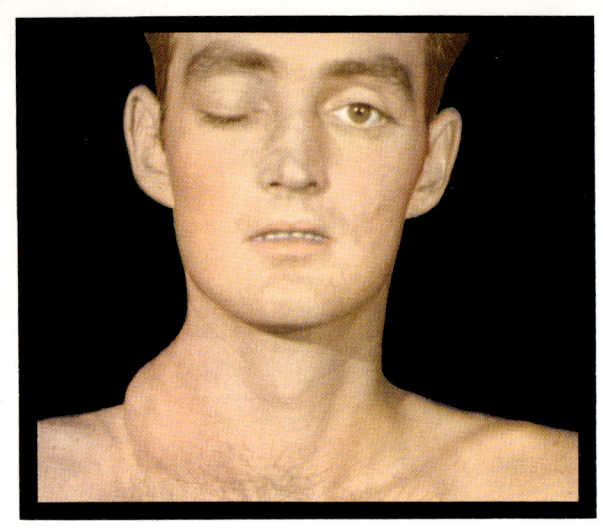

Lymphosarcoma, Lymphoblastic Type

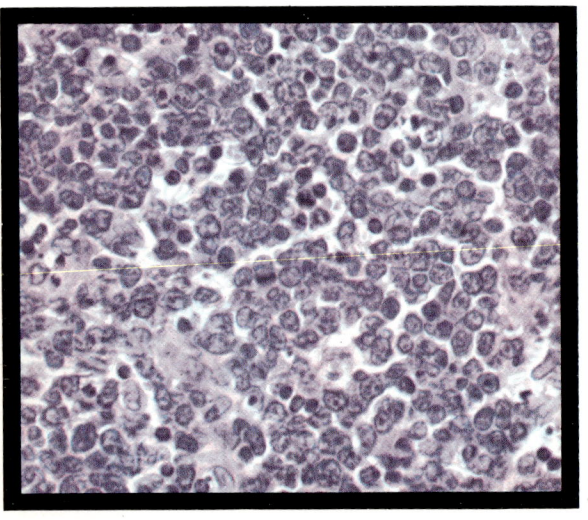

Lymphosarcoma, Lymphoblastic Type   X 400

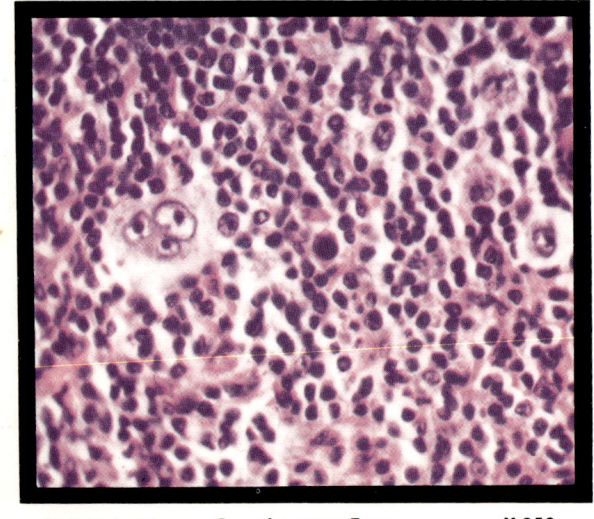

Hodgkin's Disease, Granulomatous Type   X 350

Malignant Lymphoma

Malignant lymphoma is an inclusive term for neoplasms arising from lymphoid tissue. Such neoplasms may be subclassified according to histologic pattern. The main varieties are giant follicular lymphoma, lymphosarcoma, Hodgkin's disease and reticulum cell sarcoma. There is a close relationship among these neoplasms, and one may change into another; therefore it is better to regard them as variants of a single disease process than as distinct entities. All varieties of malignant lymphoma are invariably fatal, multicentric in origin, and characterized clinically by enlarged lymph nodes. Treatment may prolong their course.

(Top) Enlargement of lymph nodes in lymphosarcoma. The large nodular mass in the supraclavicular region was nontender and moderately firm to palpation. A small lump was noted in this area 6 weeks previously. The patient died 9 weeks after the first clinical manifestations of the disease.

(Center) The predominating cells in this section are lymphoblasts. They have large nuclei in which the chromatin particles are widely dispersed. This lymphoblastic type of lymphosarcoma is more highly malignant than the lymphocytic type, which is composed of relatively mature lymphocytes. In either form of the disease the neoplastic cells may enter the peripheral blood (lymphatic leukemia).

(Bottom) Hodgkin's disease is characterized histologically by proliferation of reticuloendothelial cells. Some of these enlarge to form Dorothy Reed (Reed-Sternberg) cells. In the photomicrograph several of these special cells are seen. At left is one with a trilobed nucleus (due to fusion of 3 cells); at right several others are apparent. Hodgkin's disease may be divided into the following histologic types: paragranuloma—many small lymphocytes and a scattering of Dorothy Reed cells; granulomatous type—varying amounts of fibrous tissue in which are lymphocytes, plasma cells, eosinophils, neutrophils and numerous Dorothy Reed cells; sarcomatous type—reticulum cells predominating. The survival period is quite variable; it may be relatively long if the disease begins and remains as the paragranulomatous type.

Malignant Lymphoma (Cont.)

(Top) In this specimen the normal lymph node structures have been replaced by malignant reticulum cells. These cells have large hyperchromatic nuclei and frayed, angulated or elongated cytoplasmic processes. Many of them appear to be attached to fine strands of tissue somewhat like grapes on a stem. Reticulum cell sarcoma may become leukemic (monocytic leukemia). Sarcomatous Hodgkin's disease and reticulum cell sarcoma may appear quite similar histologically. Some pathologists believe that they are the same disease.

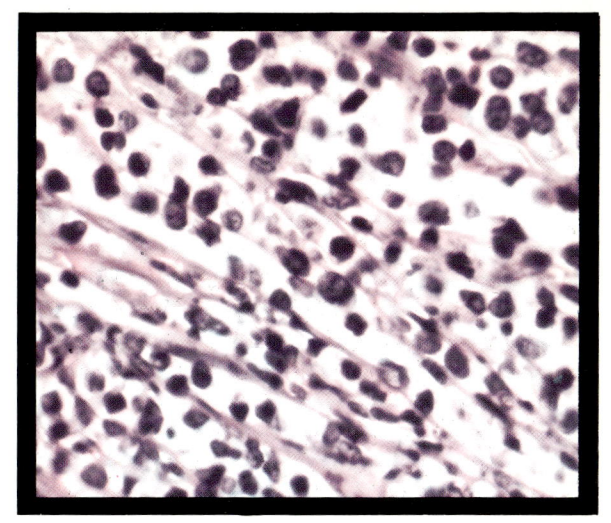

Reticulum Cell Sarcoma   X 400

Leukemia

Cells from a neoplasm of hemopoietic tissue may appear in the peripheral blood; this stage of the disease is designated leukemia and indicates a fatal prognosis. Leukemia may be designated lymphocytic, monocytic and granulocytic (myelogenous), indicating the histogenesis of the neoplasm. Lymphatic leukemia and monocytic leukemia are related to lymphosarcoma and reticulum cell sarcoma, respectively. (See malignant lymphoma, pp. 162 and 163). Each type of leukemia may be designated as acute or chronic. The acute is characterized by poorly differentiated cells, and the chronic type by well-differentiated cells. In general, the more differentiated the cells, the longer the course of the disease. The oral changes that may occur in leukemia are related to local leukemic infiltrations, thrombocytopenia, neutropenia and anemia.

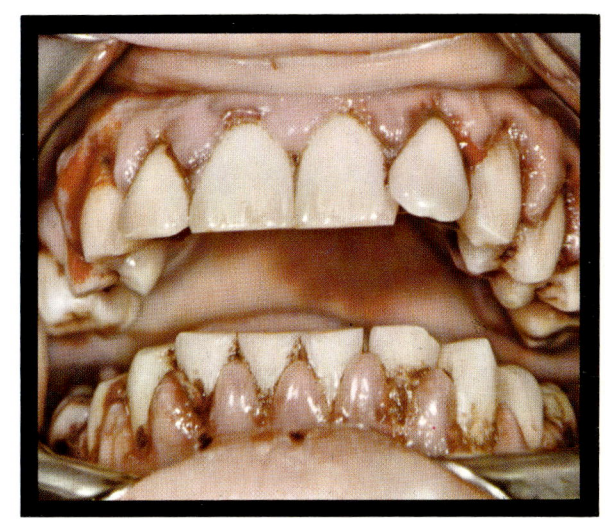

(Center) The gingival tissue in this leukemic patient is hyperplastic in many areas due to an infiltration of the abnormal cells. (See leukemic gingivitis, p. 81.) Another common oral manifestation of leukemia, gingival hemorrhage, is also apparent. This patient was not aware that he had leukemia until a blood count was done when he appeared for dental treatment.

(Bottom) In this leukemic patient the mucosa is pale, and numerous petechiae are seen in the hard and soft palates as well as in the lip. In some cases minor acts of trauma may produce ulcers that will not heal due to the diminished number of circulating neutrophils. (See agranulocytosis, p. 128.)

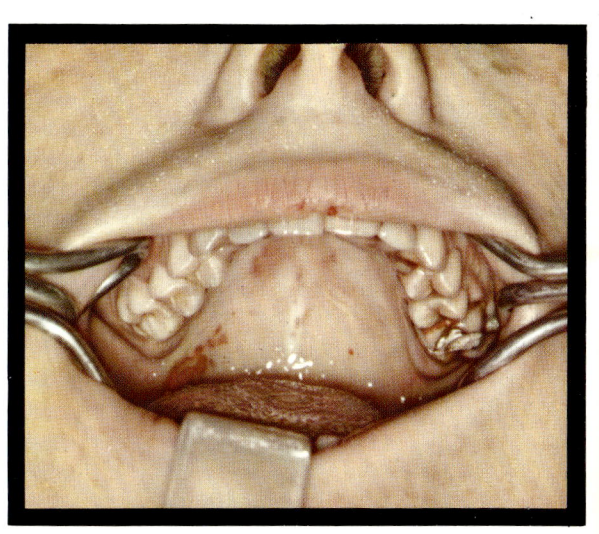

Leukemia

Leukemia

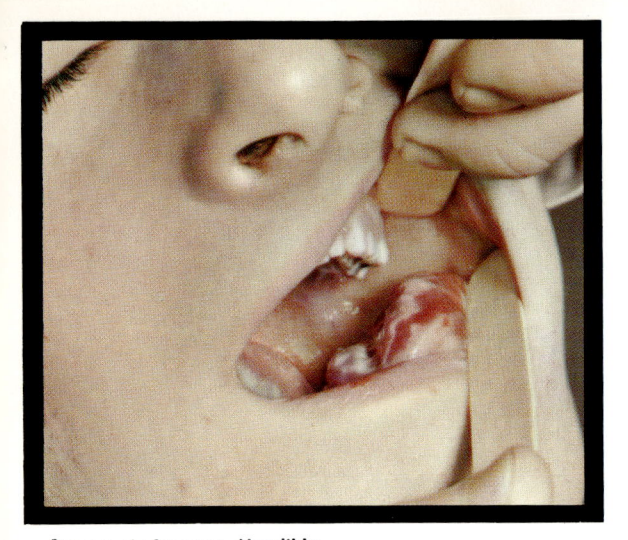

Neoplasms

Osteogenic Sarcoma, Mandible

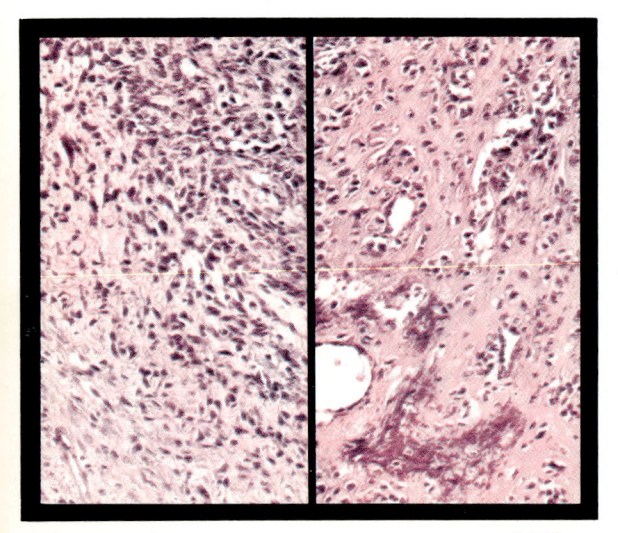

Osteogenic Sarcoma   X 100

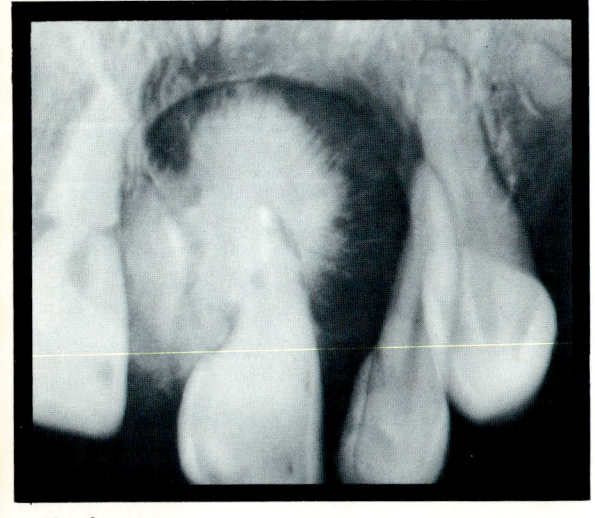

Chondrosarcoma

Osteogenic Sarcoma

In osteogenic sarcoma, which is a malignant neoplasm of bone-forming mesenchymal tissue, the bone is usually produced directly from the tumor parenchyma, but some may be formed via cartilage. This neoplasm is highly malignant and generally metastasizes to the lungs. Osteogenic sarcomas occur most frequently in the 2nd and 3rd decades. They are relatively rare in older individuals except in patients with Paget's disease. (See p. 134.)

(Top) Osteogenic sarcoma in the left mandible of a 19-year-old male. Biting on this large nodular mass has caused it to become distorted and ulcerated.

(Center) Two areas from one tumor are demonstrated in this photomicrograph. At left is proliferating connective tissue in which there are atypical spindle and stellate cells. At right, near the lower border, atypical bone is being formed directly from the malignant connective tissue.

Chondrosarcoma

Chondrosarcoma is a malignant neoplasm of mesenchymal tissue that produces atypical, poorly differentiated cartilage cells. Some bone may be produced in the neoplasm and develops directly from the connective tissue along with the cartilage. Chondrosarcoma is most prevalent in individuals 30 to 50 years of age, does not generally run a rapid course except in the jaws, and in many instances appears to develop from preexisting benign cartilaginous tumors.

(Bottom) This chondrosarcoma in the premaxilla is radiopaque centrally and radiolucent peripherally. The "sun-ray" appearance resulting from the radiopaque streaks extending from the central calcified mass is commonly considered characteristic of sclerosing osteogenic sarcoma. Histologic examination revealed a cartilaginous tumor with a marked amount of calcification and ossification. It appeared benign and was diagnosed as an osteochondroma. There was massive recurrence 4 years later, at which time biopsy revealed chondrosarcoma. Upon further sectioning and reevaluation of the first biopsy specimen, small sarcomatous areas were discovered.

Chondrosarcoma (Cont.)

(Top) In some chondrosarcomas histologic evidence of malignancy is readily apparent. In many, however, most of the cartilage cells are well differentiated, and malignant characteristics may be overlooked unless sufficient material is examined in detail. A cartilaginous neoplasm should be considered malignant if in some areas the following are apparent: large nuclei, some binucleated cells, and occasional large cells with several nuclei or clumped chromatin. In the accompanying photomicrograph all these malignant features are apparent.

Some pathologists designate malignant bone- or cartilage-producing tumors according to the main component or components. Others classify all such neoplasms as osteosarcomas.

Chondrosarcoma   X 220

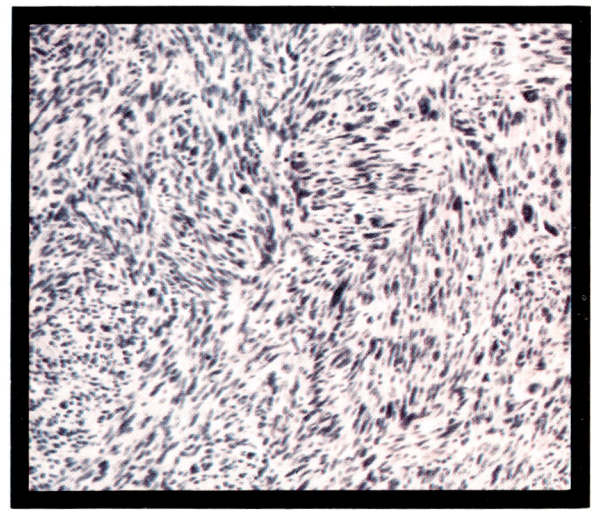

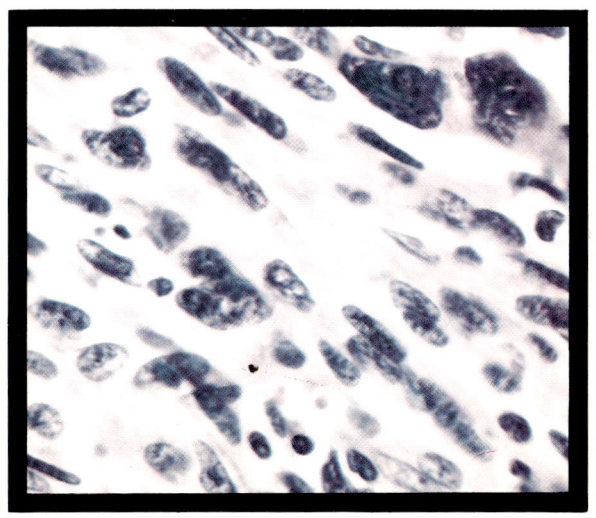

Fibrosarcoma

(Center) Fibrosarcoma is a malignant neoplasm consisting of fibroblasts. It may arise from the periosteum or from extra-osseous soft tissue. The aggressiveness of these tumors varies, but generally they are relatively slow-growing. Many fibrosarcomas are well-differentiated lesions. The one in the photomicrograph, however, is highly anaplastic. It is composed of spindle-shaped cells with hyperchromatic nuclei, many of which are exceptionally large. Throughout the specimen there are bands of tissue in which the cells are oriented in one direction, giving them a combed appearance. Some of these bands are at right angles to others. Malignant tumors of nerve or muscle may sometimes appear quite similar to this lesion. When the tissue of origin is not evident in neoplasms having such a histologic pattern, it is convenient to designate them as spindle cell sarcomas.

Fibrosarcoma   X 100

(Bottom) This is a higher magnification of the tumor in the center picture, showing the component cells in greater detail. It is apparent that most of the cells are spindle-shaped but of various sizes. In several, the chromatin material is irregularly dispersed throughout the nucleus; in other cells it is condensed and stains intensely. At upper right 2 very large, bizarre chromatin masses are seen.

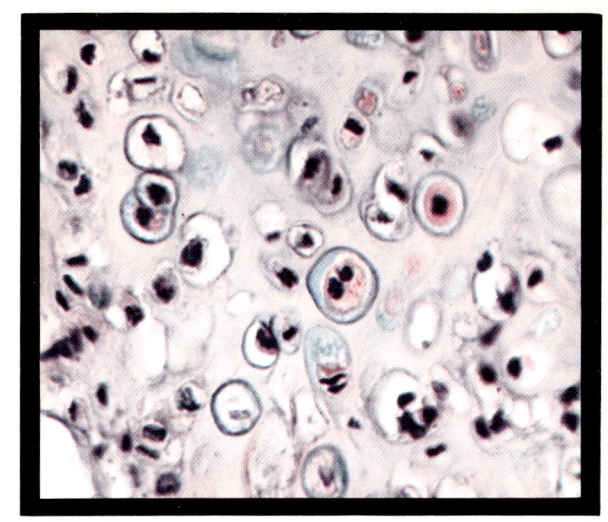

Fibrosarcoma   X 575

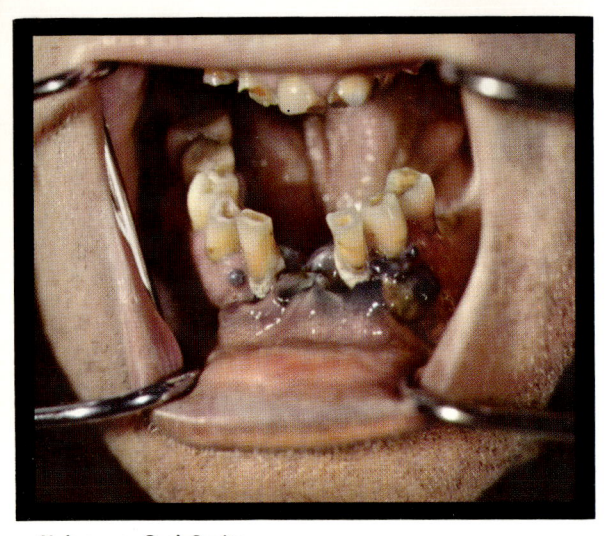

Melanoma, Oral Cavity

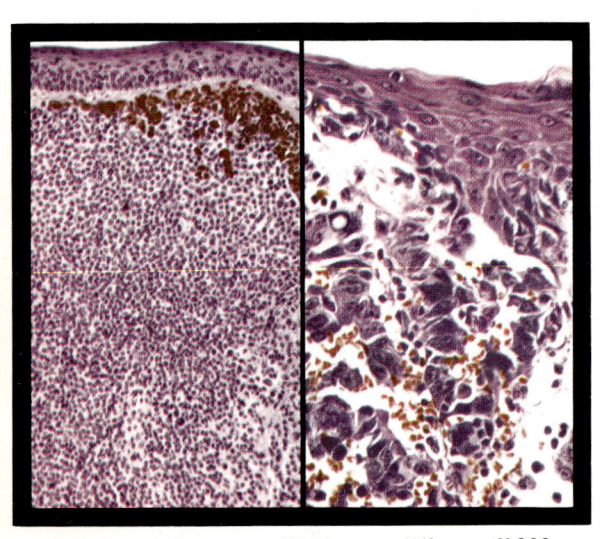

Nevus, Buccal Mucosa X 100   Melanoma X 200

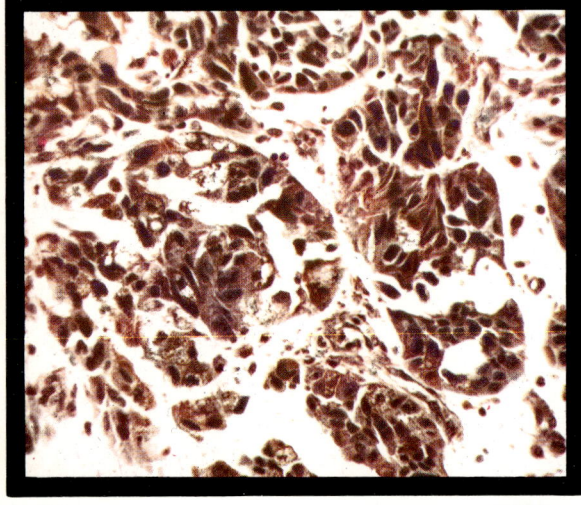

Melanoma   X 250

Melanoma

(Top) A melanoma (melanoblastoma, melanocarcinoma) is a neoplasm composed of malignant melanocytes (melanoblasts). It metastasizes early and widely. The cure rate is low. Melanoma in the skin and mucous membrane usually appears clinically as an enlarging bluish-black or slate-gray, raised lesion. The pigmented areas seen in the accompanying picture are metastatic lesions. Melanoma is seldom primary in the oral cavity.

Melanomas are to be differentiated from pigmented nevi, which are benign. The latter lesions are relatively static, may be raised or flat, and are generally of a brown color except for those designated as blue nevi. The histologic characteristics of the different types are as follows: *junctional nevus*—clumps of loosened, pigmented cells in the lower malpighian layer; *intradermal nevus*—nevus cells grouped in the corium; *compound nevus*—combination of junctional and intradermal types; *blue nevus*—heavily pigmented spindle cells deep in the corium. In many instances melanomas appear to have developed from junctional or compound nevi. The first clinical indication of malignant change is an increase in size and in the degree of pigmentation.

(Center) In the intradermal nevus at left the nevus cells form a solid sheet in the corium, though they are usually found in nests and cords. They are separated from the flattened covering epithelium by a small band of connective tissue. The superficial cells are heavily pigmented. At right is a section from a malignant lesion. The so-called junctional change (loosening of the cells), is evident in the overlying epithelium. In the corium are large, lightly pigmented cells with bizarre nuclei. These are malignant melanocytes which appear to have arisen from the overlying epithelium. The junctional change is not present in metastatic lesions.

(Bottom) In this melanoma the malignant cells are heavily pigmented. When melanin is not present (amelanotic melanoma), the diagnosis is somewhat difficult. Juvenile melanomas, which occur before puberty, appear malignant histologically but do not metastasize.

Metastasis to the Jaws

Epithelial neoplasms, especially adenocarcinoma, have a marked tendency to metastasize to bone. This is particularly true of adenocarcinomas of breast, thyroid and prostate, and of hypernephroma. The jaws, especially the mandible, may be the site of intra-osseous metastasis. This always should be considered in the patient with a history of previous treatment of malignant neoplasm. Skeletal metastasis is often late, and the lesions may therefore occur more than 5 years after treatment when it appears that the primary neoplasm has been successfully treated.

(Top) This patient presented because of looseness of the lower teeth and swelling of the labial aspect of the ridge. It was thought by the patient and his dentist that the looseness and swelling were due to periodontal disease. However, radiographs demonstrated a destructive lesion in the anterior mandible with expansion of the buccal plate. The patient had a history of bronchogenic carcinoma, and biopsy revealed that the jaw lesion was metastatic from the lung.

(Center) Radiograph showing destruction of alveolar crest by metastatic neoplasm. The irregular pattern of destruction is typical of metastatic neoplasm. Teeth, when present in the area, usually show root resorption, having "spiked" appearances.

(Bottom) This patient presented for a denture, and from the time the impression was taken until the denture was fabricated the ridge had enlarged. Radiographs showed destructive lesions throughout the maxilla. Biopsy revealed metastatic carcinoma from the breast. The patient had had a radical mastectomy 8 years previously without any intervening evidence of metastasis or recurrence. In case of such jaw enlargement one should consider neoplastic disease and metabolic disturbances such as acromegaly (p. 133), Paget's disease (p. 134) and osteitis fibrosa cystica (p. 129).

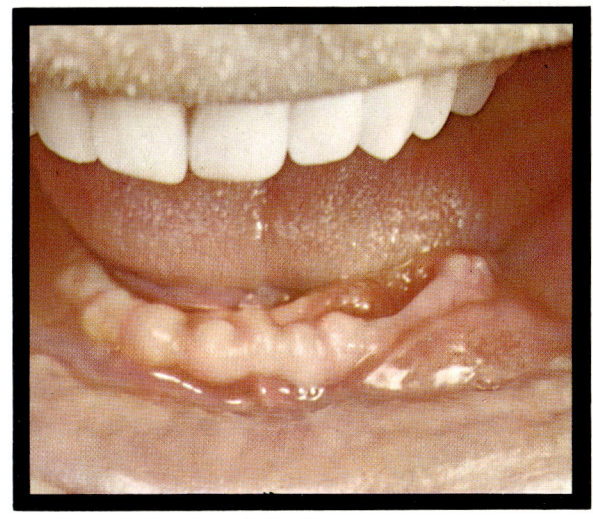

Metastatic Bronchogenic Carcinoma

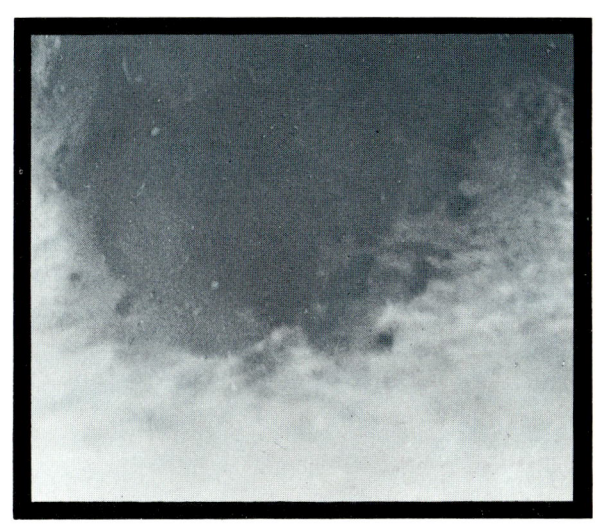

Bone Destruction, Mandible, Metastatic Neoplasm

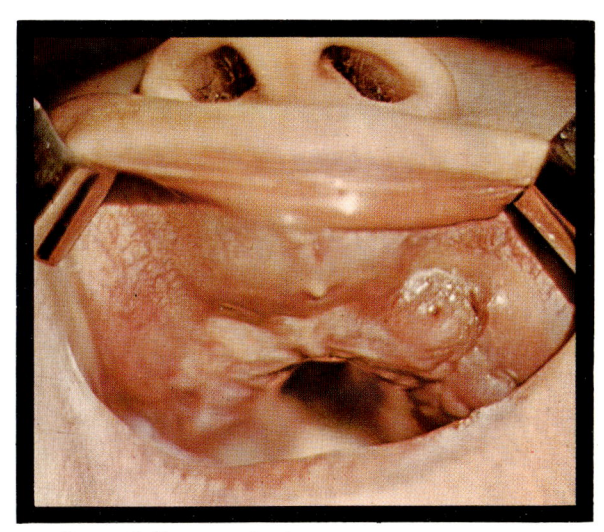

Metastatic Mammary Carcinoma

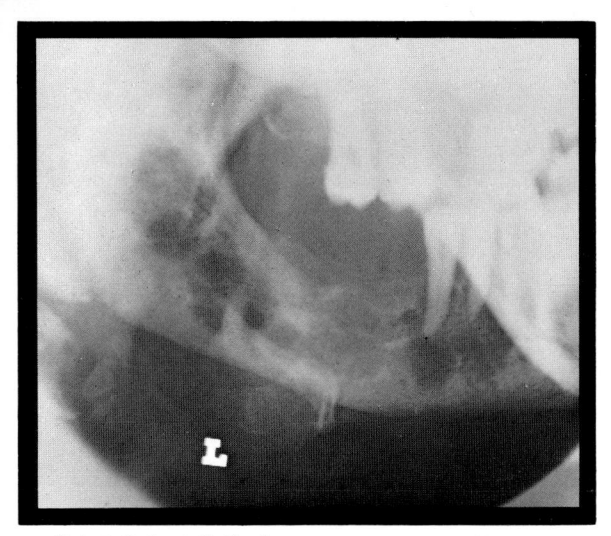

Metastatic Prostatic Carcinoma

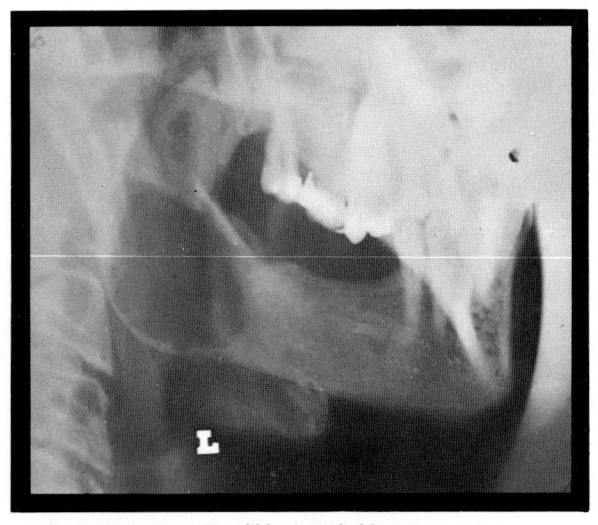

Bone Destruction, Mandible, Lymphoblastoma

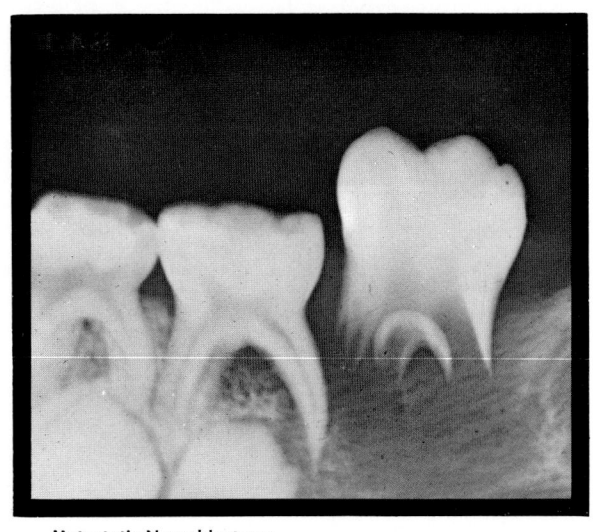

Metastatic Neuroblastoma

Metastasis to the Jaws (Cont.)

(Top) This patient had pain, numbness and looseness of the lower teeth. The lateral jaw film shows radiolucencies suggesting the pattern seen in osteomyelitis, multiple myeloma, eosinophilic granuloma, metastatic carcinoma, and possibly ameloblastoma. The patient had been treated for a carcinoma of the prostate, and biopsy of the jaw verified that this was a carcinoma metastatic from the prostate.

(Center) Patient complained of swelling in region of angle of mandible. Lateral jaw films demonstrated a unilocular cystic-appearing lesion at the angle of the mandible. This was misinterpreted as an odontogenic cyst. At surgery it was found to be a solid lesion. Histologic examination demonstrated the lesion was a lymphoblastoma. Other bones were negative.

(Bottom) A 9-year-old child had had a diagnosis of neuroblastoma of the adrenal. Metastasis to the bones was widespread, and the jaws did not escape. The 1st molar shown was very loose, and radiographs revealed a "spiking" of the incompletely formed roots, complete loss of the lamina dura and of the normal architecture of the supporting bone. The loss of bone extends to the 2nd deciduous molar. Whenever a loose permanent tooth is encountered in a young child without evident history of trauma, a malignant neoplasm, either local or metastatic, should be suspected.

Malignant neoplasms are characterized by their ability to metastasize either through the blood or lymph stream. While classically carcinomas metastasize through lymph channels and sarcomas through blood vessels, there is no hard and fast rule. Rarely, tumors may metastasize by transplantation; for example, when cells from an ovarian tumor become detached and spread through the peritoneal cavity or those from an intra-oral tumor are aspirated and become implanted in the lung. Vascular metastasis is a similar process with the cells borne by the blood or lymph. Metastasis can occur from the jaws or to the jaws.

Bibliography

1. HISTOLOGY AND EMBRYOLOGY

Histology

Ainamo, J., and Loe, H.: Anatomic characteristics of gingiva: Clinical and microscopic study of free and attached gingiva, J. Periodont. 37:5, 1966.

Avery, J. K.: Histology and embryology of the face and oral structures, in Steele, P. F.: Dimensions in Dental Hygiene, Philadelphia, Lea & Febiger, 1966.

Bailey, F. R.: Textbook of Histology, rev. by Copenhaver, W. M., ed. 15, Baltimore, Williams & Wilkins, 1964.

Bloom, W., and Fawcett, D. W.: Textbook of Histology, ed. 9, Philadelphia, Saunders, 1968.

Cutwright, D. E., and Bhaskar, S. N.: Pulpal vasculature as demonstrated by new method, Oral Surg., Oral Med. and Oral Path. 27:678, 1969.

Di Fiore, M. S. H.: An Atlas of Human Histology, ed. 2, Philadelphia, Lea & Febiger, 1963.

Farbman, A. I.: The dual pattern of keratinization in filiform papillae on rat tongue, J. Anat. 106:233, 1970.

Finn, S. B. (ed.): Biology of the Dental Pulp Organ, A Symposium, University, Alabama, University of Alabama Press, 1968.

Greep, R. O.: Histology, ed. 2, New York, Blakiston, 1966.

Ham, A. W.: Histology, ed. 6, Philadelphia, Lippincott, 1969.

Hoffman, S., McEwan, W. S., and Drew, C. M.: Scanning electron microscopy of dental enamel, J. Dent. Res. 47:842, 1968.

Hubner, G., and Goerttler, K.: Changes with age in mucosa of human tongue, Virchows Arch. Path. Anat. 345:71, 1968.

Kerr, D. A.: Histology of the oral structures, in Bunting's Oral Hygiene, ed. 3, ch. 2, Philadelphia, Lea & Febiger, 1957.

Melcher, A. H., and Bowen, W. H.: Biology of the Periodontium, New York, Academic Press, 1969.

Noyes, F. B.: Oral Histology and Embryology, rev. by Schour, I., ed. 8, Philadelphia, Lea & Febiger, 1960.

Provenca, D. V.: Oral Histology, Philadelphia, Lippincott, 1964.

Sicher, H. (ed.): Orban's Oral Histology and Embryology, ed. 6, St. Louis, Mosby, 1966.

Simpson, H. E.: Three-dimensional approach to microscopy of periodontal membrane, Proc. Roy. Soc. Med. 60:537, 1967.

Weinmann, J. P.: Bone formation and bone resorption, Oral Surg., Oral Med. and Oral Path. 8:1074, 1955.

Weinmann, J. P., and Sicher, H.: Bone and Bones. Fundamentals of Bone Biology, ed. 2, St. Louis, Mosby, 1955.

Windle, W. F.: Textbook of Histology, ed. 4, New York, McGraw-Hill, 1969.

Embryology

Arey, L. B.: Developmental Anatomy. A Textbook and Laboratory Manual of Embryology, ed. 7, Philadelphia, Saunders, 1965.

Bosma, J. F.: Symposium on Oral Sensation and Perception, Springfield, Ill., Thomas, 1967.

Boyde, A.: Development of enamel structure, Proc. Roy. Soc. Med. 60:923, 1967.

Chase, S. W.: Histogenesis of the enamel, J.A.D.A. 19:1275, 1932.

——: The nature of the enamel matrix at different ages, J.A.D.A. 22:1343, 1935.

Deakins, M.: Changes in ash, water and organic content of pig enamel during calcification, J. Dent. Res. 21:429, 1942.

Frank, R. M.: Comparative aspects of development of dental hard structures, J. Dent. Res. 42:422, 1963.

Jordan, H. E.: Textbook of Embryology, ed. 9, New York, Appleton, 1952.

Krogman, W. M.: Biologic timing and the dentofacial complex, J. Dent. Child. 35:175, 377, 328, 1968.

Logan, W. H. G., and Kronfeld, R.: Development of the human jaws and surrounding structures from birth to the age of fifteen years. J.A.D.A., 20:379, 1933.

Nuckolls, J., Saunders, J. B. de C. M., and Frisbie, H. E.: Amelogenesis, J. Am. Col. Dent. 10:241, 1943.

Orban, B., Sicher, H., and Weinmann, J. P.: Amelogenesis (a critique and a new concept), J. Am. Col. Dent. 10:13, 1943.

Patten, B. M.: Human Embryology, ed. 3, New York, McGraw-Hill, 1968.

Schaeffer, J. P.: The ontogenetic development of the human face, Dent. Cosmos 77:464, 1935.

Schour, I., and Massler, M.: Studies in tooth development. The growth pattern of human teeth, J.A.D.A. 27:1778, 1918, 1940.

Sicher, H. (ed.): Orban's Oral Histology and Embryology, ed. 6, St. Louis, Mosby, 1966.

Thomas, J. B.: Introduction to Human Embryology, Philadelphia, Lea & Febiger, 1968.

Weinmann, J. P., Wessinger, G. D., and Reed, G.: Correlation of chemical and histological investigations on developing enamel, J. Dent. Res. 21:171, 1942.

Weller, G. L.: Development of the thyroid, parathyroid and thymus glands in man, Carnegie Contrib. Embryol. 24:93, 1933.

2. DEVELOPMENTAL DISTURBANCES

Congenital Clefts of Face and Jaw

Baker, B. R.: Pits of the lip commissures in Caucasoid males, Oral Surg., Oral Med. and Oral Path. 21:56, 1966.

Bjuggren, G., Jensen, R., and Strombeck, J. O.: Macroglossia and its surgical treatment: Indications and postoperative experiences from orthodontic, phonetic and surgical points of view, Scandinav. J. Plast. and Reconstr. Surg. 2:116, 1968.

Davis, W. B.: Congenital deformities of the face, Surg. Gynec. Obstet. 61:201, 1935.

Donahue, R. F.: Birth variables and incidence of cleft palate: Part I, Cleft Palate J. 2:282, 1965.

Dorrance, G. M.: The Operative Story of Cleft Palate, Philadelphia, Saunders, 1933.

Everett, F. G., and Wescott, W. B.: Commissural lip pits, Oral Surg., Oral Med. and Oral Path. 14:202, 1961.

Fogh-Anderson, P.: Thalidomide and congenital cleft deformities, Acta Chir. Scandinav. 131:197, 1966.

Fraser, F. C., and Fainstat, T. D.: Causes of congenital defects, Am. J. Dis. Child. 82:593, 1951.

Fukuhara, T.: New method and approach to genetics of cleft lip and cleft palate, J. Dent. Res. 44 (Suppl.):259, 1965.

Graber, T. M.: Craniofacial morphology in cleft palate and cleft lip deformities, Surg. Gynec. Obstet. 88:359, 1949.

Grace, L. G.: Frequency of occurrence of cleft palates and harelips, J. Dent. Res. 22:495, 1943.

Harris, H. I.: New technic for correction of macrostomia, J. Oral Surg. 3:156, 1945.

Kemper, J. W.: The responsibility of the surgeon in treating palatal and related defects. Am. J. Orthodont. and Oral Surg. (Oral Surg. Sec.) 32:667, 1946.

King, T. S.: The anatomy of harelip in man, J. Anat. 88:1, 1954.

Knapp, M. J.: Oral tonsils: Location, distribution and histology, Oral Surg., Oral Med. and Oral Path. 29:155, 1970.

Kraus, B. S., Jordan, R. E., and Pruzansky, S.: Dental abnormalities in the deciduous and permanent dentitions of individuals with the cleft lip and cleft palate, J. Dent. Res. 45:1736, 1966.

Kreshover, S. J.: Prenatal factors in oral pathologic conditions, Oral Surg., Oral Med. and Oral Path. 13:569, 1960.

Lis, E. F., Pruzansky, S., Loepp-Baker, H. and Kobes, H. R.: Cleft lip and cleft palate: Perspectives in management, Pediat. Clin. N. Am., p. 995, November 1956.

Lyons, C. J.: Etiology of cleft palate and cleft lip and some fundamental principles in operative procedure, J.A.D.A. 17:827, 1930.

MacMahn, B., and McKeown, T.: The incidence of harelip and cleft palate related to birth, rank and maternal age, Am. J. Genetics 5:176, 1953.

Mills, L. F., Niswander, J. D., Mazaheri, M., and Brunelle, J. A.: Minor oral and facial defects in relatives of oral cleft patients, Angle Orthodont. 38:199, 1968.

Mylin, W. K., and Hagerty, R. F.: Modern concepts in treatment of unilateral cleft lip and cleft palate, Southern Med. J. 62:171, 1969.

Potter, E. L.: Pathology of the Fetus and the Newborn, ed. 2, Chicago, Year Book Publishers, 1961.

Rozenzweig, S.: Psychologic stress in cleft palate etiology, J. Dent. Res. 45:1585, 1966.

Schaumann, B. F., Peagler, F. D., and Gorlin, R. J.: Minor craniofacial anomalies among a Negro population. I. Prevalence of cleft uvula, commissural lip pits, preauricular pits, torus palatinus and torus mandibularis, Oral Surg., Oral Med. and Oral Path. 29:566, 1970.

Strean, L. P., and Peer, L. A.: Stress as an etiological factor in the development of cleft palate, Plast. Reconstr. Surg. 18:1, 1956.

Warkany, J., and Deuschle, F. M.: Congenital malformations induced in rats by maternal riboflavin deficiency: dentofacial changes, J.A.D.A. 51:139, 1955.

Webster, R. C.: Cleft palate. Part I (Collective review). Oral Surg., Oral Med. and Oral Path. 1:647, 1948.

Auricular Tags

Altmann, F.: Malformations of the auricle and the external auditory meatus. A critical review. Arch. Otolaryng. 54:115, 1951.

Costello, M. J., and Shepard, J. H.: Supernumerary external ears, Arch. Otolaryng. 29: 695, 1939.
Lewin, M. L.: Congenital malformations of the ear and mandible, Oral Surg., Oral Med. and Oral Path. 3:1115, 1950.
Streeter, C. L.: Development of the auricle in the human embryo, Carnegie Contrib. Embryol. 14:111, 1922.

Brachygnathia

Baume, L. V., Haüpl, K., and Stellmach, R.: Growth and transformation of temporomandibular joint in orthopedically treated case of Pierre Robin's syndrome, Am. J. Orthodont. 45:901, 1959.
Engel, M. B., Richmond, J., and Brodie, A. G.: Mandibular growth disturbance in rheumatoid arthritis of childhood, Am. J. Dis. Child. 78:788, 1949.
Kennedy, J. M., and Thompson, J. M.: Hypoplasia of the mandible (Pierre Robin syndrome) with complete cleft palate, Oral Surg., Oral Med. and Oral Path. 3:421, 1950.
Nisenson, Aaron: Receding chin and glossoptosis, J. Pediat. 32:397, 1948.
Peskin, S., and Laskin, D. M.: Contribution of autogenous condylar grafts to mandibular growth, Oral Surg., Oral Med. and Oral Path. 20:517, 1965.
Prowler, J. R., and Glassman, S.: Agenesis of the mandibular condyles, Oral Surg., Oral Med. and Oral Path. 7:133, 1954.
Pruzansky, S., and Richmond, J. B.: Growth of mandible in infants with micrognathia. Clinical implications, Am. J. Dis. Child. 88:29, 1954.
Randall, P., Krogman, W. M., and Jahina, S.: Pierre Robin and the syndrome that bears his name, Cleft Palate J. 2:237, 1965.
Weseman, C. M.: Congenital micrognathia, Arch. Otolaryngol. 69:31, 1959.

Hemiatrophy

Archambault, L., and Fromm, N. K.: Progressive facial hemiatrophy, Arch. Neurol. Psychiat. 27:529, 1932.
Finesilver, B., and Rosow, H. M.: Total hemiatrophy, J.A.M.A. 110:366, 1938.
Kazanjian, V. H., and Sturgis, S. H.: Surgical treatment of hemiatrophy of the face, J.A.M.A. 115:348, 1940.
Rushton, M. A.: An early case of facial hemiatrophy, Oral Surg., Oral Med. and Oral Path. 4:1457, 1951.

Hygroma Colli Congenitum

Goetsch, E.: Hygroma colli cysticum and hygroma axillare. Pathologic and clinical study and report of twelve cases, Arch. Surg. 36:394, 1938.
Sedgwick, C. E.: Hygroma colli congenitum, Surg. Clin. N. A. 33:653, 1953.
Vaughn, A. M.: Cystic hygroma of the neck, Am. J. Dis. Child. 48:149, 1934.

Cysts, Sinuses and Fistulae of the Soft Tissue

Baumgartner, C. J.: Surgery of congenital lesions of the neck, Postgrad. Med. 1:181, 1947.
Becker, S. W., and Brunschwig, A.: Sinus preauricularis, Am. J. Surg. 24:174, 1934.
Bhaskar, S. N., and Bernier, J. L.: Histogenesis of branchial cysts, Am. J. Path. 35:407, 1959.
Brintnall, E. S., Davis, J., Huffman, W. C., and Lierle, D. M.: Thyroglossal ducts and cysts, Arch. Otolaryng. 59:282, 1954.
Cataldo, E., and Berkman, M. D.: Cysts of oral mucosa in newborns, Am. J. Dis. Child. 116:44, 1968.
Colp, R.: Dermoid cysts of the floor of the mouth, Surg. Gynec. Obstet. 40:183, 1925.
Conway, H., and Jerome, A. P.: The surgical treatment of branchial cysts and fistulas, Surg. Gynec. Obstet. 101:621, 1955.
Dingman, R. O.: Congenital preauricular sinus, Arch. Otolaryng. 29:982, 1939.
Egervary, G., and Csiba, A.: Bilateral nasolabial cyst, Dent. Digest 75:504, 1969.
Erich, J. B.: Sebaceous, mucous, dermoid and epidermoid cysts, Am. J. Surg. 50:672, 1940.
Everett, F. G., and Wescott, W. B.: Commissural lip pits, Oral Surg., Oral Med. and Oral Path. 14:202, 1961.
Fromm, A.: Epstein's pearls, Bohn's nodules and inclusion cysts of oral cavity, J. Dent. Child. 34:275, 1967.
Gorlin, R. J., and Jirasek, J. E.: Oral cysts containing gastric or intestinal mucosa: Unusual embryologic accident or heterotopia, J. Oral Surg. 28:9, 1970.
Gross, R. E., and Connerley, M. L.: Thyroglossal cysts and sinuses. A study and report of 198 cases, New Eng. J. Med. 223:616, 1940.
Harding, R. L.: Congenital preauricular sinus, Am. J. Orthodont. and Oral Surg. (Oral Surg. Sect.) 28:399, 1942.
Hicks, S. P.: Embryology and pathology of branchial cleft cysts, Surg. Clin. N. Am. 33:619, 1953.

Ladd, W. E., and Gross, R. E.: Congenital branchiogenic anomalies. A report of 82 cases, Am. J. Surg. 39:234, 1938.

Mahler, W. P., and Swindle, P. F.: Etiology and vascularization of dental lamina cysts. Oral Surg., Oral Med. and Oral Path. 29:590, 1970.

Marshall, S. F.: Thyroglossal cysts and sinuses, Surg. Clin. N. Am. 33:633, 1953.

McNealy, R. W.: Cystic tumors of the neck: Branchial and thyroglossal cysts, J.A.D.A. 29:1808, 1942.

Meyer, I.: Dermoid cysts (dermoids) of the floor of the mouth, Oral Surg., Oral Med. and Oral Path. 8:1149, 1955.

Montgomery, M. L.: Congenital auricular fistula. Report of 3 cases in the same family, Surg. Clin. N. Am. 11:141, 1931.

Neel, H. B., and Pemberton, J. de J.: Lateral cervical (branchial) cysts and fistulas. Surg. 18:267, 1945.

New, G. B.: Congenital cysts of the tongue, the floor of the mouth, the pharynx and the larynx, Arch. Otolaryng. 45:145, 1947.

Pemberton, J. de J., and Stalker, L. K.: Cysts, sinuses and fistulae of the thyroglossal duct, Ann. Surg. 111:950, 1940.

Proctor, B.: Lateral vestigial cysts and fistulas of the neck, Laryngoscope 65:355, 1955.

Quinn, J. H.: Congenital epidermoid cyst of anterior half of tongue, Oral Surg., Oral Med. and Oral Path. 13:1283, 1960.

Sedgwick, C. E., and Walsh, J. F.: Branchial cysts and fistulas. A study of seventy-five cases relative to clinical aspects and treatment, Am. J. Surg. 83:3, 1952.

Warbrick, J. G., McIntyre, J. R., and Ferguson, A. G.: Aetiology of congenital bilateral fistulae of the lower lip, Brit. J. Plastic Surg. 4:254, 1952.

Ward, G. E., Hendrick, J. W., and Chambers, R. G.: Thyroglossal tract abnormalities—cysts and fistulas, Surg. Gynec. Obstet. 89:727, 1949.

Watanabe, Y., Igaku-Hakushi, M. O., and Tomida, K.: Congenital fistulas of the lower lip. Reports of five cases with special reference to the etiology, Oral Surg., Oral Med. and Oral Path. 4:709, 1951.

Tori

Christiansen, G. W., and Bradley, J. L.: Congenital bone anomalies, J. Oral Surg. 3:74, 1945.

Dorrance, G. M.: Torus palatinus, Dent. Cosmos 71:275, 1929.

Kolas, S., Halperin, V., Jefferis, K. R., Huddleston, S., and Robinson, H. B. G.: The occurrence of torus palatinus and torus mandibularis in 2,478 dental patients, Oral Surg., Oral Med. and Oral Path. 6:1134, 1953.

Miller, S. C., and Roth, H.: Torus palatinus: A statistical study, J.A.D.A. 27:1950, 1940.

Schaumann, B. F., Peagler, F. D., and Gorlin, R. V.: Minor craniofacial anomalies among a Negro population: I. Prevalence of cleft uvula, commissural lip pits, preauricular pits, torus palatinus and torus mandibularis, Oral Surg., Oral Med. and Oral Path. 29:566, 1970.

Thoma, K. H.: Torus palatinus, Internat. J. Orthodont. and Oral Surg. 23:194, 1937.

Defective Development of the Tongue

Cahn, L.: Oral amyloid as a complication of myelomatosis, Oral Surg., Oral Med. and Oral Path. 10:735, 1957.

Di Palma, J. R.: Objective and clinical study of the tongue, Arch. Intern. Med. 78:405, 1946.

Grace, R. V., and Weeks, C.: Lingual thyroid, Ann. Surg. 96:973, 1932.

Halperin, V., Kolas, S., Jefferis, K. R., Huddleston, S. O., and Robinson, H. B. G.: The occurrence of Fordyce spots, benign migratory glossitis, median rhomboid glossitis and fissured tongue in 2,478 dental patients, Oral Surg., Oral Med. and Oral Path. 6:1072, 1953.

Hopkin, G. B.: Neonatal and adult tongue dimensions, Angle Orthodont. 37:132, 1967.

Hubinger, H. L.: Bifid tongue. Report of a case, J. Oral Surg. 10:64, 1952.

Johnson, B. F., and Triedman, L.: Lingual thyroid: Review and report of typical case, Clin. Med. 75:55, 1968.

Knapp, M. J.: Pathology of oral tonsils, Oral Surg., Oral Med. and Oral Path. 29:295, 1970.

Martin, H. E., and Howe, M. E.: Glossitis rhombica mediana, Ann. Surg. 107:39, 1938.

McEnery, E. T., and Gaines, F. P.: Tongue-tie in infants and children, J. Pediat. 18:252, 1941.

Royer, R. Q., and Bruce, K. W.: Median rhomboid glossitis, Oral Surg., Oral Med. and Oral Path. 5:1287, 1952.

Schaumann, B. F., Peagler, F. D., and Gorlin, R. J.: Minor craniofacial anomalies among a Negro population. II. Prevalence of tongue anomalies, Oral Surg., Oral Med., and Oral Path. 29:729, 1970.

Shapiro, M. J.: Cysts on the base of tongue in infants, Ann. Otol., Rhin. and Laryng. 58:457, 1949.

Spitzer, R.: Partial ankyloglossia, Oral Surg., Oral Med. and Oral Path. *13*:787, 1960.
Stein, G., and Gold, H.: Correlation between gross appearance and histopathology of the tongue, Oral Surg., Oral Med. and Oral Path. *8*:1165, 1955.

Fordyce Spots

Cahn, L. R.: Fordyce's disease, Arch. Clin. and Oral Path. *2*:44, 1938.
———: Fordyce's disease. A historical review, Arch. Clin. and Oral Path. *2*:82, 1938.
Chambers, S. O.: The structure of Fordyce's disease as demonstrated by wax reconstruction, Arch. Dermat. and Syph. *18*:666, 1928.
Halperin, V., Kolas, S., Jefferis, K. R., Huddleston, S. O., and Robinson, H. B. G.: The occurrence of Fordyce spots, benign migratory glossitis, median rhomboid glossitis and fissured tongue in 2,478 dental patients, Oral Surg., Oral Med. and Oral Path. *6*:1072, 1953.

Cysts of the Jaw

Abrams, A. M., and Howell, F. V.: The calcifying odontogenic cyst, Oral Surg., Oral Med. and Oral Path. *25*:594, 1968.
Bernier, J. L., and Tiecke, R. W.: Incisive canal cyst, J. Oral Surg. *8*:254, 1950.
Boone, C. G.: Nasoalveolar cyst, Oral Surg., Oral Med. and Oral Path. *8*:40, 1955.
Bradley, J. L.: Cysts of the jaw bones, J. Oral Surg. *9*:295, 1951.
Browne, R. M.: The odontogenic keratocyst: clinical aspects, Brit. Dent. J. *128*:225, 1970.
Burket, L. W.: Nasopalatine duct structures and peculiar bony pattern observed in anterior maxillary region, Arch. Path. *23*:793, 1937.
Cohen, M. M.: Fissural cysts of the median palatine suture, Am. J. Orthodont. and Oral Surg. (Oral Surg. Sect.) *29*:442, 1943.
Conklin, W. W., and Stafne, E. C.: A study of odontogenic epithelium in the dental follicle, J.A.D.A. *39*:143, 1949.
Cross, W. G.: Lateral periodontal cyst. Report of a case, J. Periodont. *25*:287, 1954.
Fickling, B. W.: Cysts of jaw: long-term survey of types and treatment, Proc. Roy. Soc. Med. *58*:847, 1965.
Gettinger, R.: Relationship of odontogenic epithelium to cystic and other diseases of the mouth and jaw, Arch. Clin. and Oral Path. *4*:198, 1940.
Gold, L., and Christ, T.: Granular cell odontogenic cyst, Oral Surg., Oral Med. and Oral Path. *29*:437, 1970.

Gorlin, R. J., Pindborg, J. J., Clausen, F. P., and Vickers, R. A.: The calcifying odontogenic cyst—a possible analogue of the cutaneous calcifying epithelioma of Malherbe, Oral Surg., Oral Med. and Oral Path. *15*:1235, 1962.
Hammer, J. E., III, and Ketcham, A. S.: Cherubism: analysis of treatment, Cancer *23*:1133, 1969.
Hayward, J. R.: Dentigerous cysts, Am. J. Orthodont. and Oral Surg. (Oral Surg. Sect.) *32*:140, 1946.
Hill, T. J.: The epithelium in dental granulomata, J. Dent. Res. *10*:323, 1930.
Lovestedt, S. A., and Bruce, K. W.: Cysts of the incisive canal with concrements, J. Oral Surg. *12*:48, 1954.
McCrea, M. W.: Histologic studies of the occurrence of epithelium in dental granulomas, J.A.D.A. *24*:1133, 1937.
Meyer, A. W.: Median anterior maxillary cysts, J.A.D.A. *18*:1851, 1931.
Miller, J. B., and Moore, P. M.: Nasoalveolar cysts, Ann. Otol., Rhin. and Laryng. *58*:200, 1949.
Panders, A. K., and Hadders, H. N.: Solitary kerato cysts of the jaws, J. Oral Surg. *27*:931, 1969.
Priebe, W. A., Lazansky, J. P., and Wuehrmann, A. H.: The value of the roentgenographic film in the differential diagnosis of periapical lesions, Oral Surg., Oral Med. and Oral Path. *7*:979, 1954.
Robinson, H. B. G.: Classification of cysts of the jaws, Am. J. Orthodont. and Oral Surg. (Oral Surg. Sect.) *31*:370, 1945.
Robinson, H. B. G., Koch, W. E., and Kolas, S.: Radiographic interpretation of oral cysts, D. Radiogr. and Photogr. *29*:61, 1956.
Roper-Hall, H. T.: Premaxillary cysts, Brit. Dent. J. *74*:197, 1943.
Rosen, M. D.: Nasoalveolar cyst, Oral Surg., Oral Med. and Oral Path. *14*:148, 1961.
Salman, I.: Cysts of the jaws, J. Oral Surg. *9*:188, 1951.
Schlack, C. A.: Rate of occurrence of epithelial tissue in periapical lesions, U. S. Navy Med. Bull. *42*:158, 1944.
Scott, J. H.: The early development of oral cysts in man, Brit. Dent. J. *98*:109, 1955.
Shafer, W. G.: Benign tumors and cysts of the jawbones, Dent. Clinics of N. Am. p. 75, November, 1957.
Shear, M.: Histogenesis of the dental cyst, Dent. Pract. *13*:238, 1963.
Stafne, E. C., Austin, L. T., and Gardiner, B. S.: Median anterior maxillary cysts, J.A.D.A. *23*:801, 1936.

Stafne, E. C., and Millhon, J. A.: Periodontal cysts, J. Oral Surg. 3:102, 1945.
Standish, S. M., and Shafer, W. G.: Lateral periodontal cyst, J. Periodont. 29:27, 1958.
Thoma, K. H.: Diagnosis and treatment of odontogenic and fissural cysts, Oral Surg., Oral Med. and Oral Path. 3:961, 1950.
——: Facial cleft or fissural cysts, Internat. J. Orthodont. and Oral Surg. 23:83, 1937.
——: Naso-alveolar cyst, Am. J. Orthodont. and Oral Surg. (Oral Surg. Sect.) 27:48, 1941.
Toller, P.: Permeability of cyst walls in vivo: investigations with radioactive tracers, Proc. Roy. Soc. Med. 59:724, 1966.
——: Origin and growth of cysts of the jaws, Ann. Roy. Coll. Surg. England 40:306, 1967.
Wais, F. T.: Significance of findings following biopsy and histologic study of 100 periapical lesions, Oral Surg., Oral Med. and Oral Path. 11:650, 1958.

Gemination, Fusion, Dens Invaginatus and Miscellaneous Anomalies

Bolk, L.: Supernumerary teeth in molar region of man, Dent. Cosmos 56:154, 1914.
British Dental Association: The Report on Odontomes, London, John Bale, Sons & Danielsson, Ltd., 1914.
Clayton, J. M.: Congenital dental anomalies occurring in 3,557 children, J. Dent. Children 23:206, 1956.
Cook, T. J.: Supernumerary teeth, Ann. Dent. 3:140, 1936.
Flint, E. G.: Supernumerary teeth, Am. J. Orthodont. and Oral Surg. 25:135, 1939.
Glenn, F. B., and Stanley, H. R.: Dilaceration of a mandibular permanent incisor, Oral Surg., Oral Med. and Oral Path. 13:1249, 1960.
Goldman, H. M., and Bloom, J.: A collective review and atlas of dental anomalies and diseases, Oral Surg., Oral Med. and Oral Path. 2:874, 1949.
Heslop, I. H.: True gemination in posterior teeth, Brit. Dent. J. 97:93, 1954.
Hitchin, A. D., and McHugh, W. D.: Three coronal invaginations in a dilated composite odontome, Brit. Dent. J. 97:90, 1954.
Hrdlicka, A.: Normal variation of teeth and jaws, and orthodonty, Internat. J. Orthodont. and Dent. Child. 21:1099, 1935.
Hunter, H. A.: Dilated composite odontome, Oral Surg., Oral Med. and Oral Path. 4:668, 1951.
Kitchin, P. C.: Dens in dente, Oral Surg., Oral Med. and Oral Path. 2:1181, 1949.

Kronfeld, R.: Dens in dente, J. Dent. Res. 14:49, 1934.
Lau, T. C.: Odontomes of the axial core type, Brit. Dent. J. 99:219, 1955.
Miles, A. E. W.: Malformations of the teeth, Proc. Roy. Soc. Med. Sect. Odont. 47:817, 1954.
Oehlers, F. A. C.: Dens invaginatus (dilated composite odontome), Oral Surg., Oral Med. and Oral Path. 10:1204, 1957.
Osburn, R. C.: On supernumerary teeth in man and other mammals, Dent. Cosmos 54:1193, 1912.
Pitts, A. T.: Some reflections on the nature of odontomes, Brit. Dent. J. 54:217, 1933.
Rabinowitch, B. Z.: Dens in dente, Oral Surg., Oral Med. and Oral Path. 2:1480, 1949.
Rounds, F. W.: Principles and techniques of exodontia, Oral Surg., Oral Med. and Oral Path. 3:1104, 1950. (Anomalies of teeth.)
Rushton, M. A.: A collection of dilated composite odontomes, Brit. Dent. J. 63:65, 1937.
——: Partial gigantism of face and teeth, Brit. Dent. J. 62:572, 1937.
Searcy, W. M., Jr.: Dens in dente . . . with a report of bilateral anomaly, Dent. Radiog. and Photog. 21:29, 1948.
Shaw, J. C. M.: Composite odontomes, Brit. Dent. J. 53:640, 1932.
Sprawson, E.: Definition of an odontome, Brit. Dent. J. 50:775, 1929.
——: Odontomes, Brit. Dent. J. 62:177, 1937.
Stafne, E. C.: Supernumerary upper central incisors, Dent. Cosmos 73:976, 1931.
——: Supernumerary teeth, Dent. Cosmos 74:653, 1932.
Steinberg, A. G., Warren, J. F., and Warren, L. M.: Hereditary generalized microdontia, J. Dent. Res. 40:58, 1961.
Swanson, W. F., and McCarthy, F. M.: Bilateral dens in dente, J. Dent. Res. 26:167, 1947.
Tratman, E. K.: Odontomes and their relationship to each other, Brit. Dent. J. 66:580, 1939.

Ectodermal Dysplasia

Bowen, R.: Hereditary ectodermal dysplasia of the anhidrotic type, Southern Med. J. 25:481, 1932.
Brekhus, P. J., Oliver, C. P., and Montelius, G.: A study of the pattern and combinations of congenitally missing teeth in man, J. Dent. Res. 23:117, 1944.
Chaudhry, A. P., Johnson, O. N., Mitchell, D. F., Gorlin, R. J., and Barthaldi, W. L.: Hereditary enamel dysplasia, J. Ped. 54:776, 1959.

Everett, F. G., Jump, E. B., Sutherland, W. F., Savara, B. S., and Suher, T.: Anhidrotic ectodermal dysplasia with anodontia. A study of 2 families, J.A.D.A. 44:173, 1952.

Grant, R., and Falls, H. F.: Anodontia. Report of a case associated with ectodermal dysplasia of the anhidrotic type, Am. J. Orthodont. and Oral Surg. (Oral Surg. Sect.) 30:661, 1944.

Redpath, T. H., and Winter, G. B.: Autosomal dominant ectodermal dysplasia with significant dental defects, Brit. Dent. J. 126:123, 1969.

Sacket, L. M., Marans, A. E., and Hursey, R. J.: Congenital ectodermal dysplasia of the anhidrotic type, Oral Surg., Oral Med. and Oral Path. 9:659, 1956.

Thannhauser, S. J.: Hereditary ectodermal dysplasia of the "anhidrotic type," J.A.M.A. 106:908, 1936.

Upshaw, B. Y., and Montgomery, H.: Hereditary anhidrotic ectodermal dysplasia, Arch. Dermat. and Syph. 60:1170, 1949.

Hypercementosis

Gardner, B. S., and Goldstein, H.: The significance of hypercementosis, Dent. Cosmos 73:1065, 1931.

Kupfer, I. J.: Correlation of hypercementosis with toxic goiter, J. Dent. Res. 30:734, 1951.

Weinberger, A.: The clinical significance of hypercementosis, Oral Surg., Oral Med. and Oral Path. 7:79, 1954.

Odontomes

British Dental Association, Report on Odontoma, London, J. Bale Sons and Danielsson, 1914.

Browne, W. G.: Familial compound composite odontomas, Oral Surg., Oral Med., and Oral Path. 29:428, 1970.

Glickman, I., and Wuehrmann, A. H.: Compound composite odontoma, Am. J. Orthodont. and Oral Surg. (Oral Surg. Sect.) 32:173, 1946.

Gullifer, W. H.: Odontoma, Am. J. Orthodont. and Oral Surg. 24:795, 1938.

Manning, G. L., and Browne, R. M.: Dentinoma, Brit. Dent. J. 128:178, 1970.

Miles, A. E. W.: Malformations of the teeth, Proc. Roy. Soc. Med. 47:817, 1954.

Wainwright, W. W.: Complex odontoma, Am. J. Orthodont. and Oral Surg. (Oral Surg. Sect.) 31:447, 1945.

Waldron, C. W., Peterson, R. G., and Worman, H. G.: Compound composite odontome of the mandible, J. Oral Surg. 4:48, 1946.

Wilkinson, F. C.: A complex type of odontome, Brit. Dent. J. 65:99, 1938.

Enamel Dysplasia

Bauer, W. H.: Effect of periapical processes of deciduous teeth on the buds of permanent teeth, Am. J. Orthodont. and Oral Surg. (Oral Surg. Sect.) 32:232, 1947.

Boyle, P. E.: The histopathology of the human tooth-germ in congenital syphilis, J. Dent. Res. 12:425, 1932.

Bradlaw, R. V.: The dental stigmata of prenatal syphilis, Oral Surg., Oral Med. and Oral Path. 6:147, 1953.

Brauer, J. C., and Blackstone, C. H.: Dental aspects of congenital syphilis, J.A.D.A. 28:1633, 1941.

Cole, H. N.: Congenital and prenatal syphilis, J.A.M.A. 109:580, 1937.

Darling, A. I.: Some observations on amelogenesis imperfecta and calcification of dental enamel, Proc. Roy. Soc. Med. 49:759, 1956.

Dean, H. T., and Elvove, E.: Further studies on the minimal threshold of chronic endemic fluorosis, Pub. Health Rep. 52:1249, 1937.

Hoffman, M. M., Schuck, C., and Furuta, W. J.: Histologic study on effects of fluorine administered in dry and moist diets on teeth of young albino rats, J. Dent. Res. 21:157, 1942.

Kerr, D. A.: Histological changes in the enamel organ responsible for enamel hypoplasia, Am. J. Orthodont. and Oral Surg. (Oral Surg. Sect.) 30:673, 1944.

Kreshover, S. J.: The pathogenesis of enamel hypoplasia. An experimental study, J. Dent. Res. 23:231, 1944.

McKay, F. S.: The study of mottled enamel (dental fluorosis), J.A.D.A. 44:133, 1952.

Sarnat, B. G., and Schour, I.: Enamel hypoplasia (chronologic enamel aplasia) in relation to systemic disease. A chronologic, morphologic and etiologic classification, J.A.D.A. 28:1989, 1941; 29:67, 1942.

Sarnat, B. G., and Shaw, N. G.: Dental development in congenital syphilis, Am. J. Orthodont. and Oral Surg. (Oral Surg. Sect.) 29:270, 1943.

Schour, I., and Smith, M. C.: Mottled teeth. An experimental and histologic analysis, J. Am. Dent. A. 22:796, 1935.

Weinmann, J. P., Svoboda, J. F., and Woods, R. W.: Hereditary disturbances of enamel formation and calcification, J.A.D.A. 32:397, 1945.

Faulty Dentin Development

Abrams, A. M., and Groper, J.: Odontodysplasia: report of three cases, J. Dent. Child. 33:353, 1966.

Alley, T. R., and Burket, L. W.: Hereditary opalescent dentin, Oral Surg., Oral Med. and Oral Path. 6:328, 1953.

Bergman, G.: Studies on mineralized dental tissues. XIV. The incremental pattern of the dentine in a case of osteogenesis imperfecta, Oral Surg., Oral Med. and Oral Path. 13:70, 1960.

Bickel, W. H., Ghormley, R. K., Camp, J. H.: Osteogenesis imperfecta, Radiol. 40:145, 1943.

Bixler, D., Conneally, P. M., and Christen, A. G.: Dentinogenesis imperfecta: genetic variations in six-generation family, J. Dent. Res. 48:1196, 1969.

Blattner, R. J., Heys, F., and Robinson, H. B. G.: Osteogenesis imperfecta and odontogenesis imperfecta (hereditary opalescent dentin), J. Dent. Res. 21:325, 1942.

———: Osteogenesis imperfecta and odontogenesis imperfecta, clinical and genetic aspects in eighteen families, J. Pediat. 56:234, 1960.

Hodge, H. C., et al.: Hereditary opalescent dentin. III. Histological, chemical and physical studies, J. Dent. Res. 19:521, 1940.

Hursey, R. J., Witkop, C. J., Miklashek, D., and Sackett, L. M.: Dentinogenesis imperfecta in a racial isolate with multiple hereditary defects, Oral Surg., Oral Med. and Oral Path. 9:641, 1956.

Johnson, O. N., Chaudhry, A. P., Gorlin, R. J., Mitchell, D. F., and Bartholdi, W. L.: Hereditary dentinogenesis imperfecta, J. Pediat. 54:786, 1959.

Roberts, E., and Schour, I.: Hereditary opalescent dentine (dentinogenesis imperfecta), Am. J. Orthodont. and Oral Surg. 25:267, 1939.

Rushton, M. A.: A new form of dentinal dysplasia: shell teeth, Oral Surg., Oral Med. and Oral Path. 7:543, 1954.

———: Anomalies of human dentine, Brit. Dent. J. 98:431, 1955.

Skillen, W. G.: Histologic and clinical study of hereditary opalescent dentin, J.A.D.A. 24:1426, 1937.

Wilson, G. W., and Steinbrecker, M.: Hereditary hypoplasia of the dentin, J.A.D.A. 26:866, 1929.

Witkop, C. J.: Genetics and Dental Health, New York, McGraw-Hill, 1962.

Cleidocranial Dysostosis

Archer, W. H., and Henderson, S. G.: Cleidocranial dysostosis. Report of two cases, Oral Surg., Oral Med. and Oral Path. 4:1201, 1951.

Eisen, D.: Cleidocranial dysostosis with a report of four cases, Radiol. 61:21, 1953.

Kelln, E. E., Chaudhry, A. P., and Gorlin, R. J.: Oral manifestations of Crouzon's disease, Oral Surg., Oral Med. and Oral Path. 13:1245, 1960.

Millhon, J. A., and Austin, L. T.: Dental findings in four cases of cleidocranial dysostosis, Am. J. Orthodont. and Oral Surg. (Oral Surg. Sect.) 30:30, 1944.

Rankow, R. M.: Cleidocranial dysostosis. Report of two cases, J. Oral Surg. 1:352, 1943.

Winter, G. R.: Dental conditions in cleidocranial dysostosis, Am. J. Orthodont. and Oral Surg. (Orthodont. Sect.) 29:61, 1943.

3. DISEASES OF THE TEETH AND SUPPORTING STRUCTURES

Abrasion, Attrition and Erosion

Cogswell, W. F.: Bobby-pin destruction of the incisal edges of upper anterior teeth, Dent. Digest 53:386, 1947.

Davies, T. G. H., and Pedersen, P. O.: The degree of attrition of the deciduous teeth and first permanent molars of primitive and urbanised Greenland natives, Brit. Dent. J. 99:35, 1955.

Elsbury, W. B.: Hydrogen-ion concentration and acid erosion of teeth, Brit. Dent. J. 93:177, 1952.

Epstein, S., and Tainter, M. L.: Abrasion of teeth by commercial dentifrices, J.A.D.A. 30:1036, 1943.

Everett, F. G., and Kunkel, P. W.: Abrasion through the abuse of dental floss, J. Periodont. 24:186, 1953.

Gerry, R. G., Smith, S. T., and Calton, M. L.: The oral characteristics of Guamanians including the effects of betel chewing on the oral tissues. Part I, Oral Surg., Oral Med. and Oral Path. 5:762, 1952.

Guernsey, L. H.: Gastric juice as a chemical erosive agent, Oral Surg., Oral Med. and Oral Path. 6:1233, 1953.

Kitchin, P. C., and Robinson, H. B. G.: The abrasiveness of dentifrices as measured on the cervical areas of extracted teeth, J. Dent. Res. 27:195, 1948.

Lovestedt, S. A.: Dental erosions, North-West Dent. 30:43, 1951.

Robinson, H. B. G.: A clinic on the differential diagnosis of oral lesions, Am. J. Orthodont. and Oral Surg. (Oral Surg. Sect.) 32:729, 1946. (Abrasion, erosion and attrition, p. 738.)

Schour, I., and Sarnat, B. G.: Oral manifestations of occupational origin, J.A.M.A. 120:1197, 1942.

Zander, H. A.: Decalcification of teeth in cases of achlorhydria, Am. J. Orthodont. and Oral Surg. (Oral Surg. Sect.) 32:184, 1946.

Zipkin, I., and McClure, F. J.: Salivary citrate and dental erosion, J. Dent. Res. 28:613, 1949.

Stains

Ayers, P.: Green stain, J.A.D.A. 26:2, 1939.

Boyle, P. E., and Dinnerman, M.: Natural vital staining of the teeth of infants and children, Am. J. Orthodont. and Oral Surg. (Oral Surg. Sect.) 27:377, 1941.

Isaac, S., and Brudevald, F.: Discoloration of teeth by metallic ions, J. Dent. Res. 36:753, 1957.

Kitchin, P. C., and Robinson, H. B. G.: How abrasive need a dentifrice be, J. Dent. Res. 27:501, 1948.

Leung, S. W.: Naturally occurring stains on the teeth of children, J.A.D.A. 41:191, 1950.

Manley, R. S.: A structureless recurrent deposit on teeth, J. Dent. Res. 22:479, 1943.

Scofield, H. H.: Effect of tetracyclines on dentition, Med. Ann. Dist. Col. 34:56, February 1965.

Shay, D. E., Haddox, J. H., and Richmond, J. L.: An inorganic qualitative and quantitative analysis of green stain, J.A.D.A. 50:156, 1955.

Stewart, D. J.: Teeth discolored by tetracycline bleaching following exposure to daylight, Dent. Pract. 20:309, 1970.

Tank, G.: Two cases of green pigmentation of the deciduous teeth associated with hemolytic disease of the newborn, J.A.D.A. 42:302, 1951.

Vallotton, C. F.: An acquired pigmented pellicle of the enamel surface, J. Dent. Res. 24:161, 1945.

Root Fractures

Claus, E. C., and Orban, B.: Fractured vital teeth, Oral Surg., Oral Med. and Oral Path. 6:605, 1953.

Kronfeld, R.: A case of tooth fracture with special emphasis on tissue repair and adaptation following traumatic injury, J. Dent. Res. 15:429, 1936.

Losee, F. L.: Untreated root fractures. Report of 3 cases, Oral Surg., Oral Med. and Oral Path. 1:464, 1948.

Resorption, Internal and Apical

Aub, J. C., Evans, R. D., Hempelmann, L. H., and Martland, H. S.: The late effects of internally-deposited radioactive materials in man, Medicine, 31:221, 1952.

Becks, H.: Root resorptions and their relation to pathologic bone formation, Internat. J. Orthodont. and Oral Surg. 22:445, 1936.

Browne, W. G.: Idiopathic tooth resorption in association with metaplasia, Oral Surg., Oral Med. and Oral Path. 7:1298, 1954.

Goldman, H. M.: Spontaneous intermittent resorption of teeth, J.A.D.A. 49:522, 1954.

Hayes, R. L.: Idiopathic internal resorption of teeth, Oral Surg., Oral Med. and Oral Path. 13:723, 1960.

Kerr, D. A., Courtney, R. M., and Burkes, E. J.: Multiple idiopathic root resorption, Oral Surg., Oral Med. and Oral Path. 29:552, 1970.

Lepp, F. H., and Berning, H. P.: Roentgenologic differential diagnosis of progressive internal resorption of residual teeth. Fortschr. Röntgenstr. 85:159, 1956, and Year Book of Dentistry, p. 31, 1957-58.

Massler, M., and Malone, A. J.: Root resorption in human permanent teeth, Am. J. Orthodont. 40:619, 1954.

Rudolph, C. E.: A comparative study in root resorption in permanent teeth, J.A.D.A. 23:822, 1936.

Stafne, E. C., and Slocumb, C. H.: Idiopathic resorption of teeth, Am. J. Orthodont. and Oral Surg. (Oral Surg. Sect.) 30:41, 1944.

Zemsky, J. L.: Root resorption and its clinical significance, J.A.D.A. 16:520, 1929.

Cementoma

Bernier, J. L., and Thompson, H. C.: The histogenesis of the cementoma, Am. J. Orthodont. and Oral Surg. (Oral Surg. Sect.) 32:543, 1946.

Catania, A. F.: Localized osteitis fibrosa and cementoma, J. Oral Surg. 11:202, 1953.

Scannell, J. M.: Cementoma, Oral Surg., Oral Med. and Oral Path. 2:1169, 1949.

Stafne, E. C.: Periapical fibroma, J.A.D.A. 30:688, 1943.

Zegarelli, E. V., and Ziskin, D. E.: Cementomas. A report of 50 cases, Am. J. Orthodont. and Oral Surg. (Oral Surg. Sect.) 29:285, 1943.

Radiation Effect, Teeth

Bruce, K. W., and Stafne, E. C.: The effect of irradiation on the dental system as demonstrated by the roentgenogram, J.A.D.A. 41:684, 1950.

del Regato, J. A.: Dental lesions observed after roentgen therapy in cancer of the buccal cavity, pharynx and larynx, Am. J. Roentgen 42:404, 1939.

Frank, R. M., Herdly, J., and Philippe, E.: Acquired dental defects and salivary gland lesions after irradiation for carcinoma, J.A.D.A. 70:868, 1965.

Stafne, E. C., and Bowing, H. H.: The teeth and their supporting structures in patients treated by irradiation, Am. J. Orthodont. and Oral Surg. (Oral Surg. Sect.) 33:567, 1947.

Dental Caries

Arnold, F. A.: The use of fluorides in the practice of dental medicine, Oral Surg., Oral Med. and Oral Path. 3:622, 1950.

Ast, D. B., Bushel, A., Wachs, B., and Chase, H. C.: Newburgh-Kingston caries-fluorine study. VIII. Combined clinical and roentgenographic dental findings after eight years of fluoride experience, J.A.D.A. 50:680, 1955.

Becks, H., Jensen, A. L., and Millarr, C. B.: Rampant dental caries. Prevention and prognosis, J.A.D.A. 31:1189, 1944.

Brudevald, F., Hein, J. W., Bonner, J. F., Nevin, R. B., Bibby, B. G., and Hodge, H. C.: Reaction of tooth surfaces with one ppm of fluoride as sodium fluoride, J. Dent. Res. 36:771, 1957.

Bunting, R. W., and Palmerlee, F.: The role of bacillus acidophilus in dental caries, J.A.D.A. 12:381, 1925.

Burnett, G. W., and Scherp, H. W.: Accessibility of organic dentinal matrix, J. Dent. Res. 31:776, 1952.

Darling, A. I.: Studies of early lesions of enamel caries: its nature, mode of spread and points of entry, Brit. Dent. J. 105:119, 1958.

Dean, H. T.: Fluorine in the control of dental caries, J.A.D.A. 52:1, 1956.

Dean, H. T., Jay, P., Arnold, F. A., and Elvove, E.: Domestic waters and dental caries. II. Pub. Health Rep. 56:761, 1941.

Fosdick, L. S.: Enzyme inhibitors as a factor in the control of dental caries, J.A.D.A. 52:9, 1956.

Gottlieb, B., Diamond, M., and Applebaum, E.: The caries problem, Am. J. Orthodont. and Oral Surg. (Oral Surg. Sect.) 32:365, 1946.

Hadley, F. P.: A quantitative method for estimating bacillus acidophilus in saliva, J. Dent. Res. 13:415, 1933.

Jay, P.: Dental caries, in Bunting's Oral Hygiene, ed. 3, Philadelphia, Lea & Febiger, 1957.

Jay, P., and Bennett, A. S.: Role of diet in the control of dental caries, J.A.D.A. 52:18, 1956.

Kesel, R. G.: An evaluation of recent developments in caries control, Oral Surg., Oral Med. and Oral Path. 4:439, 1951.

McClure, F. J., and Muller, A., Jr.: Further observations on the cariostatic effect of phosphates, J. Dent. Res. 38:776, 1959.

Miller, W. A.: Spread of carious lesions in dentin, J.A.D.A. 78:1327, 1969.

Mitchell, D. F.: The mechanism of dental caries, J.A.D.A. 52:14, 1956.

National Research Council: A Survey of the Literature of Dental Caries, Committee on Dental Health, Publication 225, Washington, D. C., 1952.

Newbrun, E.: Sucrose: arch criminal of dental caries, J. Dent. Child. 36:239, 1969.

Orland, F. J., Blayney, J. R., Harrison, R. W., Reyniers, J. A., Trexler, P. C., Wagner, M., Gordon, H. A., and Luckey, T. D.: Use of the germfree animal technic in the study of experimental dental caries. I. Basic observations on rats reared free of all microorganisms, J. Dent. Res. 33:147, 1954.

Pigman, W.: In vitro production of experimental caries, J.A.D.A. 51:685, 1955.

Proceedings: University of Michigan workshop for evaluation of dental caries control technics, J. Dent. Res. 27:70, 1948.

Ripa, L. W.: Histology of early carious lesion in primary teeth with special reference to "prismless" outer layer of primary enamel, J. Dent. Res. 45:5, 1966.

Robinson, H. B. G.: Bacteriology of dental caries, Oral Surg., Oral Med. and Oral Path. 5:1223, 1952.

Rogosa, M., Mitchell, J. A., and Wiseman, R. F.: A selective medium for the isolation and enumeration of oral lactobacilli, J. Dent. Res. 30:682, 1951.

Soni, N. N., Silberkweit, M., and Parrish, B. A.: Microradiographic-microphotometric and polarized light study of demineralization pattern in carious lesions, Oral Surg., Oral. Med. and Oral Path. 20:321, 1965.

Weisenstein, P. R., and Green, G. E.: Clinical and bacteriologic studies of caries-immune human beings, J. Dent. Res. 36:690, 1957.

Pulp and Sequelae of Pulp Disease

Anderson, A. W., Sharav, Y., and Massler, M.: Reparative dentine formation and pulp morphology., Oral Surg., Oral Med. and Oral Path. 26:837, 1968.

Bostick, W. L.: The vascular-cellular dynamics of inflammation, Oral Surg., Oral Med. and Oral Path. 2:425, 1949.

Boulger, E. P.: Histologic study of a hypertrophied pulp, J. Dent. Res. 11:257, 1931.

Bourgoyne, J. R., and Quinn, J. H.: The periapical abscess, J. Oral Surg. 7:320, 1949.

Boyle, P. E.: Intracellular bacteria in a dental granuloma, J. Dent. Res. 14:297, 1934.

Childs, H. G., and Courville, C. B.: Thrombosis of cavernous sinus secondary to dental infection, Am. J. Orthodont. and Oral Surg. (Oral Surg. Sect.) 28:367, 402, 458, and 515, 1942.

Clarke, N. G.: The morphology of the reparative dentine bridge, Oral Surg., Oral Med. and Oral Path. 29:746, 1970.

Eisenbud, L., and Busch, S. A.: A massive acute alveolar abscess, Oral Surg., Oral Med. and Oral Path. 7:1021, 1954.

Eisenbud, L., and Klatell, J.: Acute alveolar abscess. A review of 300 hospitalized cases, Oral Surg., Oral Med. and Oral Path. 4:208, 1951.

Frey, H.: A contribution to the histopathology of pulp "polypi," especially of temporary teeth, Brit. Dent. J. 85:225, 1948.

Fullmer, H. M.: Observations on the development of oxytalan fibers in dental granulomas and radicular cysts, Arch. Path. 70:59, 1960.

Glass, R. L., and Zander, H. A.: Pulp healing, J. Dent. Res. 28:97, 1949.

Gurley, W. B., and Van Huysen, G.: Histologic response of the teeth of dogs to operative procedures, J. Dent. Res. 19:179, 1940.

Haymaker, W.: Fatal infections of central nervous system and meninges after tooth extractions, Am. J. Orthodont. and Oral Surg. (Oral Surg. Sect.) 31:117, 1945.

Hedman, W. J.: An investigation into residual periapical infection after pulp canal therapy, Oral Surg., Oral Med. and Oral Path. 4:1173, 1951.

Hill, T. J.: Pathology of the dental pulp, J.A.D.A. 21:820, 1934.

Kramer, I. R. H.: Pulp changes of non-bacterial origin, Int. Dent. J. 9:435, 1959.

Langeland, K.: Effects of various procedures on the human dental pulp, Oral Surg., Oral Med. and Oral Path. 14:210, 1961.

Lefkowitz, W., Robinson, H. B. G., and Postle, H. H.: Pulp response to cavity preparation, J. Prosh. Dent. 8:315, 1958.

Manly, E. B.: Experimental investigation into the early effects of various pulp filling materials on the human pulp, Proc. Roy. Soc. Med. 34:157, 1941.

Mills, J. S.: The evocation and production of protective secondary dentine, Australian J. Dent. 57:241, 1953.

Patterson, S. S., and Mitchell, D. F.: Calcific metamorphosis of dental pulp, Oral Surg., Oral Med. and Oral Path. 20:94, 1965.

Patterson, S. S., and Van Huysen, G.: The treatment of pulp exposures, Oral Surg., Oral Med. and Oral Path. 7:194, 1954.

Robinson, H. B. G.: Pathology of periapical infections, Oral Surg., Oral Med. and Oral Path. 4:1044, 1951.

Robinson, H. B. G., and Boling, L. R.: Anachoretic effect in pulpitis, J.A.D.A. 28:268, 1941.

Russel, A., and Fearing, S. J.: Cavernous sinus thrombosis in a diabetic, Oral Surg., Oral Med. and Oral Path. 8:372, 1955.

Second International Conference on Endodontics, Oral Surg., Oral Med. and Oral Path. 13:990, 1960.

Sicher, H.: The propagation of dental infection, in Sicher's Oral Anatomy, ed. 4, St. Louis, Mosby, 1965.

Spilka, C. J.: Pathways of dental infection, J. Oral Surg. 24:111, 1966.

Stanley, H., Zander, H., Robinson, H. B. G., and Bernier, J. L.: Pulp reaction to operative procedures, Oral Surg., Oral Med. and Oral Path. 13:329, 1960.

Stanley, H., and Swerdlow, H.: Biologic effects of various cutting methods on cavity preparation: the part pressure plays in pulpal response, J.A.D.A. 61:450, 1960.

Stuteville, O. H.: Spread of infections in head and neck, J. Internat. Coll. Surgeons 29:750, 1958.

Zander, H. A., and Glass, R. L.: The healing of phenolized pulp exposures, Oral Surg., Oral Med. and Oral Path. 2:803, 1949.

Zander, H. A., Glenn, J. F., and Nelson, C. A.: Pulp protection in restorative dentistry, J.A.D.A. 41:563, 1950.

Periodontal Disease

Adkins, K. F., Martinez, M. G., and Hartley, M. W.: Ultrastructure of giant cell lesions, Oral Surg., Oral Med. and Oral Path. 28:713, 1969.

Aisenberg, M. S.: Histology and physiology of supporting structures, J.A.D.A. 44:628, 1952.

Akiyoshi, M., and Mori, K.: Marginal periodontitis: histologic study of incipient stage, J. Periodont. 38:45, 1967.

American Dental Association Research Commission: Vincent's infection, J.A.D.A. 32:756, 1945.

Bernier, J. L., and Cahn, L. R.: The peripheral giant cell reparative granuloma, J.A.D.A. 49:141, 1954.

Bhaskar, S. N., and Orban, B.: Experimental occlusal trauma, J. Periodont. 26:270, 1955.

Bossert, W. A., and Marks, H. H.: Prevalence and characteristics of periodontal disease in 12,800 persons under periodic dental observation, J.A.D.A. 52:429, 1956.

Burket, L. W.: Systemic aspects of periodontal disease, J. Periodont. 24:7, 1953.

Cohen, B.: Morphologic factors in pathogenesis of periodontal disease, Brit. Dent. J. 107:31, 1959.

Cohen, M. M., Winer, R. A., Schwartz, S., and Shklar, G.: Oral aspects of mongolism. Part I. Periodontal disease in mongolism, Oral Surg., Oral Med. and Oral Path. 14:92, 1961.

Cooke, B. E. D.: The fibrous epulis and the fibro-epithelial polyp: their histogenesis and natural history, Brit. Dent. J. 93:305, 1952.

Cutwright, D. E.: Proliferation of blood vessels in gingival wounds, J. Periodont. 40:137, 1969.

Dummett, C. O.: Oral tissue reactions from Dilantin medication in control of epileptic seizures, J. Periodont. 25:112, 1954.

Emerson, T. G.: Hereditary gingival hyperplasia: family pedigree of four generations, Oral Surg., Oral Med. and Oral Path. 19:1, 1965.

Engel, M. B.: Hormonal gingivitis, J.A.D.A. 44:691, 1952.

Foss, C. L., Grupe, H. E., and Orban, B.: Gingivosis, J. Periodont. 24:207, 1953.

Francis, L. E., and Melville, K. I.: Effects of diphenylhydantoin (dilantin) on histamine changes in gingival tissue, J. Canad. D. A. 24:142, 1958.

Gans, B. J., Engel, M. B., and Joseph, N. R.: Electrometric studies of human gingiva in pregnancy, J. Dent. Res. 35:566, 1956.

Glavind, L., Lund, B., and Loë, H.: Relationship between periodontal state and diabetic duration, insulin dosage and retinal change. J. Periodont. 39:341, 1968.

Glickman, I.: A basic classification of "gingival enlargement," J. Periodont. 21:131, 1950.

———: Bifurcation involvement in periodontal disease, J.A.D.A. 40:528, 1950.

———: Periodontosis. Critical evaluation, J.A.D.A. 44:706, 1952.

Glickman, I., and Smulow, J. B.: Chronic desquamative gingivitis: its nature and treatment, J. Periodont. 35:397, 1964.

Gridly, M.: Gingival condition in pregnant women. A report based on the examination of the gingivae of 1,002 pregnant women, Oral Surg., Oral Med. and Oral Path. 7:641, 1954.

Hampp, E. G.: Vincent's infection—a wartime disease. Observations on the oral spirochetal flora present in Vincent's infection, Am. J. Pub. Health 35:441, 1945.

Hilming, F.: Gingivitis gravidarum, Oral Surg., Oral Med. and Oral Path. 5:734, 1952.

Hine, M. K.: Fibrous hyperplasia of gingiva, J.A.D.A. 44:681, 1952.

Holmes, C. H.: Morphology of the interdental papilla, J. Periodont. 36:455, 1965.

Kerr, D. A.: Granuloma pyogenicum, Oral Surg., Oral Med. and Oral Path. 4:158, 1951. (Includes pregnancy tumor.)

———: Herpetic gingivostomatitis, J.A.D.A. 44:674, 1952.

Lieb, A. M., Berdon, J. K., and Sabes, W. R.: Furcation involvements correlated with enamel projections from the cementoenamel junction, J. Periodont. 38:330, 1967.

Listgarten, M. A.: Electron microscopic observations on bacterial flora of acute necrotizing gingivitis, J. Periodont. 36:328, 1965.

Lundquist, G. R.: Gingivitis, J.A.D.A. 44:663, 1952.

McCarthy, F. P., McCarthy, P. L., and Shklar G.: Chronic desquamative gingivitis: a reconsideration, Oral Surg., Oral Med. and Oral Path. 13:1300, 1960.

Maier, A. W., and Orban, B.: Gingivitis in pregnancy, Oral Surg., Oral Med. and Oral Path. 2:334, 1949.

Mammel, C. K.: Peripheral and central giant cell tumors of the head region, J. Oral Surg. 8:38, 1950.

Orban, B.: Gingivitis, J. Periodont. 26:173, 1955.

———: Histology and physiology of the gingiva, J.A.D.A. 44:624, 1952.

Orban, B., and Weinmann, J. P.: Diffuse atrophy of the alveolar bone (periodontosis), J. Periodont, 13:31, 1942.

Person, P.: Metabolic studies of human alveolar bone disease, Oral Surg., Oral Med. and Oral Path. 12:610, 1959.

Phillips, R. L., and Shafer, W. G.: An evaluation of the peripheral giant cell tumor, J. Periodont. 26:216, 1955.

Pritchard, J. F.: Etiology, diagnosis and treatment of intrabony defect, J. Periodont. 38:455, 1967.

Ramfjord, S.: Experimental periodontal reattachment in rhesus monkeys, J. Periodont. 22:67, 1951.

———: The histopathology of inflammatory gingival enlargement, Oral Surg., Oral Med. and Oral Path. 6:516, 1953.

———: Local factors in periodontal disease, J.A.D.A. 44:647, 1952.

———: A rational plan for periodontal therapy, J. Periodont. 24:88, 1953.
Reader, Z. A.: Gingival hyperplasia resulting from diphenylhydantoin sodium. A review of the literature, J. Oral Surg. 8:25, 1950.
Reports of evaluating committees of 1951 periodontal workshop, J.A.D.A. 45:2, 16, 21, 26 and 33, 1952.
Ritchey, B., and Orban, B.: The periodontal pocket, J. Periodont. 23:199, 1952.
Robinson, H. B. G.: Pathology of periodontal disease, J.A.D.A. 44:636, 1952.
Russell, B. G.: Gingival changes in diabetes mellitus, Acta Path. Microbiol. Scandinav. 68:161, 1966.
Schaffer, E. M.: Biopsy studies of necrotizing ulcerative gingivitis, J. Periodont. 24:22, 1953.
Scott, T. F. M., Steigman, A. J., and Convey, J. H.: Acute infectious gingivostomatitis, J.A.M.A. 117:999, 1941.
Sorrin, S.: Chronic desquamative gingivitis, J.A.D.A. 27:250, 1940.
Stanley, H. R.: The cyclic phenomenon of periodontitis, Oral Surg., Oral Med. and Oral Path. 8:598, 1955.
Stern, L., Eisenbud, L., and Klatell, J.: Analysis of oral reactions to Dilantin-Sodium, J. Dent. Res. 22:157, 1943.
Uohara, G. I.: Histogenesis of the gingival sulcus epithelium in rat, J. Periodont. 30:326, 1959.
Waerhaug, J.: New concept of "epithelial attachment" and gingival crevice in health and disease, Australian Dent. J. 4:164, 1959.
———: Pathogenesis of pocket formation in traumatic occlusion, J. Periodont. 26:107, 1955.
Weinmann, J. P.: Periodontitis—etiology, pathology and symptomatology, J.A.D.A. 44:701, 1952.
Wentz, F. M., Anday, G., and Orban, B.: Histopathologic changes in the gingiva in leukemia, J. Periodont. 20:119, 1949.
Wentz, F. M., Maier, A. W., and Orban, B.: Age changes and sex differences in the clinically "normal" gingiva, J. Periodont. 23:13, 1952.
Whitten, J. B.: Fine structure of desquamative gingivitis, J. Periodont. 39:75, 1968.
Ziskin, D. E., and Nesse, G. J.: Pregnancy gingivitis. History, classification, etiology, Am. J. Orthodont. and Oral Surg. (Oral Surg. Sect.) 32:390, 1946.

4. DISEASES OF THE ORAL MUCOSA AND JAWS
Traumatic (Amputation) Neuroma

Cahn, L. R.: Traumatic (amputation) neuroma, Am. J. Orthodont. and Oral Surg. 25:190, 1939.

Huber, C. G., and Lewis, D.: Amputation neuromas, their development and prevention, Arch. Surg. 1:85, 1920.
Shafer, W. G., and Moorman, W. C.: Traumatic (amputation) neuroma, J. Oral Surg. 15:253, 1957.
Swanson, H. H.: Traumatic neuromas, Oral Surg., Oral Med. and Oral Path. 14:317, 1961.

Hyperplasia from Denture Irritation

Bhaskar, S. N., Beasley, J. D., and Cutwright, D. E.: Inflammatory hyperplasia of the oral mucosa: report of 341 cases, J.A.D.A. 81:949, 1970.
Fisher, A. K., and Rashid, P. J.: Inflammatory papillary hyperplasia of the palatal mucosa, Oral Surg., Oral Med. and Oral Path. 5:191, 1952.
Lambson, G. O.: Papillary hyperplasia of the palate, J. Prosth. Dent. 16:636, 1966.
Lambson, G. O., and Anderson, R. R.: Palatal papillary hyperplasia, J. Prosth. Dent. 18:528, 1967.
Robinson, H. B. G.: Neoplasms and "precancerous" lesions of the oral regions, Dent. Clinics of N. Am., p. 621, November 1957.
Sutton, R. L., Jr.: A fissured granulomatous lesion of the upper labial-alveolar fold, Arch. Dermat. and Syph. 26:425, 1932.
Sutton, R. L.: Granuloma fissuratum, Arch. Dermat. and Syph. 26:865, 1932.

Traumatic Bone Lesion

Bhaskar, S. H., Bernier, J. L., and Godby, F.: Aneurysmal bone cyst and other giant cell lesions of the jaws: report of 104 cases, J. Oral Surg. 17:30, 1959.
Gruskin, S. E., and Dahlin, D. C.: Aneurysmal bone cysts of the Jaws, J. Oral Surg. 26:523, 1968.
Jaffe, H. L.: Giant-cell reparative granuloma, traumatic bone cyst, and fibrous (fibro-osseous) dysplasia of the jaw bones, Oral Surg., Oral Med. and Oral Path. 6:159, 1953.
Olech, E., Sicher, H., and Weinmann, J. P.: Traumatic mandibular bone cysts, Oral Surg., Oral Med. and Oral Path. 4:1160, 1951.
Poyton, H. G., and Morgan, G. A.: Simple bone cyst, Oral Surg., Oral Med. and Oral Path. 20:188, 1965.
Symposium: Solitary bone cysts of the mandible, Oral Surg., Oral Med. and Oral Path. 8:903, 1955.

Thermal, Chemical and Electrical Burns

Chiru-Mocanu, M., Teodorescu, T., Ciubotaru, S., Butureanu, E., and Mialache, C.: Clinical manifestations of buccal galvanism, Rev. Stomat. 70:501, 1970.

Coven, E. M.: Burns of the oral mucosa—and their treatment, Penn. Dent. J. 46:14, 1943.

Kanner, O.: Metals and galvanic currents in the mouth, J. Dent. Res. 17:305, 1938.

Laudenbach, P., and Recoing, J.: Buccal galvanism: is it pathogenic? Rev. Stomat. 70:34, 1969.

Moritz, A. R.: Study of thermal injury. III. The pathology and pathogenesis of cutaneous burns. An experimental study, Am. J. Path. 23:915, 1947.

Reed, G. J., and Willman, W.: Galvanism in the oral cavity, J.A.D.A. 27:1471, 1940.

Reinhard, M. C., Solomon, H. A., and Goltz, H. L.: Further experiments in galvanism, J.A.D.A. 26:1846, 1939.

Schriever, W., and Diamond, L. E.: Electromotive forces and electric currents caused by metallic dental fillings, J. Dent. Res. 31:205, 1952.

Schultz, L. W., and Vazirani, S. J.: Burns of the oral cavity, Oral Surg., Oral Med. and Oral Path. 14:143, 1961.

Stumboff, A. V.: Chemical burns of the oral cavity and esophagus, Arch. Otolaryng. 52:419, 1950.

Sugarman, M. M.: Chromic acid burn, J. Periodont. 23:178, 1952.

Nicotinic Stomatitis

Cahn, L. R.: A note on the histopathology of leucoplakia of the palate, Am. J. Orthodont. and Oral Surg. (Oral Surg. Sect.) 27:35, 1941.

Chapman, I., and Redish, C. H.: Tobacco-induced epithelial proliferation in human subjects, Arch. Path. 70:133, 1960.

Cummer, C. L.: Leukoplakia (leukokeratosis) of the palate, papular form, J.A.M.A. 132:493, 1946.

Saunders, W. H.: Nicotine stomatitis of palate, Ann. Otol., Rhin. and Laryng. 67:638, 1958.

Thoma, K. H.: Stomatitis nicotina and its effect on the palate, Am. J. Orthodont. and Oral Surg. (Oral Surg. Sect.) 27:38, 1941.

Pigmentation

Bartels, H. A.: Observations on the bismuth line and hydrogen sulfide production by mouth organisms, Am. J. Orthodont. and Oral Surg. (Oral Surg. Sect.), 27:565, 1941.

Bell, C. D., Cooksey, D. E., and Nickel, W. R.: Amalgam tattoo (localized argyria), Arch. Dermat. and Syph. 66:523, 1952.

Dean, M. R.: Oral manifestations of bismuth therapy in the treatment of syphilis, J.A.D.A. 30:651, 1943.

Dormandy, T. L.: Gastrointestinal polyposis with mucocutaneous pigmentation (Peutz-Jeghers syndrome), New Eng. J. Med. 256:1093, 1186, 1957.

Dummett, C. O.: Oral tissues in vitiligo, Oral Surg., Oral Med. and Oral Path. 12:1073, 1959.

Dummett, C. O., and Barens, G.: Pigmentation of oral tissues: review of the literature, J. Periodont. 38:369, 1967.

Goldberg, H., and Goldhaber, P.: Hereditary intestinal polyposis with oral pigmentation (Jeghers' syndrome), Oral Surg., Oral Med. and Oral Path. 7:378, 1954.

Hall, T. C., McCracken, B. H., and Thorn, G. W.: Skin pigmentation in relation to adrenal cortical function, J. Clin. Endocrinol. 13:243, 1953.

Hill, W. R., and Montgomery, H.: Argyria, Arch. Dermat. and Syph. 44:588, 1941.

Jeghers, H.: Pigmentation of the skin, New Eng. J. Med. 231:88, 122, 181, 1944.

Jeghers, H., McKusick, V. A., and Katz, K. H.: Generalized intestinal polyposis and melanin spots of the oral mucosa, lips and digits. A syndrome of diagnostic significance, New Eng. J. Med. 241:993, 1031, 1949.

Kenny, J. A., and Curtis, A. C.: The physiology of pigmentation, Oral Surg., Oral Med. and Oral Path. 7:241, 1954.

Laidlaw, G. F., and Cahn, L. R.: Melanoblasts in the gum, J. Dent. Res. 12:534, 1932.

Monash, S.: Normal pigmentation of the oral mucosa, Arch. Dermat. and Syph. 26:139, 1932.

Moskow, B. S., and Tenen, C.: Familial intestinal polyposis with melanosis oris: the syndrome of Peutz and Jeghers, Oral Surg., Oral Med. and Oral Path. 13:924, 1960.

Prinz, H.: Pigmentation of the oral mucous membrane, Dent. Cosmos 74:554, 1932.

Wachstein, M., and Zak, F. G.: Bismuth pigmentation. Its histochemical identification, Am. J. Path. 22:603, 1946.

Zegarelli, E. V., Kesten, B. M., and Kutscher, A. H.: Melanin spots of the oral mucosa and skin associated with polyps, Oral Surg., Oral Med. and Oral Path. 7:972, 1954.

Radiation Effect, Soft Tissue and Bone

Bernier, J. L.: The effect of atomic radiation on the oral and pharyngeal mucosa, J.A.D.A. 36:647, 1949.

Brown, J. B., McDowell, F., and Fryer, M. P.: Surgical treatment of radiation burns, Oral Surg., Oral Med. and Oral Path. 4:1549, 1951.

Cohen, B., and Stanford, R. W.: Reviews of progress of radiation in dentistry, Brit. Dent. J. 107:81, 127, 155, 192, 236, 280, 327 and 374, 1959.

Conn, J. H., Fain, W. R., Farrell, G. W., and Sloan, R. D.: Prevention of radio-osteomyelitis in mandible and maxilla, Surg. Gynec. Obstet. 123:114, 1966.

Cook, T. J.: Late radiation necrosis of the jaw bones, J. Oral Surg. 10:118, 1952.

Cutler, M.: The problem of extractions in relation to osteoradionecrosis complicating radiotherapy for intraoral cancer, Oral Surg., Oral Med. and Oral Path. 4:1077, 1951.

Goldsmith, N. R.: Dangers of cumulative exposure to roentgen rays, J.A.D.A. 34:290, 1947.

Kashima, H. K., Kirkham, W. R., and Andrews, J. R.: Postirradiation sialadenitis; a study of clinical features, histopathologic changes and serum enzyme variations following irradiation of human salivary glands, Am. J. Roentgen. 94:271, 1965.

Low-Beer, B. V. A.: Radiation therapy and dental medicine, Oral Surg., Oral Med. and Oral Path. 4:739, 1951.

Medak, H., and Burnett, G. W.: The effect of X-ray irradiation on the oral tissues of the macacus rhesus monkey, Oral Surg., Oral Med. and Oral Path. 7:778, 1954.

Meyer, I.: Osteoradionecrosis of Jaws, Chicago, Year Book Pub., 1958.

Mohs, F. E.: Roentgen ray cancer of the hands of dentists, J.A.D.A. 45:160, 1952.

Niebel, H. H., Neenan, E. W., Walsh, R. P., and Weimer, J. B.: Removal of teeth from irradiated tissue, J. Oral Surg. 15:313, 1957.

Van den Brenk, H. A. S., Hurley, R. A., Gomez, C., and Richter, W.: Serum amylase as a measure of salivary gland radiation damage, Brit. J. Radiol. 42:688, 1969.

Wildermuth, O., and Cantril, S. T.: Radiation necrosis of the mandible, Radiol. 61:771, 1953.

Yale, S.: Studies in dental radiology, J.A.D.A. 58:36, May 1959.

Young, H. H., and Kunkel, M. G.: Diagnosis, treatment and prognosis of roentgen ray injuries to dentists, J.A.D.A. 51:1, 1955.

Drug Idiosyncrasy

Bartels, H. A.: Black hairy tongue, Oral Surg., Oral Med. and Oral Path. 7:559, 1954.

Cohen, E. L.: Aspects of allergy, Brit. Dent. J. 99:185, 1955.

Cook, T. J.: Angioneurotic edema, Am. J. Orthodont. and Oral Surg. 24:1208, 1938.

Curtis, A. C., and Taylor, H.: Allergic dematoses of importance to the dentist, Am. J. Orthodont. and Oral Surg. (Oral Surg. Sect.) 33:201, 1947.

Fisher, A. A.: Allergic sensitization of the skin and oral mucosa to acrylic denture material, J.A.M.A. 156:238, 1954.

Goldman, L., and Goldman, B.: Contact testing of the buccal mucous membrane for stomatitis venenata, Arch. Dermat. and Syph. 50:79, 1944.

Kile, R. L.: Contact dermatitis from procaine penicillin, Arch. Dermat. and Syph. 61:484, 1950.

Loveman, A. B.: Stomatitis venenata, Arch. Dermat. and Syph. 37:70, 1938.

Miller, C. R.: Sulfadiazine reactions, report of three cases, J. Oral Surg. 5:17, 1947.

Ramirez, M. A.: Oral manifestations in allergy, Dent. Items Interest 60:803, 1938.

Simms, W. B.: Oral lesions caused by antienzyme dentifrices, U. S. Armed Forces Med. J. 6:995, 1955.

Spiegel, L. H.: Penicillinase treatment of allergic penicillin reactions, J. Oral Surg. 17:27, 1959.

Thomas, J. W., and Syrop, H. M.: Allergy problems related to dentistry, Ann. Allergy 15:603, 1957.

Wolfson, S. A.: Black hairy tongue associated with penicillin therapy, J.A.M.A. 140:1206, 1949.

Leukoplakia and Solar Cheilosis

Adkins, K. F.: Diagnosis of white lesions of the oral mucosa, Australian Dent. J. 11:227, 1966.

Ayres, S.: Chronic actinic cheilitis, J.A.M.A. 81:1183, 1923.

Bernier, J. L., and Reynolds, M. C.: The relationship of senile elastosis to actinic radiation and to squamous cell carcinoma of the lip, Mil. Med. 117:209, 1955.

Blum, H. F.: Sunlight as an environmental factor in cancer of the skin, Mil. Med. 117:202, 1955.

Cowdry, E. V., and Andrew, W.: Some cytochemical and cytologic features of senile keratosis, J. Gerontol. 5:97, 1950.

Kerr, D. A.: Keratotic lesion of the oral cavity, J. Dent. Med. 13:92, 1958.

Kollar, J. A., Finley, C. W., Nabers, J. M., Ritchey, B., and Orban, B. J.: Leukoplakia, J.A.D.A. 49:538, 1954.

Laband, P. F., and Bumsted, W. D.: Premalignant lesions of the lips in soldiers returning from Korea, Oral Surg., Oral Med. and Oral Path. 8:64, 1955.

Mehta, F. S., Daftary, D. K., Stroff, B. C., and Samghvi, L. D.: Clinical and histologic study of oral leukoplakia in relation to habits, Oral Surg., Oral Med. and Oral Path. 28:372, 1969.

Mehta, F. S., Pindborg, J. J., Gupta, P. C.; and Daftary, D. K.: Epidemiologic and histologic study of oral cancer and leukoplakia among 50,915 villagers in India, Cancer 24:832, 1969.

Nicalou, S. G., and Balus, L.: Chronic actinic cheilitis and cancer of the lower lip, Brit. J. Derm. 76:278, 1964.

Pindborg, J. J., Renstrup, G., Jølst, O., and Roed-Petersen, B.: Studies in oral leukoplakia: Preliminary report on the period prevalence of malignant transformation in leukoplakia based on follow-up study of 248 patients, J.A.D.A. 76:767, 1968.

Robinson, H. B. G.: White lesions of the oral mucosa, J. Dent. Med. 17:80, 1962.

Rothman, S.: Physiology of keratinization, Oral Surg., Oral Med. and Oral Path. 7:1085, 1954.

Shafer, W. G., and Waldron, C. A.: A clinical and histopathologic study of oral leukoplakia, Surg. Gynec. Obstet. 112:411, 1961.

Silverman, S., and Ware, W. H.: Comparisons of histologic, cytologic, and clinical findings in intraoral leukoplakia and associated carcinoma, Oral Surg., Oral Med. and Oral Path. 13:412, 1960.

Sturgis, S. H., and Lund, C. C.: Leukoplakia buccalis and keratosis labialis, New Eng. J. Med. 210:996, 1934.

Szodoray, L.: Histologic characteristics of the so-called precancerous processes of the skin, Arch. Dermat. and Syph. 36:552, 1937.

Turesky, S., Glickman, I., and Provost, J.: A histochemical study of the keratotic process in oral lesions diagnosed clinically as leukoplakia, Oral Surg., Oral Med. and Oral Path. 14:442, 1961.

Waldron, C. A., and Shafer, W. G.: Current concepts of leukoplakia, Internat. Dent. J. 10:350, 1960.

White Spongy Nevus and Related Lesions

Browne, W. G., Izatt, M. M., and Redwick, J. H.: White sponge nevus of the mucosa: clinical and linkage data, Ann. Human Genetics 32:271, 1969.

Cannon, A. B.: White sponge nevus of the mucosa (naevus spongiosus albus mucosae), Arch. Dermat. and Syph. 31:365, 1935.

Cooke, B. E. D., and Morgan, V.: Oral epithelial naevi, Brit. J. Derm. 11:134, 1959.

Everett, F. G., and Noyes, H. J.: White folded gingivo-stomatosis, J. Periodont. 24:32, 1953.

Haye, K. R., and Whitehead, F. I. H.: Hereditary leukokeratosis of mucous membranes, Brit. J. Derm. 80:529, 1968.

Ludy, J. B., and Shirazy, E.: Congenital leukokeratosis mucosa oris (keratosis disseminée de muqueuse), New Internat. Clin., new series 4:38, 1941.

Stiff, R. H., and Ferraro, E.: Hereditary keratosis, Oral Surg., Oral Med. and Oral Path., 28:697, 1969.

Whitten, J. B.: The electron microscopic examination of oral mucous membranes: I. White sponge nevus, Oral Surg., Oral Med. and Oral Path. 29:69, 1970.

Witkop, C. J., Shankle, C. H., Graham, J. B., Murray, M. R., Rucknagel, D. L., and Byerly B. H.: Hereditary benign intraepithelial dyskeratosis, A.M.A. Arch. Path. 70:696, 1960.

Cysts, Stones and Inflammation of Salivary Glands

Bark, C. J., and Perzik, S. L.: Mikulicz's disease, sialoangiectasis and autoimmunity based upon a study of parotid lesions, Am. J. Clin. Path. 49:683, 1968.

Bhaskar, S. N.: Lympho-epithelial lesions of the oral cavity; report of twenty-four cases, Oral Diag. 21:120, 1966.

Bhaskar, S. N., and Bernier, J. L.: Mikulicz's disease, Oral Surg., Oral Med. and Oral Path. 13:1387, 1960.

Bourgoyne, J. R.: Sialolithiasis, Oral Surg., Oral Med. and Oral Path. 1:719, 1948.

Brook, A. H.: Recurrent parotitis in childhood, Brit. Dent. J. 127:271, 1969.

Bunim, J. J., Buchanan, W. W., and Wertlake, P. T.: Clinical, pathologic and serologic studies in Sjögren's syndrome: Combined clinical staff conference at the National Institutes of Health, Ann. Intern. Med. 61:509, 1964.

Garusi, G. F.: Sialoangiectasis: Asymptomatic forms, recurrent sialoadenitis, Sjögren's syndrome and other mesenchymal diseases, Fortschr. Roentgenstr. 98:759, 1963.

Gerry, R. G., and Seigman, E. L.: Chronic sialadenitis and sialography, Oral Surg., Oral Med. and Oral Path. 8:453, 1955.

Hall, H. D.: Diagnosis of diseases of salivary glands, J. Oral Surg. 27:15, 1969.
Hettwer, K. J., and Folsom, T. C.: Normal sialogram, Oral Surg., Oral Med. and Oral Path. 26:790, 1968.
Kaltreider, H. B. and Talal, N.: Bilateral parotid gland enlargement and hyperlipoproteinemia, J.A.M.A. 210:2067, 1969.
Lathrop, F. D.: Diseases of salivary gland, Laryngoscope 66:251, 1956.
Morse, D. R., and Hoffman, H.: Microbial diseases of the salivary glands. New York State Dent. J. 36:203, 1970.
Nathanson, N. R., and Quinn, T. W.: Ranula. A review of the literature and a report of 3 cases, Oral Surg., Oral Med. and Oral Path. 5:250, 1952.
Sela, J., and Ulmansky, M.: Mucous retention cysts of salivary glands, J. Oral Surg. 27:619, 1969.
Seldin, H. M., Seldin, S. D., and Rakower, W.: Conservative surgery for the removal of salivary calculi, Oral Surg., Oral Med. and Oral Path. 6:579, 1953.
Smith, J. B.: Obstructive submaxillary salivary adenitis caused by foreign body. Report of a case, J. Oral Surg. 7:78, 1949.
Standish, S. M., and Shafer, W. G.: The mucous retention phenomenon, J. Oral Surg., Anesth., and Hosp. Dent. Service 17:15, July 1959.
Tholen, E. F.: Sialolithiasis, J. Oral Surg. 7:63, 1949.
Thoma, K. H.: The diagnosis and treatment of salivary cysts and stones, Oral Surg., Oral Med. and Oral Path. 3:1087, 1950.
Thoma, K. H., Holland, D. J., Woodbury, H. W., Burrow, J. G., and Sleeper, E. L.: Salivary cysts, Oral Surg., Oral Med. and Oral Path. 1:17, 1948.
Whinery, J. G.: Salivary calculi, J. Oral Surg. 12:43, 1954.
White, N. S.: Sjögren's syndrome, Oral Surg., Oral Med. and Oral Path. 22:163, 1966.
Wilson, T. G.: Diseases of salivary glands, Practitioner 196:261, 1966.
Wohl, M. J., and Bloch, K. J.: Sjögren's syndrome, Postgrad. Med. 45:180, 1969.

Herpetiform and Related Lesions

Brightman, V. J., and Guggenheimer, J. G.: Herpetic paronychia—primary herpes simplex infection of the finger, J.A.D.A. 80:112, 1970.
Cahn, L.: Viral diseases of the mouth, Oral Surg., Oral Med. and Oral Path. 3:1172, 1950.
Cooke, B. E. D.: Epithelial smears in diagnosis of herpes simplex and herpes zoster affecting the oral mucosa, Brit. Dent. J. 104:99, 1958.
Dolby, A. E.: Mikulicz's recurrent oral aphthae, Brit. Dent. J. 128:579, 1970.
Dolby, A. E., and Allison, R. T.: Quantitative changes in mast cell population in Mikulicz's recurrent oral aphthae, J. Dent. Res. 48:901, 1969.
Francis, T.: Viruses as agents of disease, Oral Surg., Oral Med. and Oral Path. 1:153, 160, 1948.
Graykowski, E. A., Barile, M. F., Lee, W. B., and Stanley, H. R., Jr.: Recurrent aphthous stomatitis, J.A.M.A. 196:637, 1966.
Herriut, R. M.: Infectious nucleic acids: New dimensions in virology, Science 134:236, 1961.
Hurt, W. C.: Periadenitis mucosa necrotica recurrens, Oral Surg., Oral Med. and Oral Path. 13:750, 1960.
Kerr, D. A.: Herpetic gingivostomatitis, J. Am. Dent. A. 44:674, 1952.
———: Stomatitis and gingivitis in the adolescent and preadolescent, J.A.D.A. 44:27, 1952.
Ramfjord, S. P.: Recurrent herpetic, gingivostomatitis treated with gamma globulin, Oral Surg., Oral Med. and Oral Path. 13:165, 1960.
Robinson, H. B. G.: Vesicular lesions of the oral mucosa, New York State Dent. J. 33:523, 1967.
Scott, T. F. M.: Infection with herpes simplex virus, G. P. 12, No. 3:59, 1955.
Scott, T. F. M., Steigman, A. J., and Convey, J. H.: Acute infectious gingivostomatitis, J.A.M.A. 117:999, 1941.
Ship, I. I., Morris, A. L., Durocher, R. T., and Burket, L. W.: Recurrent aphthous ulcerations in a professional school student population, Oral Surg., Oral Med. and Oral Path. 14:30, 1961.
Strean, L. P., Williams, B. H., and Prichard, J.: Oral herpetiform lesions treated with gamma globulin, Oral Surg., Oral Med. and Oral Path. 11:226, 1958.
Weathers, D. R., and Griffin, J. W.: Intraoral ulcerations in recurrent herpes simplex and recurrent aphthae: two distinct clinical entities, J.A.D.A. 81:81, 1970.
Woodburne, A. R.: Herpetic stomatitis, Arch. Dermat. and Syph. 43:543, 1941.

Exanthems

Koplik, H.: Diagnosis of the invasion of measles; from a study of the exanthem as it appears on the buccal mucosa, Arch. Pediat. 13:918, 1896.

Kraus, B. S., Ames, M. D., and Clark, G. R.: Effects of maternal rubella on dental crown development, Clin. Pediat. 8:204, 1969.
McCarthy, P. L., and Shklar, G.: Diseases of the Oral Mucosa, New York, McGraw-Hill, 1964.

Tuberculosis

Abbott, J. N., Briney, A. T., and Denaro, S. A.: Recovery of tubercle bacilli from mouth washings of tuberculous dental patients, J. Am. Dent. A. 50:49, 1955.
Boyes, J., Jones, J. D. T., and Miller, F. J. W.: Recognition of a primary tuberculosis of mouth, Arch. Dis. Childhood 31:81, 1956.
Brodsky, R. H.: Oral tuberculous lesions, Am. J. Orthodont. and Oral Surg. (Oral Surg. Sect.) 28:132, 1942.
Bruce, K. W.: Tuberculosis of the alveolar gingiva, Oral Surg., Oral Med. and Oral Path. 7:894, 1954.
Castigliano, S. G., and Shigeoka, E.: Tuberculosis of the oral cavity, Ann. Otol., Rhin. and Laryng. 62:662, 1953.
Darlington, C. C., and Salman, I.: Oral tuberculous lesions, Am. Rev. Tuberc. 35:147, 1937.
Moore, W. J., and Hamilton, J. F.: Tuberculosis of tongue, J. Internat. Coll. Surgeons 26:135, 1956.
Shengold, M. A., and Sheingold, H.: Oral tuberculosis, Oral Surg., Oral Med. and Oral Path. 4:239, 1951.

Syphilis

Boyle, P. E.: The histopathology of the human tooth germ in congenital syphilis, J. Dent. Res. 12:425, 1932.
Captline, A. M., White, N. S., Merkow, L. P., and Snyder, S. P.: Atrophic luetic glossitis, Oral Surg., Oral Med. and Oral Path. 30:192, 1970.
Cole, H. N.: Congenital and prenatal syphilis, J.A.M.A. 109:580, 1937.
Curtis, A. C., and Slaughter, J. C.: The clinical diagnosis of dermatologic lesions of the face and oral cavity, Am. J. Orthodont. and Oral Surg. (Oral Surg. Sect.) 33:218, 1947.
Hollander, L., and Goldmann, B. A.: Syphilis of the oral mucosa, Dent. Digest 40:90, 135, 174, 1934.
Huebsch, R. F.: Gumma of the hard palate with perforation, Oral Surg., Oral Med. and Oral Path. 8:690, 1955.
Lumsden, C. E.: The viability of Treponema pallidum, Lancet 2 (253):827, 1947.
Meyer, I., and Shklar, G.: Oral manifestations of acquired syphilis: Study of 81 cases, Oral Surg., Oral Med. and Oral Path. 23:45, 1967.
Monash, S.: Aspects of syphilis of interest to the dentist, Dent. Cosmos 73:1172, 1931.
O'Leary, P. A.: Oral syphilis, J.A.D.A. 17:413, 1930.
Soloway, H. M.: Control of syphilis in pregnant women, J.A.M.A. 129:500, 1945.

Histoplasmosis

Dunlap, C. L., and Barnes, W. G.: Oral histoplasmosis, J. Missouri Dent. Assoc. 49:26, 1969.
Kemper, J. W., and Bloom, H. J.: Histoplasmosis, J. Oral Surg. 2:167, 1944.
Levy, B. M.: Oral manifestations of histoplasmosis, J.A.D.A. 32:215, 1945.
Loosli, C. G., Procknow, J. J., Grayston, J. T., and Combs, L. W.: Pulmonary histoplasmosis in a farm family. A three year follow-up, J. Lab. and Clin. Med. 43:669, 1954.
Methot, Y., Blank, F., and Masson, A. M.: Gingivitis caused by histoplasma capsulatum, Canad. M. A. J. 79:836, 1958.
Moore, M., and Jorstad, L. H.: Histoplasmosis and its importance to otorhinolaryngologists. A review with report of a new case, Ann. Otol., Rhin. and Laryng. 52:779, 1943.
Nutman, N. N.: A case of histoplasmosis with oral manifestations, Oral Surg., Oral Med. and Oral Path. 2:1562, 1949.
Palchanis, W. T.: Tuberculosis and histoplasmosis in foreign students entering our colleges, Dis. Chest. 23:552, 1953.
Parsons, R. J., and Zarafonetis, C. J. D.: Histoplasmosis in man, Arch. Intern. Med. 75:1, 1945.
Scherr, G. H.: The laboratory diagnosis of mycotic infections. 1. Histoplasmosis, Neb. State Med. J. 39:339, 1954.

Actinomycosis

Davis, M. I. J.: Analysis of forty-six cases of actinomycosis with special reference to its etiology, Am. J. Surg. 52:447, 1941.
Dorph-Petersen, L., and Pindborg, J. J.: Actinomycosis of the tongue, Oral Surg., Oral Med. and Oral Path. 7:1178, 1954.
Hertz, J.: Actinomycosis, borderline cases, J. Internat. Coll. Surgeons 34:148, 1960.
Lesney, T. A., and Traeger, K. A.: Cervical-facial actinomycosis: a postextraction complication, J. Oral Surg., Anesth., and Hosp. Dental Service 17:51, Jan. 1959.

McVay, L. V., Guthrie, F., and Sprunt, D. H.: Aureomycin in the treatment of actinomycosis, New Eng. J. Med. 245:91, 1951.

Norman, J. E. de B.: Cervicofacial actinomycosis, Oral Surg., Oral Med. and Oral Path. 29:735, 1970.

Robinson, H. B. G., and Ennever, J.: Etiology and diagnosis of actinomycosis, Oral Surg., Oral Med. and Oral Path. 1:850, 1948.

Rosebury, T., Epps, L. J., and Clark, A. R.: A study of the isolation, cultivation and pathogenicity of *Actinomyces israeli* recovered from the human mouth and from actinomycosis in man, J. Infect. Dis. 74:131, 1944.

Rosh, R., and Seldin, H. M.: Actinomycosis. Treatment of five cases, J. Oral Surg. 6:93, 1948.

Rud, J.: Cervicofacial actinomycosis, J. Oral Surg. 25:299, 1967.

Weed, L. A., and Baggenstoss, A. H.: Actinomycosis. A pathologic and bacterial study of twenty-one fatal cases, Am. J. Clin. Path. 19:201, 1949.

Candidiasis

Hermans, P. E., Ulrich, J. A., and Markowitz, H.: Chronic mucocutaneous candidiasis as a surface expression of deep-seated abnormalities, Am. J. Med. 47:503, 1969.

Osteomyelitis

Durbeck, W. E.: Mandibular osteomyelitis, its diagnosis and treatment, J. Oral Surg. 4:33, 1946.

Killey, H. C., Kay, L. W., and Wright, H. C.: Subperiosteal osteomyelitis of the mandible, Oral Surg., Oral Med. and Oral Path. 29:576, 1970.

Meyer, I.: Infectious diseases of the jaws, J. Oral Surg. 28:17, 1970.

Stuteville, O. H.: A new concept of treatment of osteomyelitis of the mandible, J. Oral Surg. 8:301, 1950.

Thoma, K. H., Holland, D. J., Woodbury, H. W., Burrow, J. G., and Sleeper, E. L.: Osteomyelitis of the jaws, Oral Surg., Oral Med. and Oral Path. 1:76, 1948.

Waldron, C. W.: Osteomyelitis of the jaws, J. Oral Surg. 1:317, 1943.

Pyogenic Granuloma

Bhaskar, S. N.: Pyogenic granuloma, J. Oral Surg. 24:391, 1966.

Eisen, D.: Granuloma, pyogenicum, Canad. Med. A. J. 42:528, 1940.

Kerr, D. A.: Granuloma pyogenicum, Oral Surg., Oral Med. and Oral Path. 4:158, 1951.

Michelson, H. E.: Granuloma pyogenicum. A clinical and histologic review of twenty-nine cases, Arch. Dermat. and Syph. 12:492, 1925.

Montgomery, D. W., and Culver, G. D.: Granuloma pyogenicum, Arch. Dermat. and Syph. 26:131, 1932.

Lichen Planus

Andreason, J. O.: Oral lichen planus: I. Clinical evaluation of 115 cases, Oral Surg., Oral Med. and Oral Path. 25:31, 1968.

Cawley, E. P., and Kerr, D. A.: Lichen planus, Oral Surg., Oral Med. and Oral Path. 5:1069, 1952.

Darling, A. I., and Crabb, H. S. M.: Lichen planus, Oral Surg., Oral Med. and Oral Path. 7:1276, 1954.

Fox, H.: Lichen planus confined to the mouth, Arch. Dermat. and Syph. 24:1071, 1931.

Pullon, P. A.: Ultrastructure of oral lichen planus, Oral Surg., Oral Med. and Oral Path. 28:365, 1969.

Shklar, G., and McCarthy, P. L.: The oral lesions of lichen planus, Oral Surg., Oral Med. and Oral Path. 14:164, 1961.

Vriezen, T. C.: Lichen planus of the oral mucosa, Nederl. T. Geneesk. III:1469, August 26, 1967.

Erythema Multiforme

Fisch, H. U.: Behçet's disease with neurologic complications in childhood, Helvet. Paediat. Acta 23:154, 1968.

Jones, R. M.: Erythema multiforme exudativum (Stevens-Johnson syndrome), Am. J. Orthodont. and Oral Surg. (Oral Surg. Sect.) 33:326, 1947.

Moe, T. I.: Vitamin B therapy in erythema multiforme, Oral Surg., Oral Med. and Oral Path. 1:485, 1948.

Moodie, W.: Erythema multiforme exudative, Brit. Dent. J. 89:239, 1950.

Rakower, W.: Erythema multiforme—Stevens Johnson syndrome, Oral Surg., Oral Med. and Oral Path. 7:750, 1954.

Robinson, A. M.: Stevens-Johnson syndrome, J. South Carolina M. A. 52:12, 1956.

Robinson, H. M., and McCrumb, F. R.: Comparative analysis of the mucocutaneous-ocular syndromes, Arch. Dermat. and Syph. 61:539, 1950.

Soll, S. N.: Eruptive fever with involvement of the respiratory tract, conjunctivitis, stomatitis, and balanitis, Arch. Intern. Med. 79:475, 1947.

Stevens, A. M., and Johnson, F. C.: A new eruptive fever associated with stomatitis and ophthalmia, Am. J. Dis. Child. 24:26, 1922.

Whinston, G. J.: Oral lesions of erythema multiforme, Oral Surg., Oral Med. and Oral Path. 5:1207, 1952.

Pemphigus

Brody, H, A., and Wuepper, K. D.: Mucous membrane pemphigoid—immunofluorescent studies, J. Dent. Res. 48:1248, 1969.

Cahn, L.: Pemphigus, Am. J. Orthodont. and Oral Surg. (Oral Surg. Sect.) 33:541, 1947.

Cooke, B. D.: Oral manifestations of bullous lesions. J. Roy. Coll. Surg. Edinburgh 15:129, 1970.

Lever, W. F.: Oral lesions in pemphigus, Am. J. Orthodont. and Oral Surg. (Oral Surg. Sect.) 28:569, 1942.

———: Pemphigus, Medicine 32:1, 1953.

Levin, H. L.: Oral manifestations and treatment of pemphigus vegetans, Oral Surg., Oral Med. and Oral Path. 9:742, 1956.

McCarthy, P. L., and Shklar, G.: Benign mucous membrane pemphigus, New Eng. J. Med. 258:726, 1958.

———: Diseases of the Oral Mucosa, New York, McGraw-Hill, 1964.

Medak, H., Burlakow, P., McGrew, E., and Tiecke, R.: The cytology of vesicular conditions affecting the oral mucosa: pemphigus vulgaris, Acta Cytol. 14:11, 1970.

Rouchon, C., Kuffer, R., and Badillet, G.: Cytodiagnosis in buccal pemphigus, Actualites Odonto-Stomat. 21:363, 1967.

Shkar, G.: Histopathology and cytology of oral lesions of pemphigus, Arch. Derm. 101:635, 1970.

Stern, L., Jr.: The diagnosis of pemphigus by its oral signs, Oral Surg., Oral Med. and Oral Path. 2:1443, 1949.

Tzanck, A.: Le cytodiagnostic immediat en dermatologie, Ann. Derm. Syph. 8:205, 1948.

Lupus Erythematosus

Andreasen, J. O.: Oral manifestations of discoid and systemic lupus erythematosus: I. Clinical investigation, Acta Odont. Scandinav. 22:295, 1964.

Bianchi, F. A., Bistue, A. R., Wendt, V. E., Puro, H. E., and Keech, M. K.: Analysis of 27 cases of progressive systemic sclerosis (including 2 with combined systemic lupus erythematosus) and a review of literature, J. Chron. Dis. 19:953, 1966.

Haserick, J. R.: Plasma L. E. test in systemic lupus erythematosus, J.A.M.A. 146:16, 1951.

Klemperer, P., Pollack, A. D., and Baehr, G.: Pathology of disseminated lupus erythematosus, Arch. Path. 32:569, 1941.

McCreight, W. G., and Montgomery, H.: Cutaneous changes in lupus erythematosus, Arch. Dermat. and Syph. 61:1, 1950.

Sugarman, M. M.: Lupus erythematosus, Oral Surg., Oral Med. and Oral Path. 6:836, 1953.

Weiss, R. S., and Swift, S.: The significance of a positive L. E. phenomenon, Arch. Dermat. and Syph. 72:103, 1955.

Geographic Tongue

Halperin, V., Kolas, S., Jefferis, K. R., Huddleston, S. O., and Robinson, H. B. G.: The occurrence of Fordyce spots, benign migratory glossitis, median rhomboid glossitis and fissured tongue in 2,478 dental patients, Oral Surg., Oral Med. and Oral Path. 6:1072, 1953.

Prinz, H.: Wandering rash of the tongue (geographical tongue), Dent. Cosmos 69:272, 1927.

Redman, R. S., Vance, F. L., Gorlin, R. J., Peagler, F. D., and Meskin, L. H.: Psychologic component in etiology of geographic tongue, J. Dent. Res. 45:1403, 1966.

Hairy Tongue

Bartels, H. A., and Maillard, E. R.: Hairy tongue, Oral Surg., Oral Med. and Oral Path. 8:659, 1955.

Pincus, P., and Boyd-Cooper, B.: Black hairy tongue. Preliminary observations on two cases, Brit. Dent. J. 65:271, 1938.

Varicose Veins, Tongue

Bean, W. D.: Caviar lesions of the tongue, in Ciba Foundation Colloquia on Ageing, ed. by Wolstenholme, G. E. W., and Cameron, M. P., vol. 1, p. 84, Boston, Little, Brown, 1955.

Hubinger, H. L.: Thrombosis of ranine vein. Report of a case, J. Oral Surg. 9:65, 1951.

Neill, D. J.: Phlebolith of a lingual vein, Brit. Dent. J. 98:250, 1955.

Telangiectasia

Bird, R. M., Hammarstein, J. F., Marshall, R. A., and Robinson, R. R.: Family reunion: study of hereditary hemorrhagic telangiectasia, New Eng. J. Med. 257:105, 1957.

Bird, R. M., and Jacques, W. E.: Vascular lesion of hereditary hemorrhagic telangiectasia, New Eng. J. Med. 260:597, 1959.

Goldstein, H. I.: Goldstein's heredofamilial angiomatosis with recurring familial hemorrhage (Rendu-Osler-Weber's disease), Arch. Intern. Med. 48:836, 1931.

Koch, H. J., Jr., Escher, G. C., and Lewis, J. S.: Hormonal management of hereditary hemorrhagic telangiectasia, J.A.M.A. 149:1376, 1952.

Madden, J. F.: Generalized angiomatosis (telangiectasia), J.A.M.A. 102:442, 1934.

Peluse, S.: Gingival hemorrhage with oral manifestations in hereditary hemorrhagic telangiectasia, Arch. Otolaryng. 44:668, 1946.

Singer, K., and Wolfson, W. Q.: Hereditary hemorrhagic telangiectasia, New Eng. J. Med. 230:637, 1944.

Syrop, H. S.: Hereditary hemorrhagic telangiectasia, Oral Surg., Oral Med. and Oral Path. 10:253, 1957.

Vitamin Deficiency

Afonsky, D.: Deficiency glossitis. A collective review, Oral Surg., Oral Med. and Oral Path. 4:482, 1951.

Dreizen, S.: Nutritional changes in the oral cavity, J. Prosth. Dent. 16:1144, 1966.

Dreizen, S., Stone, R. E., and Spies, T. D.: Oral manifestations of nutritional disorders, Dent. Clin. N. Am., p. 429, July, 1958.

Jeghers, H.: The appearance of the tongue as an index of nutritional deficiency, New Eng. J. Med. 227:221, 1942.

Johnson, W. B.: Oral symptoms and treatment of a nicotinic acid deficiency, Oral Surg., Oral Med. and Oral Path. 8:1257, 1955.

Jolliffe, N., Tisdall, F. F., and Cannon, P. R.: Clinical Nutrition, ed. 2, New York, Hoeber, 1962.

Makila, E.: Prevalence of angular stomatitis: Correlation with composition of food and metabolism of vitamins and iron, Acta Odont. Scandinav. 27:655, 1969.

Mann, A. W., Dreizen, S., and Spies, T. D.: Further studies on the effect of the correction of mechanical factors on angular cheilosis in malnourished edentulous patients, Oral Surg., Oral Med. and Oral Path. 1:868, 1948.

Spies, T. D.: Some recent advances in nutrition, J.A.M.A. 167:675, 1958.

Spies, T. D., Bean, W. B., and Huff, N. E.: Endemic riboflavin deficiency in infants and children, Am. J. Med. Sc. 200:697, 1940.

Spies, T. D., Vilter, R. W., and Ashe, W. F.: Pellagra, beriberi and riboflavin deficiency in human beings, J.A.M.A. 113:931, 1939.

Stein, G.: Correlation between gross appearance and histopathology of the tongue, Oral Surg., Oral Med. and Oral Path. 8:1165, 1955.

Carotenemia

Blankenhorn, D. H.: The infiltration of carotenoids in human atheromas and xanthomas, Ann. Intern. Med. 53:944, 1960.

Jeghers, H.: Skin changes of nutritional origin, New Eng. J. Med. 228:678, 1943.

Josephs, H. W.: Hypervitaminosis A and carotenemia, Am. J. Dis. Child. 67:33, 1944.

Pernicious Anemia

Castle, W. B.: Present status of the etiology of pernicious anemia, Ann. Intern. Med. 34:1093, 1951.

Fouts, P. J., Helmer, O. M., and Chernish, S. M.: Absorptions of radioactive B_{12} in patients with pernicious anemia after long term oral and parenteral therapy, Ann. Intern. Med. 52:29, 1960.

Glass, G. B. J., and Boyd, L. J.: Oral treatment of pernicious anemia with small doses of vitamin B_{12} combined with mucinous materials derived from the hog stomach, Blood 8:867, 1953.

Graham, R. M., and Rheault, M. H.: Characteristic cellular changes in epithelial cells in pernicious anemia, J. Lab. and Clin. Med. 43:235, 1954.

Kerr, D. A.: Oral manifestations of blood dyscrasias, J. Canad. D. A. 27:149, 1961.

Meacham, G. C., and Heinle, R. W.: Maintenance therapy of pernicious anemia with vitamin B_{12}, J. Lab. and Clin. Med. 41:65, 1953.

Schieve, J. F., and Rundles, R. W.: Response of lingual manifestations of pernicious anemia to pteroylglutamic acid and vitamin B_{12}, Oral Surg., Oral Med. and Oral Path. 2:1255, 1949.

Wallerstein, R. O., Harris, J. W., Schilling, R. F., and Castle, W. B.: Observations on the etiologic relationship of achylia gastrica to pernicious anemia, J. Lab. and Clin. Med. 41:363, 1953.

Erythroblastic Anemias

Baty, J. M., Blackfan, K. D., and Diamond, L. K.: Blood studies in infants and children. I. Erythroblastic anemia, Am. J. Dis. Child. 43:667, 1932.

Caffey, J.: The skeletal changes in the chronic hemolytic anemias (erythroblastic anemia, sickle cell anemia, and chronic hemolytic icterus), Am. J. Roentgen. 37:293, 1937.

Cooley, T. B., and Lee, P.: Erythroblastic anemia, Am. J. Dis. Child. 43:705, 1932.

Koch, L. A., and Shapiro, B.: Erythroblastic anemia, Am. J. Dis. Child. 44:318, 1932.

McFarland, W., and Pearson, H. A.: Thalassemia in "non-Mediterranean" families, Ann. Intern. Med. 53:510, 1960.

Neel, J. V., and Valentine, W. N.: The frequency of thalassemia, Am. J. Med. Sci. 209:568, 1945.

Novak, A. J.: The oral manifestations of erythroblastic (Cooley's) anemia, Am. J. Orthodont. and Oral Surg. (Oral Surg. Sect.) 30:539, 1944.

Smith, C. H.: Detection of mild types of Mediterranean (Cooley's) anemia, Am. J. Dis. Child. 75:505, 1948.

Agranulocytosis

Appleton, J. L. T.: Agranulocytosis, Dent. Cosmos 74:267, 371, 1932.

Covner, A. H., and Halpern, S. L.: Fatal agranulocytosis following therapy with "Presidon," a new sedative hypnotic agent, New Eng. J. Med. 242:49, 1950.

Hadler, A. J.: Granulocytopenia following barbiturate therapy, New Eng. J. Med. 222:755, 1940.

McMillin, J. S.: Successful use of ACTH in the treatment of agranulocytosis due to sulfadiazine, Am. J. Med. Sc: 222:392, 1951.

Robinson, H. B. G.: Stomatitis in blood dyscrasias, Internat. Dent. J. 5:327, 1955.

Sreebny, L. M., and McGrew, E. A.: Fatal agranulocytosis due to Tridione therapy, Oral Surg., Oral Med. and Oral Path. 6:1301, 1953.

Wosika, P. H., and Braun, L.: Fatal agranulocytosis occurring during treatment with thiouracil, J. Lab. and Clin. Med. 30:779, 1945.

Hyperparathyroidism

Attie, J. N., and Blum, B.: Hyperparathyroidism first suspected through a giant cell epulis, Oral Surg., Oral Med. and Oral Path. 13:482, 1960.

Black, B. M.: Hyperparathyroidism, Publication No. 173, American Lecture Series, Springfield, Ill., Thomas, 1953.

Cahn, L.: The jaws in generalized skeletal disease, Ann. Roy. Coll. Surgeons England 8:115, 1951.

Coleman, R.: Giant-cell tumor of the mandible associated with hyperparathyroidism and osteitis fibrosa cystica generalisata, Oral Surg., Oral Med. and Oral Path. 7:534, 1954.

Keating, F. R.: Hyperparathyroidism, Am. J. Orthodont. and Oral Surg. (Oral Surg. Sect.) 33:116, 1947.

———: The normal and pathologic physiology of the parathyroid glands, Am. J. Orthodont. and Oral Surg. (Oral Surg. Sect.) 33:129, 1947.

Levy, B. A.: A case of hyperparathyroidism, Oral Surg., Oral Med. and Oral Path. 5:549, 1952.

Rasmussen, H.: Parathyroid hormone, Am. J. Med. 30:112, 1961.

Schneider, W.: Hyperparathyroidism (generalized osteitis fibrosa), Oral Surg., Oral Med. and Oral Path. 6:745, 1953.

Central Giant Cell Lesions

Bhaskar, S. N., Bernier, J. L., and Godby, F.: Aneurysmal bone cysts and other giant cell lesions of the jaws, J. Oral Surg., Anesth., and Hosp. Dent. Serv. 17:30, 1959.

Jaffe, H. L.: Giant-cell reparative granuloma, traumatic bone cyst, and fibrous (fibro-osseous) dysplasia of jaw bones, Oral Surg., Oral Med. and Oral Path. 6:159, 1953.

Umiker, W., and Gerry, R. G.: Pseudo giant cell tumor (reparative granuloma) of the jaw, Oral Surg., Oral Med. and Oral Path. 7:113, 1954.

Waldron, C. A.: Fibrous and granulomatous lesions of jaw bones, Am. J. Surg. 94:877, 1957.

Histiocytosis

Blevins, C., Dahlen, D. C., Lovestedt, S. A., and Kennedy, R. L. V.: Oral and dental manifestations of histiocytosis X, Oral Surg., Oral Med. and Oral Path. 12:473, 1959.

Cox, M. E.: Eosinophilic granuloma of bone with primary oral manifestations. Report of 3 cases, Am. J. Orthodont. and Oral Surg. (Oral Surg. Sect.) 32:569, 1946.

Green, W. T., and Farber, S.: "Eosinophilic or solitary granuloma" of bone, J. Bone and Joint Surg. 24:499, 1942.

Johnson, R. P., and Mohnae, A. M.: Histiocytosis X: Report of 7 cases, J. Oral Surg. 25:7, 1967.

Jones, J. C., Lilly, G. E., and Marlette, R. H.: Histiocytosis X. J. Oral Surg. 28:461, 1970.

Lichtenstein, L.: Histiocytosis X, Arch. Path. 56:84, 1953.

Lichtenstein, L., and Jaffe, H. L.: Eosinophilic granuloma of bone, Am. J. Path. 16:595, 1940.

Ross, I. F., Broun, G. N., and Conrad, S. C.: Chronic disseminated histiocytosis X (Hand-Schüller-Christian type) with oral mucosal lesions, Oral Surg., Oral Med. and Oral Path. 9:529, 1956.

Sedano, H. O., Cernea, P., Hosxe, G., and Gorlin, R. J.: Histiocytosis X: Clinical, radiologic and histologic findings with special attention to oral manifestations, Oral Surg., Oral Med. and Oral Path. 27:760, 1969.

Sleeper, E. L.: Eosinophilic granuloma of bone. Collective review, Oral Surg., Oral Med. and Oral Path. 4:896, 1951.

Talley, D. B.: Schüller-Christian's disease with reports of cases, J. Oral Surg. 6:303, 1948.

Scleroderma

Bevans, M.: Pathology of scleroderma, with special reference to the changes in the gastrointestinal tract, Am. J. Path. 21:25, 1945.

Butler, J. J.: Scleroderma, G. P. 12:103, 1955.

Kemp-Harper, R. A., and Jackson, D. C.: Progressive systemic sclerosis, Brit. J. Radiol. 38:825, 1965.

Rosenthal, I. H.: Generalized scleroderma (hidebound disease, its relation to the oral cavity, with case history and dental restoration), Oral Surg., Oral Med. and Oral Path. 1:1019, 1948.

Shearn, M. A.: Sjögren's syndrome in association with scleroderma, Ann. Intern. Med. 52:1352, 1960.

Smith, D. B.: Scleroderma: its oral manifestations, Oral Surg., Oral Med. and Oral Path. 11:865, 1958.

Stafne, E. C.: Dental roentgenologic manifestations of systemic disease, Radiol. 58:820, 1952.

Stafne, E. C., and Austin, L. T.: A characteristic dental finding in acrosclerosis and diffuse scleroderma, Am. J. Orthodont. and Oral Surg. (Oral Surg. Sect.) 30:25, 1944.

Traiger, J.: Scleroderma, Oral Surg., Oral Med. and Oral Path. 14:117, 1961.

Fibrous Dysplasia

Albright, F., Butler, A. M., Hampton, A. O., and Smith, P.: Syndrome characterized by osteitis fibrosa disseminata, areas of pigmentation and endocrine dysfunction, with precocious puberty in females, New Eng. J. Med. 216:727, 746, 1937.

Berger, A., and Jaffe, H. L.: Fibrous (fibro-osseous) dysplasia of jaw bones, J. Oral Surg. 11:3, 1953.

Bruce, K. W., Bruwer, A., and Kennedy, R. L. J.: Familial intraosseous fibrous swellings of the jaws ("cherubism"), Oral Surg., Oral Med. and Oral Path. 6:995, 1953.

Carson, I. H.: Polyostotic fibrous dysplasia, Oral Surg., Oral Med. and Oral Path. 7:524, 1954.

Cooke, B. E. D.: Benign fibrous enlargements of the jaws, Brit. Dent. J. 102:1 and 49, 1957.

Glickman, I.: Fibrous dysplasia in alveolar bone, Oral Surg., Oral Med. and Oral Path. 1:895, 1948.

Gold, L.: Classification and pathogenesis of fibrous dysplasia of the jaw, Oral Surg., Oral Med. and Oral Path. 8:628, 725, 1955.

Hammer, J. E., III, Scofield, H. H., and Cornyn, J.: Benign fibro-osseous jaw lesions of periodontal membrane origin: Analysis of 249 cases, Cancer 22:861, 1968.

Lichtenstein, L., and Jaffe, H. L.: Fibrous dysplasia of bone, Arch. Path. 33:777, 1942.

McCune, D. J., and Bruch, H.: Osteodystrophia fibrosa, Am. J. Dis. Child. 54:806, 1937.

Robinson, H. B. G.: Osseous dysplasia, a reaction to injury, J. Oral Surg. 14:3, 1956.

Schlumberger, H. G.: Fibrous dysplasia of single bones (monostotic fibrous dysplasia), Mil. Surgeon 99:504, 1946.

Shafer, W. G.: Benign tumors and cysts of the jaw bones, Dent. Clin. N. Am., p. 693, 1957.

Acromegaly

Bailey, P., and Davidoff, L. M.: Concerning the microscopic structure of the hypophysis cerebri in acromegaly, Am. J. Path. 1:185, 1925.

Coggeshall, C., and Root, H. F.: Acromegaly and diabetes mellitus, Endocrinol. 26:1, 1940.

Goldberg, M. B., and Lisser, H.: Acromegaly. A consideration of its course and treatment, J. Clin. Endocrinol. 2:477, 1942.

Hamwi, G. J., Skillman, T. G., and Tufts, K. C.: Acromegaly, Am. J. Med. 29:690, 1960.

Hurxthal, L. M., Hare, H. F., Horrax, G., and Poppen, J. L.: The treatment of acromegaly, J. Clin. Endocrinol. 9:126, 1949.

Sacherman, R. H.: Complete denture prosthesis for a case of acromegaly, J. Pros. Dent. 5:186, 1955.

Paget's Disease

Brooke, R. I.: Giant-cell tumor in patients with Paget's disease, Oral Surg., Oral Med. and Oral Path., *30*:230, 1970.

Byatt, W. J., and Ash, S.: Progressive advanced case of osteitis deformans, J. Oral Surg. *10*: 143, 1952.

Glickman, I.: Paget's disease in the maxilla, mandible, and palate, Am. J. Orthodont. and Oral Surg. (Oral Surg. Sect.) *29*:591, 1943.

Jaffe, H. L.: Paget's disease of bone, Arch. Path. *15*:83, 1933.

Lucas, R. B.: Jaws and teeth in Paget's disease of bone, J. Clin. Path. *8*:195, 1955.

Rosenkrantz, J. A., Wolf, J., and Kaicher, J. J.: Paget's disease (osteitis deformans). Review of one hundred eleven cases, Arch. Intern. Med. *90*:610, 1952.

Snapper, I.: Medical Clinics on Bone Diseases. A Text and Atlas, ed. 2, p. 159, New York, Interscience, 1949.

Sornberger, C. F., and Smedal: The mechanism and incidence of cardiovascular changes in Paget's disease (osteitis deformans). A critical review of the literature with case studies, Circulation *6*:711, 1952.

Stafne, E. C., and Austin, L. T.: A study of dental roentgenograms in cases of Paget's disease (osteitis deformans), osteitis fibrosa cystica and osteoma, J.A.D.A. *25*:1202, 1938.

Tillman, H. H.: Paget's disease of bone with characteristic changes in the mandible and selective sparing of the maxilla, Oral Surg., Oral Med. and Oral Path. *14*:69, 1961.

Woodward, H. Q.: Long term studies of the blood chemistry in Paget's disease of bone, Cancer *12*:1226, 1959.

Yamane, G. M., and Fleuchaus, P. T.: Paget's disease (osteitis deformans), Oral Surg., Oral Med. and Oral Path. *7*:939, 1954.

5. NEOPLASMS

General References

Bernier, J. L., and Tiecke, R. W.: The biopsy, J. Oral Surg. *8*:342, 1950.

Brandow, E. C., Volk, B. M., and Olson, K. B.: Significance of lump in neck, Postgrad. Med. *22*:401, 1957.

Cameron, C. S.: Cancer: Retrospect and prospect, Oral Surg., Oral Med. and Oral Path. *6*:11, 1953.

Dingman, R. O.: The importance of biopsy in oral diagnosis, J. Oral Surg. *6*:204, 1948.

Dingman, R. O., and Hayward, J. R.: Diagnosis of oral tumors, J. Oral Surg. *7*:217, 1949.

Hertz, J.: Oral precancerous lesions, Oral Surg., Oral Med. and Oral Path. *9*:687, 1956.

Jones, J. H., and Coyle, J. I.: Squamous cell carcinoma of the lip: Study of the interface between neoplastic epithelium and underlying mesenchyma, J. Dent. Res. *48*:702, 1969.

Meyer, I., and Shklar, G.: Multiple malignant tumors involving the oral mucosa and the gastrointestinal tract, Oral Surg., Oral Med. and Oral Path. *13*:295, 1960.

Moertel, C. G., Dockerty, M. V., and Baggenstoss, A. H.: Multiple primary malignant neoplasms, Cancer *14*:238, 1961.

Pindborg, J. J.: Oral submucous fibrosis as a precancerous condition, J. Dent. Res. *45*:546, 1966.

Rovin, S.: Assessment of negative oral cytology diagnosis. J.A.D.A. *74*:759, 1967.

Sandler, H. C., Stahl, S. S., Cahn, L. R., and Freund, H. R.: Exfoliative cytology for detection of early mouth cancer, Oral Surg., Oral Med. and Oral Path. *13*:994, 1960.

Strong, M. S., Vaughan, C. W., and Incze, J. S.: Toluidine blue in the diagnosis of oral cancer, Dent. Survey *45*:27, 1969.

Symposium: Tumors of the oral regions, Dent. Clin. N. Am., pp. 619-758, November 1957.

Umiker, W. O., Lampe, I., Rapp, R., and Hiniker, J. J.: Oral smears in the diagnosis of carcinoma and premalignant lesions, Oral Surg., Oral Med. and Oral Path. *13*:897, 1960.

Young, J. K.: The biopsy procedure: A plea for better case histories, Oral Surg., Oral Med. and Oral Path. *5*:1200, 1952.

Papilloma and Verruca

Bunting, H., Strauss, M. J., and Banfield, W. G.: The cytology of skin papillomas that yield virus-like particles, Am. J. Path. *28*:985, 1952.

Frank, I.: Papilloma of the tonsil, Ann. Otol., Rhin. and Laryng. *47*:715, 1938.

Henner, R.: Papilloma of the tonsil and uvula, Arch. Otolaryng. *35*:810, 1942.

Kingery, L. B.: The etiology of common warts, J.A.M.A. *76*:440, 1921.

Kohlmoos, H. W.: Papilloma of the larynx in children, Arch. Otolaryng. *62*:242, 1955.

Fibroma, Lipoma and Myxoma

Adair, F. E., Pack, G. T., and Farrior, J. H.: Lipomas, Am. J. Cancer *16*:1104, 1932.

Astaff, A.: Myxofibroma, Oral Surg., Oral Med. and Oral Path. 6:247, 1953.

Bruce, K. W., and Roger, R. O.: Lipoma of the oral cavity, Oral Surg., Oral Med. and Oral Path. 7:930, 1954.

Geschickter, C. F.: Lipoid tumors, Am. J. Cancer 21:617, 1934.

Geschickter, C. F., and Lewis, D.: Tumors of connective tissue, Am. J. Cancer 25:630, 1935.

Harbert, F., Gerry, R. G., and Dimmette, R. M.: Myxoma of the maxilla, Oral Surg., Oral Med. and Oral Path. 2:1414, 1949.

Hovnanian, A. P.: Myxoma of the maxilla, Oral Surg., Oral Med. and Oral Path. 6:927, 1953.

Smith, F.: Lipoma of the tongue, J.A.M.A. 108:522, 1937.

Stout, A. P.: Myxoma, the tumor of primitive mesenchyme, Ann. Surg. 127:706, 1948.

Wells, H. G.: Adipose tissue, a neglected subject, J.A.M.A. 114:2177, 2284, 1940.

Zimmerman, D. C., and Dahlin, D. C.: Myxomatous tumors of jaws, Oral Surg., Oral Med. and Oral Path. 11:1069, 1958.

Benign Tumors of Osseous Origin

Chaudhry, A. P., Burke, R. J., Stoesz, A. R., and Gorlin, R. J.: Benign neoplastic fibro-osseous lesion of the mandible, Oral Surg., Oral Med. and Oral Path. 13:716, 1960.

Geschickter, C. F., and Copeland, M. M.: Tumors of Bone, ed. 3, Philadelphia, Lippincott, 1949.

Hara, H. J.: Ossifying fibroma of the superior maxilla, Arch. Otolaryng. 40:180, 1944.

Hayward, J.: Malignant giant cell tumor of the mandible: report of a case, J. Oral Surg., Anesth., and Hosp. Dent. Serv. 17:75, July 1959.

Jaffe, H. L.: Tumors and Tumerous Conditions of the Bones and Joints, Philadelphia, Lea & Febiger, 1958.

Jaffe, H. L., and Lichtenstein, L.: Chondromyxoid fibroma of bone, Arch. Path. 45:541, 1948.

———: Solitary benign endochondroma of bone, Arch. Surg. 46:480, 1943.

Lichtenstein, L.: Bone Tumors, ed. 3, St. Louis, Mosby, 1965.

Phemister, D. B., and Grimson, K. S.: Fibrous osteoma of the jaws, Ann. Surg. 105:564, 1937.

Shafer, W. G.: Benign tumors and cysts of the jawbones, Dent. Clinics N. Am., p. 693, November 1957.

Smith, A. G., and Zavaleta, A.: Osteoma, ossifying fibroma, and fibrous dysplasia of facial and cranial bones, Arch. Path. 54:507, 1952.

Waldron, C. A.: Fibrous and granulomatous lesions of jaw bones, Am. J. Surg. 94:877, 1957.

Wilkinson, F. C., and Pollak, E.: Benign bone forming tumours of the jaws, Brit. Dent. J. 77:341, 1944.

Neurilemoma

Baetz, F. O., and Shackelford, J.: A schwannoma of the inferior alveolar nerve, J. Oral Surg. 9:331, 1951.

Bruce, K. W.: Solitary neurofibroma (neurilemmoma, schwannoma) of the oral cavity, Oral Surg., Oral Med. and Oral Path. 7:1150, 1954.

Couch, C. D.: Neurilemmoma of the head and neck, J. Oral Surg. 12:19, 1954.

Crawford, W. H., Jr., Korchin, L., Gresovich, F. J., Jr.: Neurilemomas of oral cavity, J. Oral Surg. 26:651, 1968.

Foot, N. C.: Histology of tumors of the peripheral nerves, Arch. Path. 30:772, 1940.

Schroff, J.: Solitary neurofibroma of the oral cavity (neurilemmoma; neurinoma), J.A.D.A. 32:199, 1945.

Stout, A. P.: The peripheral manifestations of the specific nerve sheath tumor (neurilemmoma), Am. J. Cancer 24:751, 1935.

Neurofibroma

Ayres, W. W., Delaney, A. J., and Backer, M. H.: Congenital neurofibromatous macroglossia associated in some cases with von Recklinghausen's disease, Cancer 5:721, 1952.

Baden, E., Pierce, H. E., and Jackson, W. F.: Multiple neurofibromatosis with oral lesions, Oral Surg., Oral Med. and Oral Path. 8:263, 1955.

Borkenhagen, R., and Vazirani, S.: Multiple neurofibromatosis in a family, Oral Surg., Oral Med. and Oral Path. 9:269, 1956.

Crowe, F. W., Schull, W. J., and Neel, J. V.: A Clinical, Pathological and Genetic Study of Multiple Neurofibromatosis, Springfield, Ill., Thomas, 1956.

Martin, H., and Graves, C. L.: Plexiform neurofibroma (von Recklinghausen's disease) invading the oral cavity, Am. J. Orthodont. and Oral Surg. (Oral Surg. Sect.) 28:694, 1942.

Rappaport, H. M.: Neurofibromatosis of the oral cavity. Report of a case, Oral Surg., Oral Med. and Oral Path. 6:599, 1953.

Stillman, F. S.: Neurofibromatosis, J. Oral Surg. 10:112, 1952.

Myoblastoma

Aparicio, S. R., and Lamsden, C. E.: Light and electron microscope studies on the granular cell myoblastoma of the tongue, J. Path. 97: 399, 1969.

Bangle, R.: A morphological and histochemical study of the granular-cell myoblastoma, Cancer 5:950, 1952.

Bauer, W. H., and Bauer, J. D.: The so-called "congenital epulis," Oral Surg., Oral Med. and Oral Path. 6:1065, 1953.

Bhaskar, S. N., and Akamine, R.: Congenital epulis (congenital granular cell fibroblastoma), Oral Surg., Oral Med. and Oral Path. 8:517, 1955.

Bloom, D., and Ginzler, A. M.: Myoblastoma. Report of a case of myoblastoma of the lip followed by multiple tumors of the skin, Arch. Dermat. and Syph. 56:648, 1947.

Crane, A. R., and Tremblay, R. G.: Myoblastoma, Am. J. Path. 21:357, 1945.

Fust, J. A., and Custer, R. P.: On the neurogenesis of so-called granular cell myoblastoma, Am. J. Clin. Path. 19:522, 1949.

Hagen, J. O., Soule, E. H., and Gores, R. J.: Granular cell myoblastoma of the oral cavity, Oral Surg., Oral Med. and Oral Path. 14:454, 1961.

Hershfus, L., and Wolter, J. G.: Granular cell myoblastoma of the oral cavity, Oral Surg., Oral Med. and Oral Path. 29:341, 1970.

Kerr, D. A.: Myoblastic myoma, Oral Surg., Oral Med. and Oral Path. 2:41, 1949.

Pleasants, J. E., and Hinds, E. C.: Granular cell myoblastoma. Report of a case in newborn, Oral Surg., Oral Med. and Oral Path. 8:698, 1955.

Ross, R. C., Miller, T. R., and Foote, F. W.: Malignant granular-cell myoblastoma, Cancer 5:112, 1952.

Angiomas

Bellinger, D. H.: Blood and lymph vessel tumors involving the mouth, J. Oral Surg. 2:141, 1944.

Geshickter, C. F., and Keasbey, L. E.: Tumors of blood vessels, Am. J. Cancer 23:568, 1935.

Kauffman, S. L., and Stout, A. P.: Hemangiopericytoma in children, Cancer 13:695, 1960.

Kemper, J. W., and Bloom, H. J.: Lymphangiomatous macroglossia, Am. J. Orthodont. and Oral Surg. (Oral Surg. Sect.) 30:718, 1944.

Rigg, J. P., and Waldapfel, R.: Lymphangiomas of the tongue, Am. J. Orthodont. and Oral Surg. (Oral Surg. Sect.) 27:128, 1941.

Ward, G. E., and Covington, E. E.: Hemangiomas of the skin, J.A.M.A. 114:2069, 1940.

Watson, W. L.: Blood and lymph vessel tumors in children, J. Pediat. 15:401, 1939.

Watson, W. L., and McCarthy, W. D.: Blood and lymph vessel tumors. A report of 1,056 cases, Surg. Gynec. Obstet. 71:569, 1940.

Young, F.: Vascular birthmarks, J. Pediat. 14: 671, 1939.

Neoplasms of Odontogenic Origin

Aisenberg, M. S.: Adamantinohemangioma, Oral Surg., Oral Med. and Oral Path. 3:798, 1950.

——: Histopathology of ameloblastomas, Oral Surg., Oral Med. and Oral Path. 6:1111, 1953.

Anderson, H. C., Kim, B., and Minkowitz, S.: Calcifying epithelial odontogenic tumor of Pindborg, Cancer 24:585, 1969.

Bernier, J. L.: Ameloblastoma. Review of 34 cases, J. Dent. Res. 21:529, 1942.

Bernier, J. L., and Tiecke, R. W.: Adenoameloblastoma, J. Oral Surg. 8:259, 1950.

Cahn, L. R.: The dentigerous cyst is a potential adamantinoma, Dent. Cosmos 75:889, 1933.

Carr, R. F., Halperin, V., Wood, C., Krust, L., and Schoen, J.: Recurrent ameloblastic fibroma, Oral Surg., Oral Med. and Oral Path. 29:85, 1970.

Colby, R. A.: Odontogenic tumors, Dent. Clin. N. Am. p. 91, November 1957.

Frissell, C. T., and Shafer, W. G.: Ameloblastic odontoma, Oral Surg., Oral Med. and Oral Path. 6:1129, 1953.

Gardner, D. G., Michaels, L., and Liepa, E.: Calcifying epithelial odontogenic tumor: An amyloid-producing neoplasm, Oral Surg., Oral Med. and Oral Path. 26:812, 1968.

Giansanti, J. S., Somerson, A., and Waldron, C. A.: Odontogenic adenomatoid tumor (adenoameloblastoma), Oral Surg., Oral Med. and Oral Path. 30:69, 1970.

Goldberg, G. M., and Eshbaugh, D. E.: Squamous cell nests of the pituitary gland as related to the origin of craniopharyngiomas, Arch. Path. 70:293, 1960.

Gorlin, R. J., Chaudhry, A. J., and Pindborg, J. J.: Odontogenic tumors, Cancer 14:73, 1961.

James, P. L., and Fisher, P. L.: Melanotic ectodermal tumor of infancy, Brit. Dent. J. 108: 335, 1970.

Kemper, J. W., Root, R. W.: Adamanto-odontoma, Am. J. Orthodont. and Oral Surg. (Oral Surg. Sect.) 30:709, 1944.

Kronfeld, R.: Adamantinoma, J.A.D.A. *17*:681, 1930.

Phillipsen, H. P., and Birn, H.: Adenomatoid odontogenic tumor: Ameloblastic adenomatoid tumor or adenoameloblastoma, Acta Path. Microbiol. Scandinav. *75*:375, 1969.

Pincock, L. D., and Bruce, K. W.: Odontogenic fibroma, Oral Surg., Oral Med. and Oral Path. *7*:307, 1954.

Pindborg, J. J.: A calcifying epithelial odontogenic tumor, Cancer *11*:838, 1958.

———: Ameloblastic sarcoma in the maxilla, Cancer *13*:917, 1960.

———: The calcifying epithelial odontogenic tumor: Review of literature and report of an extra-osseous case, Acta Odont. Scandinav. *4*:419, 1966.

Potdar, G. G.: Ameloblastoma of the jaw as seen in Bombay, India, Oral Surg., Oral Med. and Oral Path. *28*:297, 1969.

Robinson, H. B. G.: Ameloblastoma. Review of 379 cases, Arch. Path. *23*:831, 1937.

———: Histologic study of the ameloblastoma, Arch. Path. *23*:664, 1937.

Robinson, H. B. G., and Lefkowitz, W.: Ameloblastomatous potentiality of odontogenic epithelium demonstrated in tissue culture, Oral Surg., Oral Med. and Oral Path. *11*:630, 1958.

Robinson, H. B. G., and Wallace, W. R. J.: Solid to cystic degeneration in an ameloblastoma, Arch. Path. *28*:207, 1939.

Sharp, G. S., Bullock, W. K., and Binkley, F. C.: Ameloblastoma of the jaws, Oral Surg., Oral Med. and Oral Path. *8*:1013, 1955.

Small, I. A., and Waldron, C. A.: Ameloblastomas of the jaws, Oral Surg., Oral Med. and Oral Path. *8*:281, 1955.

Stafne, E. C.: Epithelial tumors associated with developmental cysts of the maxilla, Oral Surg., Oral Med. and Oral Path. *1*:887, 1948.

Tiecke, R. W., and Bernier, J. L.: Adenoameloblastoma, Oral Surg., Oral Med. and Oral Path. *9*:1304, 1956.

Waldron, C. A., Thompson, C. W., and Conner, W. A.: Granular cell ameloblastic fibroma, Oral Surg., Oral Med. and Oral Path. *16*:1202, 1963.

Neoplasms of Salivary Gland Origin

Ash, J. E.: Mixed tumors of the salivary gland type, Am. J. Orthodont. and Oral Surg. (Oral Surg. Sect.) *33*:509, 1947.

Bardwill, J. M., Reynolds, C. T., Ibanez, M. L., and Luna, M. A.: Report of 100 tumors of minor salivary glands, Am. J. Surg. *112*:493, 1966.

Bauer, W. H., and Bauer, J. D.: Classification of glandular tumors of salivary glands, Arch. Path. *55*:328, 1952.

Bernier, J. L.: Mixed tumors of the lip, J. Oral Surg. *4*:193, 1946.

———: Muco-epidermoid tumors of the salivary glands. A report of 3 cases, J. Oral Surg. *4*:153, 1946.

Bhaskar, S. N., and Bernier, J. L.: Mikulicz's disease, Oral Surg., Oral Med. and Oral Path. *13*:1387, 1960.

Bhaskar, S. N., and Weinmann, J. P.: Tumors of the minor salivary glands, Oral Surg., Oral Med. and Oral Path. *8*:1278, 1955.

Blanck, C., Eneroth C.-M., and Jakobsson, P. A.: Oncocytoma of the parotid gland: Neoplasm or nodular hyperplasia, Cancer *25*:919, 1970.

Buxton, R. W., Maxwell, J. H., and French, A. J.: Surgical treatment of epithelial tumors of the parotid gland, Surg. Gynec. Obstet. *97*:401, 1953.

Cheyne, V. D., Tiecke, R. W., and Horne, E. V.: A review of so-called mixed tumors of the salivary glands including an analysis of fifty additional cases, Oral Surg., Oral Med. and Oral Path. *1*:359, 1948.

Cohen, M. A., and Batsakis, J. C.: Warthin's tumor revisited, Mich. Med. J. *67*:1341, 1968.

Crocker, D. J., Cavalaris, C. J., and Finch, R.: Intra-oral minor salivary gland tumors, Oral Surg., Oral Med. and Oral Path. *29*:60, 1970.

Dhawan, I. K., Bhargava, S., Nayak, N. C., and Gupta, R. K.: Central salivary gland tumors of jaws, Cancer *26*:211, July 1970.

Eneroth, C.-M., and Zajicek, J.: Aspiration biopsy of salivary gland tumors. IV. Morphologic studies on smears and histologic sections from 45 cases of adenoid cystic carcinoma, Acta Cytol. *13*:59, February 1969.

Epker, B. N., and Henny, F. A.: Clinical, histopathologic and surgical aspects of intra-oral minor salivary gland tumors: Review of 90 cases, J. Oral Surg., *27*:792, 1969.

Fine, G., Marshall, R. B., and Horn, R. C.: Tumors of minor salivary glands, Cancer *13*: 653, 1960.

Foote, F. W., and Frazell, E. L.: Tumors of the major salivary glands, Cancer *6*:1065, 1953.

Frable, W. J., and Elzay, R. P.: Tumors of minor salivary glands, Cancer *25*:932, 1969.

Gerughty, R. M., Scofield, H. H., Brown, F. M., and Hennigar, G. R.: Malignant mixed tumors of salivary gland origin, Cancer *24*:471, 1969.

Hellwig, C. A.: Mixed tumors of salivary glands, Arch. Path. 40:1, 1945.
Kerr, D. A.: Warthin's tumor (papillary cystadenoma lymphomatosum), Am. J. Orthodont. and Oral Surg. (Oral Surg. Sect.) 33:552, 1947.
———: Epithelial neoplasms of the salivary glands: their histology and their behavior, J. Oral Surg., Anesth., and Hosp. Dent. Serv. 17:3, July, 1959.
Luna, M. A., Stimson, P. G., and Bardwill, J. M.: Minor salivary gland tumors of the oral cavity: Review of 68 cases, Oral Surg., Oral Med. and Oral Path. 25:71, 1968.
Martin, H., and Ehrlich, H. E.: Papillary cystadenoma lymphomatosum (Warthin's tumor) of the parotid salivary gland, Surg. Gynec. and Obstet. 79:611, 1944.
McFarland, J.: The histopathologic prognosis of salivary gland mixed tumors, Am. J. Med. Sc. 203:502, 1942.
McGavran, M. H., Bauer, W. C., and Ackerman, L. V.: Sebaceous lymphadenoma of the parotid salivary gland, Cancer 13:1185, 1960.
McGurk, F. M., Main, J. H. P., and Orr, J. A.: Adenolymphoma of the parotid gland. Brit. J. Oral Surg. 57:23, 1970.
Meyer, I., and Shklar, G.: Pseudoadamantine adenocarcinoma of submaxillary gland, Cancer 13:270, 1960.
Meza-Chávez, L.: Oxyphilic granular cell adenoma of the parotid gland (oncocytoma). Report of 5 cases and study of oxyphilic granular cells (oncocytes) in normal parotid glands, Am. J. Path. 25:523, 1949.
———: Sebaceous glands in normal and neoplastic parotid glands and possible significance of sebaceous glands in respect to the origin of tumors of the salivary glands, Am. J. Path. 25:627, 1949.
Ridenhour, C. E., and Spratt, J. S., Jr.: Epidermoid carcinoma of skin involving the parotid gland, Am. J. Surg. 112:504, 1966.
Rounds, C. E., and Goldman, H. M.: Adenoid cystic basal cell carcinoma (adenocarcinoma), Oral Surg., Oral Med. and Oral Path. 4:303, 1951.
Ruebner, B., and Bramhall, J. L: Malignant papillary cystadenoma lymphomatosum, Arch. Path. 69:110, 1960.
Smith, A. G., Broadbent, T. R., and Zavaleta, A. A.: Tumors of oral mucous glands, Cancer 7:224, 1954.
Stewart, F. W., Foote, F. W., and Becker, W. F.: Mucoepidermoid tumors of salivary glands, Ann. Surg. 122:820, 1945.

Thompson, A. S., and Bryant, H. C., Jr.: Histogenesis of papillary cystadenoma lymphomatosum (Warthin's tumor) of the parotid salivary gland, Am. J. Path. 26:807, 1950.
Vellios, F., and Shafer, W. G.: Tumors of intraoral accessory salivary glands, Surg. Gynec. and Obstet. 108:450, 1959.
Vickers, R. A., Gorlin, R. J., and Smart, E. A.: Lymphoepithelial lesions of the oral cavity; report of four cases, Oral Surg., Oral Med. and Oral Path., 16:1214, 1963.
Warthin, A. S.: Papillary cystadenoma lymphomatosum, J. Cancer Res. 13:116, 1929.
Wawro, N. W., and McAdams, G.: Cylindromata of major and minor salivary gland origin, Arch. Surg. 68:252, 1954.
Welsh, R. A., and Meyer, A. T.: Mixed tumors of human salivary glands: Histiogenesis, Arch. Path. 85:433, 1968.

Basal Cell Carcinoma

Anderson, D. E., and Cook, W. A.: Jaw cysts and basal cell nevus syndrome, J. Oral Surg. 24:15, 1966.
Blum, H. F.: Sunlight as a causal factor in cancer of the skin of man, J. Nat. Cancer Inst. 9:247, 1948.
Foot, N. C.: Adnexal carcinoma of the skin, Am. J. Path. 23:1, 1947.
Gorlin, R. J., and Goltz, R. W.: Multiple nevoid basal cell epithelioma, jaw cysts, and bifid rib, New Eng. J. Med. 262:908, 1960.
Lever, W. F.: Pathogenesis of benign tumors of cutaneous appendages and of basal cell carcinoma, Arch. Dermat. and Syph. 57:679, 709, 1948.
McKelvy, L. E., Albright, C. R., and Prazak, G.: Multiple hereditary familial epithelial cysts of the jaws with the associate anomaly of trichoepithelioma, Oral Surg., Oral Med. and Oral Path. 13:111, 1960.
Teloh, H. A., and Wheelock, M. C.: Histogenesis of basal cell carcinoma, Arch. Path. 48:447, 1949.
Traenkle, H. L.: Epithelioma adenoides cysticum, trichoepithelioma, and basal cell cancer, Arch. Dermat. and Syph. 42:822, 1940.

Squamous Cell Carcinoma

Arthur, J. F., and Fenner, M. L.: Influence of histologic grading on prognosis in carcinoma of the tongue: Computer analysis of 299 cases, Clin. Radiol. 17:384, 1966.

Bernier, J. L., and Clark, M. L.: Squamous cell carcinoma of the lip, Mil. Surg. *109*:379, 1951.

Cady, B., and Catlin, D.: Epidermoid carcinoma of the gum: 20-year survey, Cancer *23*:551, 1969.

Cady, B., and Hutter, R. V. P.: Nonepidermoid cancer of the gum, Cancer *23*:1318, 1969.

Erich, J. B.: Treatment of carcinoma of the lips, Oral Surg., Oral Med. and Oral Path. *1*:505, 1948.

Gibbel, M. I., Cross, J. H., and Ariel, I. M.: Cancer of the tongue. A review of 330 cases, Cancer *2*:411, 1949.

Gorlin, R. J.: Bowen's disease of the mucous membrane of the mouth, Oral Surg., Oral Med. and Oral Path. *3*:35, 1950.

Greene, G. W., and Bernier, J. L.: Spindle cell squamous carcinoma of the lip, Oral Surg., Oral Med. and Oral Path. *12*:1008, 1959.

Martin, H., MacComb, W. S., and Blady, J. V.: Cancer of the lip, Ann. Surg. *114*:226, 341, 1941.

Mehta, F. S., Pindborg, J. J., Gupta, P. C., and Daftary, D. K.: Epidemiologic and histologic study of oral cancer and leukoplakia among 50,915 villagers in India, Cancer *24*:832, 1969.

Mills, C. A., and Porter, M. M.: Tobacco smoking habits and cancer of the mouth and respiratory system, Cancer Res. *10*:539, 1950.

O'Brien, P. H., and Catlin, D.: Cancer of cheek, Cancer *18*:1392, 1965.

Schork, C. J.: Neoplasms of the head, Oral Surg., Oral Med. and Oral Path. *1*:779, 1948.

Sharp, G. S.: Cancer of the lip, Oral Surg., Oral Med. and Oral Path. *1*:516, 1948.

Tiecke, R. W., and Bernier, J. L.: Statistical and morphological analysis of four hundred and one cases of intraoral squamous cell carcinoma, J.A.D.A. *49*:684, 1954.

Wildermuth, O., and Cantril, S. T.: Problems in the diagnosis of cancer with dental symptoms, J.A.D.A. *40*:385, 1950.

Willis, R. A.: Further studies on the mode of origin of carcinomas of the skin, Cancer Res. *5*:469, 1945.

———: The mode of origin of tumors. Solitary localized squamous cell growths of the skin, Cancer Res. *4*:630, 1944.

Woodbury, H. W.: Diagnosis of oral epidermoid carcinoma, Oral Surg., Oral Med. and Oral Path. *1*:67, 1948.

Carcinoma of the Nasopharynx

Cutler, M.: Radiosensitive intra-oral tumors, Arch. Surg. *18*:2303, 1929.

Martin, H., and Morfit, H. M.: Cervical lymph node metastasis as the first symptom of cancer, Surg. Gynec. Obstet. *78*:133, 1944.

Quick, D., and Cutler, M.: Transitional cell epidermoid carcinoma, Surg. Gynec. Obstet. *45*:320, 1927.

Simmons, M. W., and Ariel, I. M.: Carcinoma of the nasopharynx, Surg. Gynec. Obstet. *88*:763, 1948.

Thompson, E. A.: Lymphoepithelioma of the nasopharynx, Arch. Otolaryng. *54*:390, 1951.

Multiple Myeloma

Bruce, K. W., and Royer, R. Q.: Multiple myeloma occurring in the jaws. A study of 17 cases, Oral Surg., Oral Med. and Oral Path. *6*:729, 1953.

Calhoun, N. R.: Plasmacytoma of mandible, Oral Surg., Oral Med. and Oral Path. *14*:385, 1961.

Calman, H. I.: Multiple myeloma. Report of a case first observed in the maxilla, Oral Surg., Oral Med. and Oral Path. *5*:1302, 1952.

Carson, C. P., Ackerman, L. V., and Maltby, J. D.: Plasma cell myeloma: a clinical, pathologic and roentgenologic review of 90 cases, Am. J. Clin. Path. *25*:849, 1955.

Ewing, M. R., and Foote, F. W.: Plasma-cell tumors of the mouth and upper air passages, Cancer *5*:499, 1952.

Kaye, R. L., Martin, W. J., Campbell, D. C., and Lipscomb, P. R.: Long survival in disseminated myeloma with onset as a solitary lesion: two cases, Ann. Intern. Med. *54*:535, 1961.

Lichtenstein, L., and Jaffe, H. L.: Multiple myeloma. A survey based on thirty-five cases, Arch. Path. *44*:207, 1947.

Stout, A. P., and Kenny, F. R.: Primary plasma-cell tumors of the upper air passages and oral cavity, Cancer *2*:261, 1949.

Whitlock, R. I. H., and Hughes, N. C.: Solitary myeloma of mandible, Oral Surg., Oral Med. and Oral Path. *13*:23, 1960.

Malignant Lymphoma and Leukemia

Barnfield, W. F.: Leukemia and dental procedures, Am. J. Orthodont. and Oral Surg. (Oral Surg. Sect.) *31*:329, 1945.

Bersack, S. R.: Hodgkin's disease—incidence and prognosis, Arch. Intern. Med. *73*:232, 1944.

Custer, R. P.: An Atlas of Blood and Bone Marrow, p. 243, The leukemias, Philadelphia, Saunders, 1949.

Custer, R. P., and Bernhard, W. G.: The interrelationship of Hodgkin's disease and other lymphatic tumors, Am. J. Med. Sc. *216*:625, 1948.
Duffy, J. H., and Driscoll, E. J.: Oral manifestations of leukemia, Oral Surg., Oral Med. and Oral Path. *11*:5, 1958.
Eisenbud, L., and Kotch, R.: Hodgkin's "sarcoma" of the cheek, Oral Surg., Oral Med. and Oral Path. *7*:213, 1954.
Friedberg, S. A., and Hass, G. M.: Lymphomas of the nasopharynx and pharynx, Arch. Otolaryng. *60*:677, 1954.
Moloney, W. C.: Clinical significance of oral lesions in acute leukemia, New Eng. J. Med. *222*:577, 1940.
Pitcock, J. A., Bauer, W. C., and McGavran, M. H.: Hodgkin's disease in children, Cancer *12*:1043, 1959.
Robinson, H. B. G.: Stomatitis in blood dyscrasias, Int. Dent. J. *5*:327, 1955.
Rosenberg, S. A., Diamond, H. D., and Craver, L. F.: Lymphosarcoma: the effects of therapy and survival in 1,269 patients in a review of 30 years' experience, Ann. Intern. Med. *53*:877, 1960.
Seldin, H. M., Seldin, S. D., and Rakower, W.: Oral lymphosarcoma, J. Oral Surg. *12*:3, 1954.
Silverman, L. M.: Lymphosarcoma of gingivae, Oral Surg., Oral Med. and Oral Path. *8*:1108, 1955.
Steg, R. F., Dahlin, D. C., and Gores, R. J.: Malignant lymphoma of mandible and maxillary region, Oral Surg., Oral Med. and Oral Path. *12*:128, 1959.
Symposium: Leukemia, Am. J. Med. *28*:671, 1960.
Warthin, A. S.: The genetic neoplastic relationships of Hodgkin's disease, aleukemic and leukemic lymphoblastoma, and mycosis fungoides, Ann. Surg. *93*:153, 1931.

Sarcomas

Broders, A. C., Hargrave, R., and Meyerding, H. W.: Pathological features of soft tissue fibro-sarcoma, Surg. Gynec. Obstet. *69*:267, 1939.
Cholnoky, T.: Round-cell, Spindle-cell, and neurogenic sarcoma of the lip, Am. J. Cancer *22*:548, 1934.
Coley, B. L., and Harrold, C. C.: An analysis of fifty-nine cases of osteogenic sarcoma and survival for five years or more, J. Bone and Joint Surg. *32-A*:307, 1950.
Coventry, M. B., and Dahlin, D. C.: Osteogenic sarcoma: a critical analysis of 430 cases, J. Bone and Joint Surg. *39-A*:741, 1957.
Cragh, L., Dahlin, D., and Erich, J.: Osteogenic sarcoma of the jaws and facial bones, Am. J. Surg. *96*:496, 1958.
DeVore, D. T., and Waldron, C. A.: Malignant peripheral nerve tumors of the oral cavity, Oral Surg., Oral Med. and Oral Path. *14*:56, 1961.
Dutz, W., and Stout, A. P.: Kaposi's sarcoma in infants and children, Cancer *13*:684, 1960.
Geschickter, C. F.: Osteogenic sarcoma, Arch. Surg. *24*:602, 798, 1932.
Johnson, L. C.: A general theory of bone tumors, Bull. New York Acad. Med. *29*:164, 1953.
Lichtenstein, L., and Jaffe, H. L.: Chondrosarcoma of bone, Am. J. Path. *19*:553, 1943.
MacDonald, I., and Budd, J. W.: Osteogenic sarcoma, Surg. Gynec. Obstet. *77*:413, 1943.
Moore, O., and Grossi, C.: Embryonal rhabdomyosarcoma of the head and neck, Cancer *12*:69, 1959.
O'Neal, L. W., and Ackerman, L. V.: Chondrosarcoma of bone, Cancer *5*:551, 1952.
Phemister, D. B.: Chondrosarcoma of bone, Surg. Gynec. Obstet. *50*:216, 1930.
Stabbe, G. D., and Dargeon, H. W.: Embryonal rhabdomyosarcoma of head and neck in children and adolescents, Cancer *3*:826, 1950.
Stout, A. P.: Fibrosarcoma. The malignant tumor of fibroblasts, Cancer *1*:30, 1948.
Waldron, C. A.: Primary and secondary malignant tumors of the jaw bones, Dent. Clin. N. Am. p. 721, 1957.

Melanoma and Nevus

Allen, A. C., and Spitz, S.: Malignant melanoma. A clinicopathological analysis of the criteria for diagnosis and prognosis, Cancer *6*:1, 1953.
Buckley, D. B., and Russell, J. G.: Intra-oral blue nevus, Brit. Dent. J. *127*:288, 1969.
Chaudhry, A. P., Hampel, A., and Gorlin, R. J.: Primary malignant melanoma of the oral cavity: a review of 105 cases, Cancer *11*:923, 1958.
Greene, G. W., Haynes, J. W., Dozier, M., Blumberg, J. M., and Bernier, J. L.: Primary malignant melanoma of the oral mucosa, Oral Surg., Oral Med. and Oral Path. *6*:1435, 1953.
Howell, J. B., and Caro, M. R.: The basal cell nevus, Arch. Derm. *79*:67, 1959.
Kernen, J. A., and Ackerman, L. V.: Spindle cell nevi and epithelioid cell nevi (so-called juvenile melanomas) in children and adults, Cancer *13*:612, 1960.

Kindel, D. J.: Fallacies in the management of the pigmented mole, G.P. 23:87, 1961.

Kjaerheim, A., Martinez, M. G., and Montes, L. F.: Blue nevus of the oral cavity (an electron microscopic study), Oral Surg., Oral Med. and Oral Path. 29:718, 1970.

Masson, P.: My conception of cellular nevi, Cancer 4:9, 1951.

McWhorter, H. E., and Woolner, L. B.: Pigmented nevi, juvenile melanomas, and malignant melanomas in children, Cancer 7:564, 1954.

Scofield, H. H.: The blue (Jadassohn-Tiecke) nevus: a previously unreported intraoral lesion, J. Oral Surg., Anesth., and Hosp. Dent. Serv. 17:4, January 1959.

Trodahl, J. N., and Sprague, W. G.: Benign and malignant melanotic lesions of the oral mucosa, Cancer 25:812, 1970.

Metastatic Neoplasms to Oral Region

Aisenberg, M. S., and Inman, C. L.: Tumors that have metastasized to the jaws, Oral Surg., Oral Med. and Oral Path. 9:1210, 1956.

Blake, H., and Blake, F. S.: Breast carcinoma metastatic to maxilla, Oral Surg., Oral Med. and Oral Path. 13:1099, 1960.

Bosco, H. F.: Metastatic adenocarcinoma of mandible, Oral Surg., Oral Med. and Oral Path. 11:86, 1958.

Campelia, C. M., and Boyle, P. E.: Embyronal carcinoma primary in the mandible of a child with involvement of tooth pulp, Am. J. Orthodont. and Oral Surg. (Oral Surg. Sect.) 29:299, 1943.

Castigliano, S. G., and Rominger, C. J.: Metastatic malignancy of jaws, Am. J. Surg. 87:496, 1954.

Dunlap, C. L., and Robinson, H. B. G.: Metastatic retinoblastoma of the mandible, Oral Surg., Oral Med. and Oral Path. 26:76, 1968.

Goldstein, I. H., and Goldstein, M. C.: Jaw metastasis in chondroblastic osteogenic sarcoma, Am. J. Orthodont. and Oral Surg. (Oral Surg. Sect.) 29:57, 1943.

Gottlieb, M.: Metastatic carcinoma of the upper jaw from primary bronchogenic tumor, J.A.D.A. 24:1075, 1937.

Ivy, R. H., and Curtis, L.: Metastasis of tumors of rectum to mandible, Ann. Dent. 3:133, 1936.

Kronfeld, R., and Weinmann, J. P.: Metastatic adenocarcinoma in lower jaw bone, Arch. Path. 29:683, 1940.

Mallett, S. P.: A renal-cell metastatic carcinoma involving the mandible and submaxillary gland, Oral Surg., Oral Med. and Oral Path. 14:4, 1961.

Mercer, R. D., Lammert, A. C., Anderson, R., and Hazard, J. B.: Choriocarcinoma in mother and infant, J.A.M.A. 166:482, 1958.

Shklar, G., and Meyer, I.: Malignant tumors metastatic to mouth and jaws, Oral Surg., Oral Med. and Oral Path. 20:350, 1965.

Skillen, W. G.: Case of metastatic carcinoma of jaws, J.A.D.A. 17:1088, 1930.

Van Huysen, G., and Wallace, W. R. J.: Tumor metastasis to jaw, leading to recognition of primary tumor of ovary, Dental Cosmos 74:53, 1932.

Vogt, L. G.: Metastatic hypernephroma simulating dental cysts of lower jaw, Röntgenpraxis 11:99, 1939.

Zorokhovich, I. I.: Metastasis of thyroid adenoma to lower jaw, Vestnik khir. 45:239, 1936.

Index

Abnormalities, developmental. *See* Anomalies
Abrasion, betel-nut, 57
  bobby-pin, 56
  dentifrice, 56
  sand, 57
  of teeth, 56, 57
  tobacco, 57
  toothpick, 56
Abscess(es), in actinomycosis, 117
  cutaneous, 75
  definition of, 71
  of face, 75, 117, 118
  gingival, 74
  in osteomyelitis, 118
  periapical, 74
  pericemental, 85
  periodontal, 74, 85
  pulp, 71
Acanthosis, 2
Accessory teeth, 40
Achlorhydria, 128
Acid, decalcification of teeth by, 58
Acinus, mixed, 4
  mucous, 4
  serous, 4
Acromegaly, 133
Actinic cheilosis, 106, 107, 155
Actinomyces bovis, 117
Actinomyces israeli, 117
Actinomycosis, 117
Adamantinoma. *See* Ameloblastoma
Addison's disease, pigmentation in, 98, 99
Adenoameloblastoma, 148
Adenocarcinoma, acidophilic cell, 153
  acinic cell, 153
  papillary, 153
Adenoid cystic basal cell carcinoma, 152
Adenoma, acinic cell, 136, 151
  oxyphilic cell, 151
  of parathyroid glands, 129
  pituitary, 133
  pleomorphic, 150, 151
  serous cell, 136
Adenomatoid odontogenic tumor, 148
Agranulocytic angina, 128
Agranulocytosis, 128
Albright's syndrome, 132
Allergy, 102, 103
Amalgam, tattoo, 98
Ameloblastic adenomatoid tumor, 148
Ameloblastoma, 147, 148
Ameloblasts, 15, 16
Amelogenesis imperfecta, 46, 47, 49
Amputation neuroma, 93

Anemia, Cooley's, 128
  Mediterranean, 128
  pernicious, 128
Anesthesia, trauma during, 94
Aneurysm, arteriovenous, 144
Angina, agranulocytic, 128
Angioma(s), 19, 25, 144, 145, 148
Angioneurotic edema, 103
Anhidrosis, 41
Anisocytosis, 128
Ankyloglossia, 24
Anodontia, 41
Anomalies, definition of, 17
  lips, 18
  palate, 18, 23
  teeth, 37-53
  tongue, 24-27
Antibiotics, reaction to, 102, 103
Aplasia of enamel, 46
Apposition, dentin, enamel, 14
Argyrosis, 98
Arrectores pilorum, 2
Arteriovenous aneurysm, 194
Aspirin burn, 96
Atabrine, pigmentation from, 98
Attached gingiva, 3
Attrition, 58
Aurantiasis cutis, 127
Auricular tags, 18
Avitaminosis, 126, 127
Axis-cylinder, 8

Bacilli, tubercle, 112, 113
Balanitis, 122
Basal cell carcinoma, 154
  pseudoadenomatous, 152
Basal cell nevoid syndrome, 154
Basaloid mixed tumor, 152
Bence-Jones protein, 161
Benign lymphoepithelial lesion, 109
Beriberi, 126
Bifid tongue, 24
Biopsy, 92, 105, 135, 157
Biotin, 126
Bismuth, pigmentation from, 98
Biting, of cheeks, 92, 93
  of lips, 94
  of thread, 56
  of tongue, 92
Blue nevus, 166
Blue sclerae, 51, 53
Bone, "absorbent-cotton" appearance of, 134
  alveolar, 6
  cancellous, 7
  cells of, 7
  compact, 7
  "hair-on-end" arrangement of, 128
  intercellular substance of, 7

Bone—(*Continued*)
  marrow, 7
  mosaic pattern of, 134
  Paget's, 134
  remodeling of, 7
  "sun-ray" appearance of, 164
  trabecular, 7
Brachygnathia, 19
Branchial arches, 12
Branchial cleft cyst, 20
Brown pellicle, 59
Brown tumor, 90, 129
Bruxism, 58
Bulla(e), in erythema multiforme, 122
  in pemphigus, 123
Burn(s), chemical, 96
  thermal, 96
  x-ray, 101
Butterfly pattern, in lupus erythematosus, 123

Cafe au lait spots, 142
Calcification, of pulp, 69
  of teeth, abnormal, 46-53
  normal, 14, 16
Calcifying epithelial odontogenic tumor, 148
Calcifying odontogenic cyst, 36
Calcinosis, 129
Calculus(i), in periodontal disease, 84, 85
  renal, 129
  salivary, 109
Cancer, 135, 152-168
Candidiasis, 117
Candidosis, 117
Carcinoma, adenocarcinoma, 135, 153, 167, 168
  adenocystic, of salivary glands, 152
  adenoid basal cell, 152
  basal cell, 154
  bronchogenic, 167
  "in situ," 158
  intra-epithelial, 158
  mammary, 167
  melanocarcinoma, 166
  metastatic to jaws, 167, 168
  mucoepidermoid, 152
  of nasopharynx, 160, 161
  of oral mucosa, 155-159
  oxyphilic cell, 153
  prostatic, 168
  of salivary glands, 152, 153
  of skin, 154
  squamous cell, of alveolar ridge, 157
  of buccal mucosa, 157
  of lip, 155

Carcinoma, squamous cell—(Cont.)
  metastatic, 160
  microscopic features of, 158, 159
  of mouth floor, 157
  of palate, 157
  of salivary glands, 152, 153
  of tongue, 156
  verruciform, 156, 159
  transitional cell, 161
Caries, dental, 64-67
  backward, 65
  bacterial plaques in, 64, 66, 67
  control of, 67
  of dentin, 65-67
  of enamel, 64, 65
  etiology of, 55, 64, 66
  immunity to, 64
  interproximal, 64
  pit and fissure, 65
  secondary, 65
  undermining, 65
Carotene, 127
Carotenemia, 127
Carotenodermia, 127
Cartilage, in cyst wall, 30
  histology of, 7
  Meckel's, 10, 11
  in mixed tumors, 151
  neoplasms of, 141, 164, 165
Cavernous sinus thrombosis, 75
Cell(s) basal, 2
  Dorothy Reed, 162
  epithelioid, 113
  foreign body giant, 9
  inflammatory, 8-9
  Langhans' giant, 113
  L.E., 123
  mononuclear, large, 9
  mucous, 4
  myoepithelial, 2
  plasma, 8
  prickle, 2
  Reed-Sternberg, 162
  resting-wandering, 9
  reticuloendothelial, 9
  scavenger, 9
  Schwann, 8
  serous, 4
  target, 128
Cellulitis, 73, 75
Cementifying fibroma, 133
Cementoma, 62
Cementosis, 62
Cementum, acellular, 6
  cellular, 6
Cervical loop, 15
Chancre, 114
Cheek, traumatic ulcer of, 92
Cheek-chewing lesions, 92, 93
Cheilosis, actinic, 106, 107, 155
  angular, 126, 127
  solar, 106, 107, 155

Chickenpox, 111
Cholesterol crystals, 9, 36
Chondroma, 141
Chondrosarcoma, 164, 165
Christian's disease, 130, 131
Clasmatocytes, 9
Cleft(s), of cheek, 18
  of lip, 18
  of palate, 18
  of tongue, 24
Cleidocranial dysostosis, 54
Collagenous fibers, 8
Compound nevus, 166
Concrescence, 42
Conjunctivitis, 122
Connective tissue, mature, 8
  young, 8
Cooley's anemia, 128
Copula, 12
Corium, 2
Cornea, vascularization of, 126
Crevice, gingival, 3, 76
Cutaneous appendages, 2
Cylindroma, 152
Cyst(s), branchial cleft, 20
  calcifying odontogenic, 36
  definition of, 17
  dentigerous, central, 31
    lateral, 31
  dermoid, 21
  epidermoidal, 21
  eruption, 31
  extravasation, of jaws, 95
  fissural, 28, 29
  follicular, 31, 33
  globulomaxillary, 29
  hemorrhagic, of jaws, 95
  in hyperparathyroidism, 129
  incisive canal, 30
  median palatine, 28
  mucous retention, 108
  nasoalveolar, 29
  nasopalatine duct, 30
  periapical, 34-36, 73
  periodontal, apical, 34-36, 73
    lateral, 32
    residual, 35
  primordial, 33
  radicular, periapical, 34-36, 73
  thyroglossal duct, 22
  tonsillocyst, 20
  traumatic, of jaws, 95

Debris of Malassez, 16, 32, 34, 73, 148
Demilune, serous, 4
Dens in dente, 38, 39
Dens invaginatus, 38, 39
Dental caries. See Caries, dental
Dental lamina, 14, 147
Dental sac, 14
Denticles, in odontoma, 45
  in pulp, 69

Dentigerous cyst, 31, 148
Dentin, cross section of, 6
  longitudinal section of, 6
  matrix, 15, 16
  opalescent, 50, 51, 53
  secondary, 68
Dentinal dysplasia, 52, 53
Dentinal fibers, 6
Dentinal tubules, 6
Dentinogenesis imperfecta, 50, 51, 53
Denture allergy, 102
Denture irritation, 94, 95
Dermatitis, in erythema multiforme, 122
  in lichen planus, 121
  in lupus erythematosus, 123
  in pemphigus, 123
  from penicillin, 103
  from procaine, 102
  from roentgen rays, 63, 101
  in syphilis, 115
  from vitamin deficiency, 126
Dermis, 2
Dermoid cyst, 21
Development, of face, 12
  of neck, 12
  of teeth, 14-16
  of thyroid gland, 13
  of tongue, 12, 13
Diaphragm, epithelial, 16
Dilaceration, 43
Dilantin gingival enlargement, 80, 81
Disease, Gaucher's, 130
  Hand-Schüller-Christian, 130, 131
  Hodgkin's, 156
  Letterer-Siwe, 130, 131
  Lobstein's, 53
  Marie and Sainton's, 54
  Niemann-Pick, 130
  Osler-Rendu-Weber, 125
  Paget's, of bone, 134
  periodontal, 76-90
  von Reckinghausen's, of bone, 129
  of nerves, 142
Distomolars, 40
Dorothy Reed cells, 162
Drug idiosyncrasy, 102, 103
Duct(s), nasopalatine, 30
  salivary gland, histology of, 4
    obstruction of, 108
    stones in, 109
  thyroglossal, 13, 22
Dwarfism, of teeth, 40
Dyskeratosis, malignant, 105
Dysplasia, dentin, 52
  ectodermal, 41
  enamel, 46-49
  epithelial, 104, 105, 106
  fibrous, 132, 133

Ear, malformation of, 18
  pits of, 21
Ectodermal dysplasia, 41
Enamel, aplasia of, 46
  decalcified, 6
  drops, 43
  dysplasia, 46-49
  ground section of, 6
  hypocalcification of, 46-49
  hypoplasia of, 46-49
  lamella, 66
  matrix, 6, 15, 16, 44
  mottled, 49
  pearls, 43
Enameloma, 43
Endoneurium, 8
Endothelial leukocytes, 9
Enlargement, gingival, 79-81
  Dilantin, 80, 81
  hereditary, 80
  hormonal, 79
  leukemic, 81, 163
Eosinophilic granuloma of bone, 130
Eosinophils, 8
Epidermis, layers of, 2
Epidermoidal cyst, 21
Epineurium, 8
Epistaxis, 125
Epithelial attachment, 3, 16, 83-85
  cuff, 83, 84
  rests, 16, 32, 34, 73, 148
Epithelioid cell, 113
Epithelium, ectodermal, 12
  entodermal, 12
  inner enamel, 15
  outer enamel, 15
  pseudostratified ciliated columnar, 3
  reduced enamel, 16
  respiratory, 3
  stratified squamous, 2
Epulis, congenital, of newborn, 143
  fibrous (fibroid), 89
  fissuratum, 94
  giant cell, 90
Erosion, acid, 58
  idiopathic, 58
Eruption, retarded, 54
Erythema multiforme, 122
Erythroblastosis fetalis, 59
Exanthems, 111
Extravasation cyst, 95

Face, abscess of, 75
  clefts of, 18
  development of, 12
  hemiatrophy of, 19
Facies, mongoloid, 128
Fetus, human, head structures in, 10, 11
Fibers, collagenous, 8

Fibers—(Continued)
  dentinal, 6
  muscle, 5
  periodontal, 6
Fibroameloblastoma, 149
Fibroblasts, 8
Fibrocytes, 8
Fibroepithelial polyp, 138
Fibrolipoma, 139
Fibroma, 138
  cementifying, 133
  irritation, 138
  odontogenic, 149
  ossifying, 132, 141
  periapical, 62
Fibromatosis, hereditary, gingival, 80
Fibro-osseous dysplasia, 132
Fibro-osteoma, 141
Fibropapilloma, 138
Fibrosarcoma, 165
Fibrous dysplasia, 132, 133
Fibrous (fibroid) epulis, 89
Fissural cysts, 28, 29
Fissure tongue, 26, 27
Fistula(e), definition of, 17
  thyroglossal duct, 22
Floss, dental, injury from, 56
Fluorosis, endemic dental, 49
Follicular cyst, 31, 33
Foramen cecum, 5, 13
Fordyce, granules, 27
  spots, 27
Fracture of roots, repair of, 60
Free gingiva, 3, 76
Furrowed tongue, 26, 27
Fusion, 37

Galvanism, 97
Gaucher's disease, 130
Gemination, 37
Geographic tongue, 124
Giant cell, epulis, 90
  Langhans', 113
  lesion, central, 129
  osteoclastic, 7
  reparative granuloma, 90
Gigantism, pituitary, 133
  of teeth, 40
Gill slits, 12
Gingiva, abscess of, 74
  enlargement of, 79-81, 163
  hyperplasia of, 79-81
  inflammation of. See Gingivitis
  normal, 3, 76
  pigmentation of, 98, 99
Gingival enlargement, 79-81, 163
  Dilantin, 80, 81
  hereditary, 80
  hormonal, 79
  leukemic, 81, 163
  of pregnancy, 79
  pubertal, 79

Gingivitis, atrophic senile, 82
  desquamative, 82
  Dilantin, 80, 81
  herpetic, 77
  hyperplastic, simple, 80
  leukemic, 81
  marginal, 76, 77
  necrotizing, ulcerative, 78
  pregnancy, 79
  pubertal, 79
  simple, 76, 77
  Vincent's, 78
Gingivosis, 82
Gland(s), accessory salivary, 4
  anterior lingual, 5
  of von Ebner, 4
  mucous, 4
  parathyroid, 12
    adenoma of, 129
  parotid, 4
  pituitary, adenoma of, 133
  salivary, 4
    inflammation of, 109
    neoplasms of, 136, 150-153
  sebaceous, 2
    ectopic, 27
  serous, 4
  sublingual, 4
  submaxillary, 4
  sweat, 2
  thyroid, development of, 13, 22
Globulomaxillary cyst, 29
Glossitis, atrophic, in pernicious anemia, 128
  in syphilis, 115
  in vitamin B deficiency, 126
  fiery-red, 126
  luetic, 115
  median rhomboid, 24
  migratory, 27, 124
  in vitamin deficiency, 126
Gnathoschisis, 18
Granular cell ameloblastoma, 148
Granules, Fordyce, 27
Granuloma(s), dental, 73
  eosinophilic, of bone, 130
  giant cell reparative, 90
  gravidarum, 90
  pyogenicum, 119
  specific infectious, 112-117
Grooved tongue, 26, 27
Gumma, 115

Hair follicle, 2
Hairy tongue, 102, 124, 125
Hand-Schüller-Christian disease, 130, 131
Hemangioendothelioma, benign, 144, 145
Hemangioma, 25, 144, 145
  capillary, 144
  cavernous, 25, 144
  hypertrophicum, 144, 145

Hemiatrophy, 19
Hemorrhage, gingival, in leukemia, 81, 163
   in Osler-Rendu-Weber disease, 125
Hemorrhagic cyst, 95
Hemosiderin-containing macrophages, 9
Hereditary opalescent dentin, 50, 51, 53
Heredity, in amelogenesis imperfecta, 46
   in cleft lip and palate, 18
   in cleidocranial dysostosis, 54
   in dentinogenesis imperfecta, 50-53
   in ectodermal dysplasia, 41
   in Mediterranean anemia, 128
   in neoplasia, 135
   in Osler-Rendu-Weber disease, 125
Herpes, primary infection, 77
   recurrent, 110
Herpetic gingivostomatitis, 77
Herpetiform lesions, recurrent, 110
Hertwig's sheath, 16
Histiocytes (Histocytes), 9
Histiocytoses, 130, 131
Histodifferentiation, 14
Histoplasma capsulatum, 116
Histoplasmin skin test, 116
Histoplasmosis, 116
Hodgkin's disease, 161
Howship's lacunae, 7
Hutchinson's teeth, 48
Hydrochloric acid, tooth decalcification from, 58
Hygroma colli congenitum, 19
Hypercalcemia, 129
Hypercalcinuria, 129
Hypercementosis, 42, 62, 134
Hyperkeratosis, 2
Hyperostoses, 23
Hyperparathyroidism, primary, 129
Hyperphosphaturia, 129
Hyperplasia, from denture irritation, 94, 95
   Dilantin, 80, 81
   gingival, 79-81
   leukemic, 81, 163
   papillary, palate, 95
   pseudoepitheliomatous, 2
Hypocalcification, of enamel, 46, 47, 49
Hypochromia, 128
Hypophosphatemia, 129
Hypoplasia, of clavicles, 54
   of enamel, 46-49

Incisive canal cyst, 30
Index, lactobacillus, 67
Infection(s), specific, 77, 110-117
   Vincent's, 78
Inflammation, 9
   of bone marrow, 118
   of gingiva. See Gingivitis
   periapical, 34-36, 73, 74
   of pulp. See Pulpitis
   of salivary glands, 109
   of tongue. See Glossitis
Inflammatory cells, 8, 9
Initiation of tooth development, 14
Injuries, to periodontium, from masticatory force, 87, 88
   soft tissue, from chewing, 92-94
   to teeth, from foreign substances, 56, 57
Involucrum, 118
Irradiation. See Radiation
Irritation, from dentures, 94, 95
   "fibroma," 138

Jaundice, 59, 127
Jaw(s), cysts of, 28-36, 73, 95, 129
   fibrous dysplasia of, 132, 133
   giant cell lesion of, 90, 129
   neoplasms of, 140, 141, 146-149, 153, 161, 164, 167, 168
      metastatic to, 167, 168
   osteomyelitis of, 118
   Paget's disease of, 134
   radionecrosis of, 101
   underdevelopment of, 19, 63
Jeghers' syndrome, 99
Junctional nevus, 166

Keratohyalin granules, 2
Keratosis, congenital, 107
   focal, 104, 105
Koplik's spots, 111

Lactobacillus, 67
   count, 67
Lamellae, enamel, 66
Lamina dura, loss of, 129, 134
   widening of, 131
Lamina propria, 3
Langhans' giant cell, 113
Lanugo hair, 10
L.E. cells, 123
Letterer-Siwe disease, 130, 131
Leukemia, gingivitis in, 81, 163
   lymphocytic, 163
   monocytic, 163
   myelogenous, 163
   oral changes in, 81, 163
Leukocytes, 8, 9
Leukoplakia, 104-106
   opinions concerning, 104
Lichen planus, 120, 121
Linea alba, 93
Lingual goiter, 22
Lingual thyroid, 22

Lingual varicosities, 125
Lip(s), angioneurotic edema of, 103
   carcinoma of, 155
   chancre of, 114
   clefts of, 18
   herpetic infection of, 77, 110
   increase in vertical markings of, 126
   melanosis of, 99
   mixed tumor of, 150
   mucocele of, 108
   pigmentation of, 99
   pits, commissural, 18
      congenital, 18
      paramedian, 18
   traumatic ulcer of, 94
Lipoma, 139
Lues, 114, 115
Lumpy jaw. See Actinomycosis
Lupus erythematosus, 123
Lymphadenitis, tuberculous, 112
Lymphadenopathy, metastatic, 160
Lymphangioma, 19, 145
   circumscriptum, 145
   cysticum, 19, 145
   simplex, 145
Lymphocytes, 8
Lympho-epithelioma, 160, 161
Lymphoepithelial lesion, benign, 109
Lymphoid tissue, 5, 20
Lymphoma, giant follicular, 162
   malignant, 162, 163, 168
Lymphosarcoma, 162, 163, 168

Macrocytosis, 128
Macrodontia, 40
Macroglossia, 25, 133, 145
Macrophages, hemosiderin-containing, 9
   lipid-containing, 9
Macrostomia, 17, 18
Magenta tongue, 126
Malassez, debris of, 16, 32, 34, 73, 148
Malnutrition, vitamin B complex, 126, 127
Mandibular arch, 12
McCall's festoons, 87
Measles, 111
Median palatine cyst, 28
Median rhomboid glossitis, 24
Medicamentosa, stomatitis, 102, 103
Mediterranean anemia, 128
Megalodontia, 40
Melanoma, 166
   amelanotic, 166
   juvenile, 166
Melanosis gingivae, 99
   lip, 99
Melanotic progonoma, 148

Mesiodens, 40
Microcytosis, 128
Microdontia, 40
Micrognathia, 19
Microstomia, 17
Migratory glossitis, 124
"Mirror-image" nuclei, 162
Mixed tumor(s), basaloid, 152
  of salivary glands, benign, 150, 151
  malignant, 152, 153
Molars, bud, 48
  mulberry, 48
Mongoloid facies, 128
Moniliasis, 117
Morphodifferentiation, 14
Mottled enamel, 49
Mucocele, 108
Mucoepidermoid carcinoma, 152
Mucous membrane, 3
Mucous patch, 114
Mulberry molars, 48
Multiple myeloma, 161
Muscle, skeletal, 5
Myelin, 8
Myeloma, multiple, 161
  plasma cell, 161
Myoblastoma, 143
Myoepithelial cells, 2
Myofibrils, 5
Myoma, myoblastic, 143
Myxoma, 139

Nasoalveolar cyst, 29
Nasopalatine duct cyst, 30
Nasopharyngeal cancer, 160, 161
Necrosis, caseation, 112
  coagulation, 78
  in osteomyelitis, 118
  of pulp, 72
  radiation, 101
Neoplasm(s), benign, 136-151
  classification of, 135
  definition of, 135
  etiology of, 135
  malignant, 152-168
  of odontogenic origin, 146-149
  of salivary glands, 136, 150-153
Nerve(s), axis-cylinder of, 8
  endoneurium of, 8
  epineurium of, 8
  fasciculi of, 8
  mandibular, 8
  myelin of, 8
  neoplasms of, 142
  neurilemma of, 8
  perineurium of, 8
  sheath of Schwann of, 8
Neurilemoma, 142
Neuroblastoma, 168
Neurofibroma, 142
  granular cell, 143

Neurofibromatosis, 142
Neuroma, traumatic (amputation), 93
Neutropenia, malignant, 128
Neutrophils, 8
  hypersegmented, 128
Nevus, pigmented, blue, 166
  compound, 166
  intradermal, 166
  junctional, 166
  vascular. See Angioma
  white sponge, 107
Nicotinic stomatitis, 97
Niemann-Pick disease, 130
Normoblasts, 128
Normochromia, 128

Occlusion, trauma from, 83, 87, 88
Odontoameloblastoma, 149
Odontoblasts, 6, 7, 15
Odontodysplasia, 53
Odontogenic fibroma, 149
Odontogenic neoplasms, 146-149
Odontoma, mixed soft, 45
  simple calcified, 45
  simple soft, 45
  Also see Odontome
Odontome, complex composite (mixed), 45
  compound composite, 45
  dens invaginatus, 38, 39
  dilated composite, 45
  geminated, 45
Oncocytes, 136
Oncocytoma, benign, 151
  malignant, 153
Ossifying fibroma, 141
Osteitis deformans, 134
  fibrosa cystica, 129
  radiation, 101
Osteoblasts, 7
Osteochondroma, 141
Osteochondromyxoma, 140, 141
Osteoclasts, 7
Osteocytes, 7
Osteogenesis imperfecta, 53
Osteogenic sarcoma, 164
Osteoma, 140
Osteomyelitis, 118
Osteopsathyrosis idiopathica, 53
Osteoradionecrosis, 101

Paget's disease of bone, 134
Palate, cleft of, 18
  cysts of, 28-30
  denture irritation of, 95
  effect of tobacco on, 97
  perforation of, 115
Pallor, circumoral, 126
Papilla(e), atrophy of, 126
  circumvallate, 4, 5, 26
  dental, 15

Papilla(e)—(*Continued*)
  dermal, 2
  filiform, 5
    elongation of, 102, 124, 125
  foliate, 5
    inflammation of, 26
  fungiform, 5
    enlargement of, 126
  interdental, 76
  palatine, 30
  vallate, 4, 5, 26
Papillary cystadenoma lymphomatosum, 136
Papilloma, 137
Parakeratosis, 2
Paramolars, 40
Parathyroid adenoma, 129
Parotid gland, 4
Parulis, 55, 74
Pearl, enamel, 43
  epithelial, 158
Pellagra, 126
Pellicle, brown, 59
Pemphigus, 123
Penicillin, reaction to, 103
Periadenitis mucosa necrotica recurrens, 111
Perichondrium, 7
Perineurium, 8
Periodontal abscess, 85
Periodontal cyst, 32, 34-36, 73
Periodontal disease, 76-90
  pocket formation in, 84-86
Periodontal membrane, 6
  thickening of, 131
Periodontal pockets, 84-86
Periodontitis, 83-88
Periodontosis, 83
Perlèche, 127
Pernicious anemia, 128
Peutz-Jeghers syndrome, 99
Pharyngeal pouches, 12
Phlebectasia, oral, 125
Phlegmon, 75
Pierre Robin syndrome, 19
Pigmentation, in Addison's disease, 98
  in Albright's syndrome, 131
  from amalgam, 98
  atabrine, 98
  bismuth, 98
  carotenoid, 127
  circumoral, 99
  melanin, 99
  physiologic, 99
  in scleroderma, 131
  from silver, 98
Pindborg tumor, 148
Pink tooth, 55, 61
Pituitary adenoma, 133
Plaque, dentobacterial, 64, 66, 67
Plasma cells, 8, 161

Pleomorphic adenoma, 150, 151
Pocket, periodontal, 84-86
Poikilocytosis, 128
Polyblasts, 9
Polymorphonuclear neutrophils, 8
Polyp, fibroepithelial, 138
  pulp, 72
Polyposis, intestinal, 99
Preauricular sinus, 21
Predentin, 6
Pregnancy, gingival enlargement in, 79
  tumor, 90
Premalignancy, changes suggestive of, 105
Primordial cyst, 33
Procaine dermatitis, 101
Process(es), lateral nasal, 12
  maxillary, 12
  medial nasal, 12
  palatine, 18, 28
Pseudoepitheliomatous hyperplasia, 2, 143
Pubertal gingival enlargement, 79
Pulp, 7
  abscess, 71
  calcification of, 69
  capping, 68
  denticles in, 69
  healing of, 68
  hyperemia of, 70
  inflammation of. See Pulpitis
  necrosis of, 72
  nodules, 69
  polyp, 72
  stones, 69
Pulpitis, 70-72
  chronic ulcerative, 71
  hyperplastic, 72
  sequelae of, 73-75
  simple focal, 70
  suppurative, focal, 71
  total, 71
Pyogenic granuloma, 119

Radiation, effect of, on developing teeth, 63
  on erupted teeth, 63
  on soft tissue and bone, 100, 101
  mucositis, 100
  osteitis, 101
Radicular cyst, lateral, 32
  periapical, 34-36, 73
Radiodermatitis, 101
Ranula, 108
Rathke's pouch, 149
Ray fungus. See Actinomyces israeli
von Recklinghausen's disease, of bone, 129
  of nerves, 142
Reduced enamel epithelium, 16

Reed-Sternberg cells, 162
Repair, of fractured root, 60
  of pulp, 71
Resorption, periapical, 62
  root, from inflammation, 62
    from malignant neoplasm, 62, 153, 167, 168
    from orthodontic treatment, 62
    in Paget's disease, 62
  of teeth, external, 61
    idiopathic, 61
    internal, 61
Rete pegs, 2
Reticuloendothelioses, 130, 131
Reticulum cell sarcoma, 162, 163
Riboflavin deficiency, 126
Robin syndrome, 19
Rodent ulcer. See Carcinoma, basal cell
Root(s), dwarfed, 39
  fracture, 60
  repair of, 60
  resorption of. See Resorption, root
  segmented, 39
Rubella, 111
Rubeola, 111

Saddle nose, 115
Salivary calculi, 109
Salivary glands, 4
  cysts of, 108
  inflammation of, 109
  neoplasms of, 136, 150-153
Salivary stones, 109
Sarcoma, chondrosarcoma, 164, 165
  fibrosarcoma, 165
  Hodgkin's, 162, 163
  osteogenic, 164
  in Paget's disease, 134
  reticulum cell, 162, 163
  spindle cell, 165
Satellite bubo, 114
Schwann cell, 8, 142
Schwann sheath, 8
Schwannoma, 142
Scleroderma, 131
Scrofula, 112
Scrotal tongue, 26, 27
Sebaceous glands, 2
  ectopic, 27
Sebum, 2
Sequestrum, 118
Sheath of Schwann, 8
"Shell teeth," 53
Sialadenitis, 109
Sialolithiasis, 109
Sinus, definition of, 17
  lateral cervical, 20
  preauricular, 21
  thyroglossal duct, 22
Sjögren's syndrome, 109

Skin, 2
  appendages of, 2
  corium of, 2
  dermis of, 2
  epidermis of, 2
Solar cheilosis, 106, 107, 155
Split papule, 114
Sponge nevus, 107
Squamous cell carcinoma. See Carcinoma, squamous cell
Squamous epithelium, stratified, 2
Stain, Brown and Brenn, 67
  Giemsa's, 116
  mucicarmine, 152
  of teeth, brown pellicle, 59
    extrinsic, 59
    green, 59
    intrinsic, 59
    in congenital porphyria, 59
    tetracycline, 59
    tobacco, 57, 59
  Warthin-Starry-Kerr, 114
  Ziehl-Neelsen, 113
Staphyloschisis, 18
Stellate reticulum, 15
Stevens-Johnson syndrome, 122
Stillman's clefts, 87
Stomatitis, herpetic, 77, 104, 105
  medicamentosa, 102, 103
  nicotinic, 97
  venenata, 102, 103
Stones, pulp, 69
  salivary, 109
Stratum corneum, 2
Stratum germinativum, 2
Stratum granulosum, 2
Stratum intermedium, 15
Stratum spinosum, 2
Sturge-Weber syndrome, 144
Sublingual gland, 4
Submaxillary gland, 4
Sulfur granules, 117
"Sun-ray" appearance of bone, 164
Supernumerary teeth, 40
Sweat glands, 2
Syndrome, Albright's 132
  basal cell nevoid, 154
  Jeghers', 99
  Peutz-Jeghers, 99
  Pierre Robin, 19
  Robin, 19
  Sjögren's, 109
  Stevens-Johnson, 122
  Sturge-Weber, 144
Syphilis, acquired, 114, 115
  congenital, 48, 115
  dental defects in, 48

Target cells, 128
Taste buds, 5
Teeth, abrasion of, 56, 57
  absence of, 41

Teeth—(*Continued*)
  anomalies of, 37-53
  attrition of, 58
  calcification of, 14, 16
  caries of. *See* Caries, dental
  concrescence of, 42
  development of, 14-16
  dilaceration of, 43
  dwarfism of, 40
  erosion of, 58
  eruption of, normal, 14, 16
    retarded, 54
  fracture of, 60
  fused, 37
  geminated, 37
  gigantism of, 40
  Hutchinson's, 48
  hypercementosis of, 42
  hypocalcification of, 46, 47, 49
  hypoplasia of, 46-49
  maturation of, 14, 16
  mottled, 49
  mulberry, 48
  opalescent, 50, 51, 53
  radiation effect on, 63
  resorption of. *See* Resorption
  "shell," 53
  stains of, 59
  supernumerary, 40
Telangiectasia, hereditary hemorrhagic, 125
Tetracycline staining, 59
Thalassemia, major, 128
  minor, 128
Thrombocytopenia, 163
Thrombophlebitis, 75
Thrush, 117
Thyroglossal duct, 13
  cyst, 22
Tobacco, abrasion from, 57
  stain from, 57, 59
  stomatitis from, 97
Tomes' fibers, 6
Tongue, bifid (cleft), 24
  carcinoma of, 156

Tongue—(*Continued*)
  development of, 12, 13
  fissured (furrowed, grooved, scrotal), 26, 27
  geographic, 27, 124
  hairy, 101, 124, 125
  histology of, 5
  inflammation of. *See* Glossitis
  magenta, 126
  papillae of, 5
  smooth, 126
  syphilitic, 115
  thyroid tissue in, 22
  traumatic ulcer of, 92
  varicosities of, 125
Tonguetie, 24
Tonsil, palatine, 12
Tonsillocyst, 20
Torus mandibularis, 23
Torus palatinus, 23
Trauma, during anesthesia, 94
  cheek, 92
  lip, 94
  tongue, 92
Traumatic bone lesion, 95
Traumatic neuroma, 93
Traumatism, occlusal, 83, 87, 88
Trench mouth, 78
Treponema pallidum, 48, 114, 115
Triad, Christian's, 150
Tubercle, 113
  bacillus, bovine, 112
  human, 112, 113
Tuberculosis, 112, 113
Tuberculum impar, 12, 13, 24
Tumor(s). *See* Neoplasms
  adenoid cystic basal cell carcinoma, 152
  adenomatoid odontogenic, 148
  brown, 90, 129
  calcifying epithelial odontogenic, 148
  giant cell, central, 90, 129
    peripheral, 90
  mixed, 150, 151

Tumor(s)—(*Continued*)
  mucoepidermoid, 152
  Pindborg, 148
  pregnancy, 90
  Warthin's, 136

Ulcer, herpetic, recurrent, 110, 111
  rodent. *See* Carcinoma, basal cell
  traumatic, cheek, 91
    lip, 94
    tongue, 92
  tuberculous, 112
Ulceromembranous gingivitis, 78
Uranoschisis, 18
Urine, Bence-Jones protein in, 161
  excess of calcium in, 129
  excess of phosphorus in, 129

Varicella, 111
Varicosities, lingual, 125
Verocay body, 142
Verruca vulgaris, 137
Vesicles, in primary herpes, 77
  in recurrent herpes, 110, 111
Vincent's infection, 78
Virus, herpes simplex, 77, 110, 111
Vitamin B complex deficiency, 126, 127
Vitamin B_{12}, 126, 128
von Recklinghausen's disease, of bone, 129
  of nerves, 142

Waldeyer's ring, 112
Wart, 137
Warthin's tumor, 136
White folded gingivostomatitis, 107
White sponge nevus, 107
Wickham's striae, 120, 121

Xanthosis cutis, 127
Xerostomia, 63

Ziehl-Neelsen stain, 113
Zymogen granules, 4